Prentice Hall
HANDBOOK
LABORATOR
DIAGNOSTIC TESTS
with Nursing Implications

Prentice Hall

HANDBOOK OF LABORATORY & DIAGNOSTIC TESTS
with Nursing Implications

SIXTH EDITION

Joyce LeFever Kee, RN, MSN
Associate Professor Emerita
College of Health and Nursing Sciences
University of Delaware

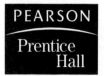

PEARSON
Prentice
Hall

Upper Saddle River, New Jersey 07458

Library of Congress Cataloging-in-Publication Data

Kee, Joyce LeFever.

    Handbook of laboratory & diagnostic tests : with nursing implications / Joyce LeFever Kee.—6th ed.

    p. ; cm.

    Rev. ed. of: Prentice Hall's handbook of laboratory & diagnostic tests/Joyce LeFever Kee. 5th ed. 2004.

    Includes bibliographical references and index.

    ISBN-13: 978-0-13-514278-3 (alk. paper)

    ISBN-10:   0-13-514278-4 (alk. paper)

    1. Diagnosis, Laboratory—Handbooks, manuals, etc. 2. Diagnosis,

Noninvasive—Handbooks, manuals, etc. 3. Nursing—Handbooks, manuals, etc.

    [DNLM: 1. Laboratory Techniques and Procedures—Handbooks. 2. Laboratory

Techniques and Procedures—Nurses' Instruction. 3. Diagnostic Tests,

Routine—Handbooks. 4. Diagnostic Tests, Routine—Nurses' Instruction. QY 39 K26h 2008]

    I. Title: Handbook of laboratory and diagnostic tests. II. Kee, Joyce LeFever.

Prentice Hall's handbook of laboratory & diagnostic tests. III. Title.

    RB38.2.K44 2008

    616.07'5—dc22
                                               2007048240

Notice: Care has been taken to confirm the accuracy of information presented in this book. The authors, editors, and the publisher, however, cannot accept any responsibility for errors or omissions or for consequences from application of the information in this book and make no warranty, express or implied, with respect to its contents.

    The authors and publisher have exerted every effort to ensure that drug selections and dosages set forth in this text are in accord with current recommendations and practice at time of publication. However, in view of ongoing research, changes in government regulations, and the constant flow of information relating to drug therapy and drug reactions, the reader is urged to check the package inserts of all drugs for any change in indications of dosage and for added warnings and precautions. This is particularly important when the recommended agent is a new and/or infrequently employed drug.

Publisher: Julie Levin Alexander	**Cover Designer:** Cheryl Asherman
Publisher's Assistant: Regina Bruno	**Director of Marketing:** Karen Allman
Editor-in-Chief: Maura Connor	**Senior Marketing Manager:** Francisco Del
Acquisitions Editor: Pamela Fuller	Castillo
Editorial Assistant: Jennifer Aranda	**Marketing Coordinator:** Michael Sirinides
Managing Production Editor: Patrick Walsh	**Marketing Assistant:** Anca David
Production Liaison: Cathy O'Connell	**Composition:** TexTech International
Production Editor: Satishna Gokuldas	**Printer/Binder:** Bind-Rite Graphics/Robbinsville
Manufacturing Manager: Ilene Sanford	**Cover Printer:** Phoenix Color Corp./Hagerstown
Senior Art Director: Maria Guglielmo	**Cover Photo:** Getty Images/Image Source Black

Pearson Education Ltd.	Pearson Education Australia Pty. Limited
Pearson Education Singapore, Pte. Ltd.	Pearson Education North Asia Ltd.
Pearson Education Canada, Ltd.	Pearson Educacíon de Mexico, S.A. de C.V.
Pearson Education—Japan	Pearson Education Malaysia, Lte. Ltd.
	Pearson Education, Upper Saddle River, New Jersey

PEARSON
Prentice
Hall

10 9 8 7 6 5 4 3 2

ISBN-13: 978-0-13-514278-3
ISBN-10:   0-13-514278-4

I dedicate this book to my three children
Eric, Katherine, and Wanda

CONTENTS

NOTICE OF PRIVACY PRACTICES

HEALTH INSURANCE PORTABILITY AND ACCOUNTABILITY ACT (HIPAA)

HIPAA, also known as "Notice of Privacy Practices," was first passed as an act on August 21, 1996. The details of the act and regulations were published on December 28, 2000. All agencies, including medical care personnel and facilities (physicians, care givers, and institutions), laboratory and diagnostic facilities, pharmacy, and others, were required to comply with the act by April 14, 2003.

Clients sign a form to protect their medical information and laboratory test results from public disclosure without permission. This act provides the clients with more control over their health information and test results. It sets boundaries on the use and release of health records. It establishes appropriate safeguards to protect the privacy of health information. Also, this privacy act informs clients how their health information may be used.

More information regarding HIPAA can be obtained on the Internet: http://www.cdc.gov/mmwr/preview/mmwhtmt/m2c411a1.htm.

PREFACE

Each day hundreds of thousands of laboratory and diagnostic tests are performed. Longevity and high technology further the use of sensitive tests to monitor the well-being of all clients and to make specific diagnoses.

As a health provider, you have the critical responsibility of staying current with the many facets of high-quality client care. *Handbook of Laboratory & Diagnostic Tests with Nursing Implications,* sixth edition, gives information about the commonly ordered laboratory and diagnostic tests, along with nursing implications and client teaching. It gives quick, pertinent information about the tests, emphasizing their purposes, the procedures, the clinical problems associated with disease entities, and drugs related to abnormal test results, as well as nursing implications together with client teaching. Reference values are given for children, adults, and the elderly.

Because the reference text is a handbook in pocket form, it can be easily carried to clinical settings. This text is appropriate for students in various types of nursing and nonnursing programs, including medical technology programs, baccalaureate and nursing programs, associate degree programs, diploma programs, and practical nursing programs. This book is most valuable to the nurse practitioner, registered nurse, student nurse, and licensed practical nurse in hospital settings, including specialty areas such as intensive care units, emergency rooms, clinics, health care provider offices, and independent nursing practices.

THE SIXTH EDITION

The sixth edition of the handbook lists more than 500 laboratory and diagnostic tests, including 30 new tests that have been added to this edition. These are the major additions and revisions:

- New laboratory and diagnostic tests have been added, such as antisperm antibody test, apolipoproteins, bioterrorism organisms (anthrax, bolulism, and smallpox), brain natriuretic peptide, breast cancer genetic testing, breast cancer tumor prognostic markers, cancer tumor markers (CA 15-3, CA 19-9, CA 27.29, CA 50, and

CA 125), marijuana testing, cardiovascular disease genetic test, C-peptide, fecal fat, N-telopeptide, osteocalcin, leukoagglutinin test, rubeola antibodies, troponins, electronystagmography, endoscopic ultrasound, oculovestibular reflex study, pericardial fluid analysis, peritoneal fluid analysis, and video capsule endoscopy.

- Many of the previous laboratory and diagnostic tests have been updated, such as arterial blood gases, human immunodeficiency virus (HIV), bilirubin tests, cryoglobin, glucose results, prostate-specific antigen (PSA) (total and percent free PSA), cardiac catheterization, echocardiography, colonoscopy, endoscopic retrograde cholangiopancreatography (ERCP), esophageal studies, computed tomography (CT), magnetic resonance imaging (MRI), mammography, nuclear scan, pulmonary function tests, positron emission tomography (PET), Pap smear, stress/exercise tests, and ultrasonography.

- The introduction has been rewritten by Professor Helen T. Yates. It includes the importance of specimen collection, types of specimens, site and time of collection, collection types, labeling and handling, transport of specimen, laboratory measurements, and critical (panic) values.

- The inside front cover lists the approved wording for abbreviations by The Joint Commission (TJC), originally known as Joint Commission on Accreditation of Healthcare Organization (JCAHO).

- Lists of all laboratory and diagnostic tests with page numbers are found at the beginning of Part One, Laboratory Tests, and Part Two, Diagnostic Tests.

- Laboratory test values have been updated, as needed, to current values. Reference values may differ among institutions. These values are guidelines; persons should check with their institutions' laboratory policies and reference values for the tests.

- Part Three, School Health Services: Education, Screening, and Testing has been updated. It includes the nurse's function in educating, screening, and testing school children.

- Part Four, Therapeutic Drug Monitoring, has been updated to include drugs for HIV monitoring.

- Appendix A, Health Problems with Laboratory and Diagnostic Tests, names forty (40) frequently identified health problems and includes the laboratory and diagnostic tests that are usually suggested.

- Appendix B, Laboratory Test Values for Adults and Children, has been updated to include the new laboratory tests. Other laboratory test values have been updated as needed.

ORGANIZATION

Each test is presented in the following sequence: name(s) of test; reference values and normal findings for adults, children, and elderly; description of the test; purpose(s); clinical problems related to the test and the effects of any medication on test results; procedure; factors affecting laboratory and diagnostic test results; and nursing implications with client teaching.

There are four parts within the text—Part One: Laboratory Tests; Part Two: Diagnostic Tests; Part Three: School Health Services; and Part Four: Therapeutic Drug Monitoring. Also included are two appendices. Appendix A, Health Problems with Laboratory and Diagnostic Tests, lists laboratory and diagnostic tests usually ordered for diagnosing common health problems. Appendix B, Laboratory Test Values for Adults and Children, provides an alphabetical list of tests found in the text as well as tests that are frequently ordered. It includes the types of specimens, such as blood, plasma, serum, urine, and feces, as well as the color-top tube used for collections of venous blood.

Joyce LeFever Kee, RN, MSN

ACKNOWLEDGMENTS

I would like to extend my sincere thanks and deep appreciation to the following people: Dr. Warren Butt, for updating the colonoscopy, ERCP, esophageal studies, and developed endoscopic ultrasound and video capsule endoscopy; Dr. Rani Beharry for updating cardiac catheterization; Ellen B. Boyda for updating arterial blood gases test and Pap smear; Susan L. Chudzik for updating Stress/Exercise tests, echocardiography, PET; Dr. Sharon W. Gould for updating the ultrasonography tests, Dr. Stephen Grahovac for updating CT and MRI; Cindy Knotts for updating Nuclear scan tests; David Sestili for updating the pulmonary function tests; Katherine Pereira-Ogan for checking and updating nursing implications for the diagnostic tests; Helen Tang Yates for the Introduction and for assisting with the laboratory tests. Anne S. Biddle, for updating the section on School Health Services: Education, Screening, and Testing; and Ronald J. LeFever, for updating Therapeutic Drug Monitoring (TDM) tests.

Also my appreciation goes to Don Passidomo, Head Librarian, Veterans Administration Medical Center, Wilmington, Delaware, for his assistance with researching the materials; and to Pamela Fuller, nursing editor, and Melisa Baez, editorial assistant at Pearson Education. To my husband, Edward, go my love and appreciation for his support.

Joyce LeFever Kee, RN, MSN

CONTRIBUTORS AND CONSULTANTS

Rani Beharry, MD
Cardiac Catheterization Department
Christiana Care Health Services
Newark, Delaware
  Cardiac catheterization

Anne S. Biddle, RN, BSN, NCSN
School Nurse, Newark Charter
School Newark, Delaware
  Part III: School Health Services:
    Education, Screening, and
    Testing

Ellen B. Boyda, BSN, MSN, FNP
Family Nurse Practitioner and
Instructor,
Widener College Chester,
Pennsylvania
  Arterial blood gases,
    Pap smear

Warren Butt, MD
Gastroenterology
Christiana Care Health Services
Newark, Delaware
  Colonoscopy
  ERCP
  Esophageal Studies, Endoscopic
    Ultrasound, Video Capsule
    Endoscopy

Susan L. Chudzik, RN, MSN, CCNRP
Cardiology Department Christiana
Care Health Services
Newark, Delaware
  Stress/exercise tests
  Echocardiography
  Positron emission tomography
    (PET)

Sharon W. Gould, MD
Director of Radiology Residency
Program Christiana Care
Health Services
Newark, Delaware
  Ultrasonography

Stephen Grahovac, MD
Department of Radiology
Christiana Care Health Services
Newark, Delaware
  Computed tomography (CT)
  Magnetic resonance imaging
    (MRI)

Cindy Knotts, BS, CNMT
Supervisor Nuclear Medicine
Christiana Care Health Services
Newark, Delaware
  Nuclear scans

Ronald J. Lefever, BS, RPh
Pharmacist, Medical College of
Virginia
Richmond, Virginia
*Therapeutic drug monitoring
(TDM)*

**Katherine Pereira-Ogan, BSN,
MSN, BC**
Nurse Manager
Christiana Care Health Services
Newark, Delaware
*Nursing implications–diagnostic
tests*

**David C. Sestili, CRT, RPFT,
LRCP**
Technical and Research coordinator
Pulmonary Laboratory
Temple University Hospital
Philadelphia, Pennsylvania
Pulmonary function tests

Leigh N. Sibert, RN, BSN, CS
Clinical Nurse Specialist, Advanced
Practice Nurse
Cardiology Consultants,
P.A. Wilmington, Delaware
*Pacemaker monitoring
Transtelephonic*

Jane Purnell Taylor, RN, MSN
Associate Professor
Neumann College
Aston, Pennsylvania
*HIV
Fetal nonstress test
Fetoscopy*

Helen Tang Yates, BS, MS
Professor Emerita Medical
Technology
University of Delaware
Newark, Delaware
*Introduction, laboratory
tests*

REVIEWERS

Kathleen Lent Becker, MS, CRNP
Assistant Professor,
Coordinator Adult Nurse
Practitioner Program
The Johns Hopkins University
Baltimore, Maryland

Jennifer Duhon, MS, RN
Assistant Professor
Illinois Central College
Peoria, Illinois

Nini W. Dyogi, MSN, RN, CCRN
Assistant Professor
Riverside Community College
Riverside, California

Tonya Ford, BSN
Assistant Professor
Kentucky Community and
Technical College System
Versailles, Kentucky

Kelly Gosnell, MSN, RN
Assistant Professor
Ivy Tech Community College of
Indiana
Terre Haute, Indiana

Cynthia Hartman, MSN, RN
Professor of Nursing Technology
Marion Technical College
Marion, Ohio

**Alethea N. Hill, MSN, RN-C,
CRNP**
Clinical Assistant Professor
University of South Alabama
Mobile, Alabama

Jo Ann King, MSN, RN, CNS
Associate Professor
Elizabethtown Community and
Technical College
Elizabethtown, Kentucky

**Margaret Lewandowski, MSN,
CNS, FNP**
Assistant Professor
University of St. Francis
Joliet, Illinois

Christine Markut, DNSc, RNC
Associate Professor
Villa Julie College
Stevenson, Maryland

Arleen M. Stahl, PhD, CNS, RN
Professor
University of St. Francis
Joliet, Illinois

INTRODUCTION

THE IMPORTANCE OF SPECIMEN COLLECTION

Nurses participate actively in laboratory-testing protocols for clients. In addition to ordering laboratory tests, either on requisition slips or electronically, nursing input is extremely critical to ascertain valid and reliable laboratory test results. As the role of caregiver and teacher, the nurse must communicate with the client, physician, and laboratory personnel to obtain information that might affect test results. Nursing responsibilities include explaining the laboratory test, ensuring that both the client and staff follow the procedure, assessing clinical findings with laboratory test results, noting pertinent information on the laboratory requisition slip (e.g., drugs the client is taking that might affect tests results), and collecting the specimen. In some clinical settings, such as ICU, ER, CCU, the nurses also perform some laboratory procedures classified by Clinical Laboratory Improvement Act (CLIA) as "Waivered Tests."

Collection of specimen is the focus of this section. The following paragraphs present an overview of the various aspects of specimen collection: the types of specimens, the collection sites, the effect of the client's position and activity on test results, the importance of the time of collection, drug interference, labeling and handling of specimens, types of collection tubes, and the types of reported laboratory measurement.

Types of Specimens. The types of specimens that are used for laboratory studies are blood; urine (random or 24-h collection); cerebrospinal fluid (CSF); feces; sputum; tissue or biopsy samples from surgery; and synovial, pleural, peritoneal, and wound exudate. Because blood is the most frequently analyzed specimen, its collection will be outlined below.

When blood is withdrawn in a plain container, it clots. The fluid that can be separated from the clotted blood is called *serum*. The term *serum* is often used interchangeably with *plasma*. When an anticoagulant is added to a collection container, *no* clot is formed. The clear fluid is known as plasma, which contains the protein *fibrinogen*, a component that is converted to the substance that composes the clot, *fibrin*.

Most tests (e.g., electrolyte levels) use serum from clotted blood. If a laboratory test requires plasma or whole blood, the tube used to collect the blood must contain an anticoagulant so that the blood does not clot. The stoppers of the collection tubes are color coded to indicate whether they will be used as serum (red top) or plasma (lavender, green, gray, or blue top).

Site of Collection. Because blood is most commonly drawn from a vein, the venous source does not have to be indicated on the laboratory slip; however, if the blood is drawn from an artery or capillary, this should be recorded on the slip. This is important when one evaluates the laboratory results, since the reference values are established using venous blood. Arterial and capillary blood may have different reference values, for example, blood gases. The legs and feet are not used for venipuncture because of the risk of exacerbating circulatory conditions.

When collecting the blood sample, the tourniquet should not be left on for longer than a minute. It can cause fluid shift from the vessel to the tissue spaces, leading to hemoconcentration and resulting in erroneous results. After collection, the blood specimen should be gently inverted several times to mix with the anticoagulant if in the tube. Shaking the tube can damage the red blood cells (RBCs) and resulting in hemolysis, which can cause an inaccurate test result.

Client Position and Activity. Standing or recent ambulation causes body fluid to most frequently shift from the vascular to the tissue spaces. Vascular hemoconcentration could result, affecting the concentration of proteins, enzymes, albumin, globulin, cholesterol, triglycerides, calcium, and iron. It take 20 to 30 min for fluid levels to reestablish equilibrium after this shift in position. Exercise just before specimen collection can also cause false results; this is especially true with enzyme testing.

Time of Collection. A time for routine blood collection needs to be established. Early morning before breakfast is the best time for blood collection because food and fluid will not affect test results. Fasting, however, is required only for a few laboratory tests, such as glucose, lipid studies, potassium, vitamin B_{12}, folate, and thyroid studies. For fasting specimens, the client is requested to fast for 8 to 12 h.

Drug Interference. Due to the growing number of drugs taken by clients, there is an increased chance that the laboratory results will be affected. This is especially true if drugs are taken over a period of time and at high doses. Drugs affecting test results should be noted on the laboratory slip. Drugs with a short half-life are withheld until the blood is drawn and thereby do not adversely affect the laboratory test result.

Labeling and Handling. Laboratory requisitions are designed specifically by an institution. The laboratory requisition slip should include the following information: the client's full name, age, sex, room location, and possible diagnosis; the physician's name; the test being requested (indicated by a check mark); the date; the time of collection; and any special notation (such as drugs). Another type of identification such as the client's social security number or medical record number may be required. In computerized laboratories, a bar-code label may be applied.

Specimen Transport. Proper handling and prompt transport of the specimen to the laboratory is vitally important. The goal for proper transport and handling is to maintain the integrity of the specimen as close to the in vivo state as possible. When a blood specimen is not processed promptly, hemolysis can occur, causing inaccurate results; when a urine specimen sits longer than 30 min, the pH of the urine becomes alkaline as a result of bacterial growth.

Collection Tubes. Tubes have color-coded stoppers that indicate the type of additive in the tube. The additives include anticoagulants such as oxalates, citrates, ethylenediaminetetraacetic acid (EDTA), and heparin. Blood-serum specimens are obtained in a red-top tube that does not contain chemical additive. However, there is a gel in the tube that hastens clotting and provides a barrier between the blood and serum. Examples of the laboratory groups and color-top tubes follow.

Red. No additive, clotted blood. Serum is obtained from the clotted blood mass. Laboratory test groups that use red-top tubes are chemistries (electrolytes, proteins, enzymes, lipids, hormones); drug monitoring; radioimmunoassay (RIA) methods; serology; and blood banking. Hemolysis should be avoided.

Lavendel. The anticoagulant additive is EDTA. Laboratory test groups that use lavender-top tubes are hematologic tests (complete blood cell count [CBC], platelet count) and certain chemistries.

Green. The anticoagulant additive is heparin. Laboratory test groups that use green-top tubes are arterial blood gases and the lupus erythematosus (LE) test. Although electrolyte levels are usually obtained from serum (red-top tube), a green-top tube may be substituted. In a STAT situation, one need not to wait for the blood to clot (red-top tube). The heparinized tube would allow the laboratory to centrifuge and separate the blood and plasma immediately.

Blue. The anticoagulant additive is citrate. Laboratory groups that use blue-top tubes are coagulation studies (prothrombin time [PT], international normalized ratio [INR], activated partial thromboplastin time [APTT], partial thromboplastin time [PTT], and hemoglobin levels).

Gray. The anticoagulant additive is sodium fluoride. The laboratory test for glucose uses gray-top tubes. The additive has a dual function as an anticoagulant and for prevention of glycolysis, thus preserving the glucose concentration in the in vivo state.

NOTE. The proper selection and usage of the color-coded collection tube is critical in meeting the reliability of the test results. The additives must be compatible with the laboratory procedure. The nurse should always check with the institution's collection manual.

TYPES OF REPORTED LABORATORY MEASUREMENTS

International System of Units. The World Health Organization (WHO) recommends that the medical and scientific community throughout the world adopt the *Système International d'Unités* (SI units) to establish a common international language for communicating laboratory measurements. Most clinical laboratories in Canada, Australia, and Western Europe, and some in the United States, are now using SI units. Currently both metric and SI units are usually reported.

Reference Values. Reference values (expected values) are based on "apparently healthy" individuals and the equipment and methods used in laboratories. Owing to differences in the methods and equipment used, these values may vary among institutions.

Critical (Panic) Values. At times a client's test results may fall outside the range of reference values, and a decision must be made as to whether the physician should be notified. Most laboratories have a list of critical values. When a client's results exceed the values on this list, the physician or charge nurse must be notified immediately. The critical value policy and list are specific to each institution.

CLINICAL LABORATORY DATA WAREHOUSE

Clinical laboratory data warehouse is the saving and using of data obtained from the laboratory database. Building a data warehouse provides a representation of laboratory values for the population. The results of the tests for a few hundred people do not adequately represent the laboratory reference values for a large client population. A data warehouse of laboratory values of clients collected over numerous years is considered more effective in evaluating the population-based reference values. This method is less expensive than the traditional recruiting of volunteers for testing to determine laboratory "norms." The warehouse data includes five to ten times more people for the laboratory values/intervals. It provides a range according to age and sex better than the traditional method for obtaining laboratory values. The young male has a higher alanine aminotransferase (ALT) level than the adult. Elevated alkaline phosphatase (ALP) is usually higher in teenagers because of bone growth. By using warehouse laboratory data, accuracy for diagnosis and treatment of diseases will be enhanced.

Descriptive interpretations are included for immunological procedures.

Helen Tang Yates

ONE

Considerations for Use of Laboratory Tests

This introductory section on laboratory tests serves a twofold orientation—to disseminate essential information and to show the basic organizational format of the individual tests.

As you know, results of laboratory tests provide the basis for diagnosis, treatment, and progress of a disease condition or health status, or both. The laboratory test is a multiphased process: identifying need for test; ordering test; generating the laboratory requisition; physical and educational preparation of the client and family; collection, labeling, and care of specimen(s); and health teaching. Naturally, the complexity of this process is dependent on many variables. For purposes of being a handy reference, general directions common to most laboratory tests related to reference values, description, purpose, clinical problems and drug effects, procedure, factors affecting laboratory results, and nursing implications with client teaching will be addressed. Only facts specific to a given test will be listed with each test. The explanations following the headings for laboratory tests help in their clarification.

Reference Values.   Laboratory test values can differ among laboratories; therefore, it is important to know your institution's laboratory values. The reference values given are comparably the same in most laboratories.

Description.   Information is provided about each laboratory test and its purpose(s).

Purpose(s).   The purpose(s) for the laboratory tests is (are) given.

Clinical Problems. The disease entities that are associated with decreased and increased test results are listed according to decreasing frequency of occurrence. Drugs that may cause false negatives or positives could result in a misleading test report. Drugs the client is taking that could affect test results should be recorded.

Procedure.   Many procedures for laboratory tests are the same. The following are helpful suggestions applicable to most tests.

1. Follow institutional policy and procedure, which may include a signed consent form.
2. Collect recommended amount of specimen (blood, urine, etc.).
3. Avoid using arm/hand with intravenous (IV) fluids for drawing venous blood specimen.
4. Clearly label specimen container with client's identifying information.
5. Note significant drug data on label or requisition, or both.
6. Avoid hemolysis; do not shake blood specimens.
7. Observe strict aseptic technique when collecting and handling each specimen.
8. Do not enforce fluid restrictions unless otherwise indicated.
9. Collect 24-h urine specimens:
   a. Have client void prior to test, discard urine, and then save all urine for 24 h.
   b. Refrigerate urine or keep on ice unless preservatives are added or otherwise indicated.
   c. Instruct client *not* to urinate directly into the container.
   d. Instruct client to avoid getting toilet paper and feces in urine specimens.
   e. Label the urine collection bottle/container with the client's name, date, and exact time of collection (e.g., 7/12/09, 7 AM to 7/13/09, 7:01 AM).
10. List drugs and food the client is taking that could affect test results.
11. When possible, hold medications and foods that could cause false test results until after the test. Before holding drugs, check with the health care provider. This may not be practical or possible; however,

if client takes medication and laboratory test is abnormal, this should be brought to the health care provider's attention.

12. Promptly send specimen to the laboratory.

Factors Affecting Laboratory Results

- Various factors that could affect test results should be identified. Drugs that affect test results are given in Clinical Problems; therefore, they are not repeated here.

Nursing Implications.   Common nursing implications that may not be repeated with each laboratory test are as follows:

1. Be knowledgeable about laboratory and diagnostic tests.
2. Provide time and be available to answer questions. Be supportive to client and family.
3. Follow procedure that is stated for each test. Label specimens with client information.
4. Relate test findings to clinical problems and drugs. Test may be repeated to confirm a suspected problem.
5. Report abnormal results to the health care provider.
6. Compare test results with other related laboratory and/or diagnostic tests.

Client Teaching

7. Explain purpose and procedure of each test to the client and family.
8. Encourage clients to keep medical appointments for follow-up.
9. Provide health teaching related to clinical problem.

List of Laboratory Tests

LABORATORY TESTS

ACETAMINOPHEN (SERUM)

TYLENOL, TEMPRA, DATRIL, LIQUIPRIN, PARACETAMOL, PANADOL, ACETA

Reference Values

Adult: Therapeutic: 5–20 mcg/ml, 31–124 μmol/l (SI units)

Toxic: Greater than 50 mcg/ml, 305 μmol/l (SI units), greater than 200 mcg/ml, possible hepatotoxicity

Child: Same as adult

Description.   Acetaminophen has antipyretic and nonnarcotic effects similar to aspirin. Acetaminophen does not inhibit platelet aggregation nor does it produce gastric distress and bleeding. It only has a weak anti-inflammatory response.

Acetaminophen is absorbed by the gastrointestinal tract and metabolized in the liver to active metabolites. Peak action time for acetaminophen occurs in 1 to 2½ h and the half-life is 3 h. Overdose of acetaminophen can be extremely dangerous since it may lead to hepatotoxicity. If a single dose of 10 g or 30 tablets (325 mg each) of acetaminophen is ingested, liver damage is likely to occur. With a serum acetaminophen level greater than 200 mg/ml in 4 h or greater than 50 mg/ml in 12 h, hepatotoxicity is likely to result.

Purposes
- To determine if the therapeutic acetaminophen dose is within therapeutic range
- To check for acetaminophen toxicity

Clinical Problems

Decreased level: High-carbohydrate meal

Drugs that may decrease acetaminophen value: Anticholinergics, cholestyramine (Questran)

Increased level: Acetaminophen overdose, liver disease
Drugs that may increase acetaminophen value: Chloramphenicol (Chloromycetin), phenobarbital

Procedure

- No food or fluid restriction is required.
- Collect 3 to 5 ml of venous blood in a red-top tube.
- Record dose and time drug was taken on the laboratory requisition slip.

Nursing Implications

- Keep the acetaminophen bottle tightly closed, out of reach of children, and away from the light.
- Suggest to the health care provider to order liver function tests and serum acetaminophen periodically for clients on long-term acetaminophen therapy. Liver damage may result when taking large doses of the drug for days, weeks, or months.
- Observe for signs and symptoms of hepatotoxicity—vomiting, jaundice, clay-colored stool, itching, epigastric or abdominal pain, diarrhea, and abnormal liver function tests.

Client Teaching

- Explain to the client that the purpose of the test is to monitor therapeutic drug level and to determine if a toxic serum acetaminophen level is present.
- Instruct the client to take the prescribed dosage. Usually the drug should not be taken for more than 10 days unless prescribed by the health care provider.
- Instruct the client to keep acetaminophen products out of the reach of children. If a child ingests large amounts of the drug, call the poison control center immediately, give syrup of ipecac if indicated by the center, and take the child to the emergency room. Acetylcysteine (Mucomyst) has been used as an antidote for adults within 16 h after drug overdose.

ACID PHOSPHATASE (ACP) (SERUM)

PROSTATIC ACID PHOSPHATASE (PAP)

Reference Values
Adult: Less than 2.6 ng/ml; 0–5 units/l range; varies according to the method used; 0.2–13 international unit/l (SI units)
Child: 6.4–15.2 units/l

Description.   The enzyme ACP is found in the prostate gland and in semen in high concentration. It is found in lesser extent in bone marrow, red blood cells (RBCs), liver, and spleen. The highest rise in serum ACP/PAP occurs in prostatic cancer. In benign prostatic hypertrophy (BPH), the rise is also above normal level. Prostate-specific antigen (PSA) is a more sensitive test for diagnosing prostatic cancer than ACP/PAP.

Purpose
- To compare ACP/PAP test with other laboratory tests for diagnosing prostatic cancer, BPH

Clinical Problems
Decreased level: Down syndrome
Drugs that may decrease ACP value: Fluorides, oxalates, phosphates, alcohol
Increased level: Carcinoma of the prostate, prostate palpation or surgery, Paget's disease, cancer of the breast and bone, multiple myeloma, osteogenesis imperfecta, benign prostatic hypertrophy, sickle cell anemia, cirrhosis, chronic renal failure, hyperparathyroidism, myocardial infarction.
Drugs that may increase ACP value: Androgens in females, clofibrate

Procedure
- No food or fluid restriction is required.
- Collect 5 to 7 ml of venous blood in a red-top tube. Avoid hemolysis. ACP is rich in blood cells.

- Take blood specimen to the laboratory *immediately*. ACP is heat- and pH-sensitive. If the specimen is exposed to air and left at room temperature, there will be a decrease in activity after 1 h.

Nursing Implications

- Recognize clinical problems associated with an elevated serum ACP level. A high serum ACP/PAP level occurs with metastasized prostatic cancer.
- Indicate on the laboratory slip if the client had a prostate examination 24 h before the test. Prostatic massage or extensive palpation of the prostate can elevate the serum ACP/PAP.
- Check the serum ACP/PAP following treatment for carcinoma of the prostate gland. With surgical intervention the serum level should drop in 3 to 4 days; following successful estrogen therapy it should drop in 3 to 4 weeks. If serum ACP/PAP has not been ordered, a reminder or suggestion to the health care provider may be necessary.
- Encourage client to express concerns about prostatic problem.

ADENOVIRUS ANTIBODY (SERUM)

Reference Values

Adult and Child: Negative. Positive: fourfold titer increase in paired sera

Description.   The adenovirus frequently is presented among school-aged children and military recruits; many may be asymptomatic. Adenovirus can be responsible for upper respiratory tract disease, cystitis (hemorrhagic), and keratoconjunctivitis. Transmission may be by direct or indirect contact (there are 41 different types of adenoviruses).

Purpose

- To determine the cause of upper respiratory tract disease and pharyngitis

Clinical Problems

Positive: Adenoviral infections of the upper respiratory tract, hemorrhagic cystitis, pharyngitis, keratoconjunctivitis

Procedure

- No food or fluid restriction is required.
- Collect 3 to 5 ml of venous blood in a red-top tube. Avoid hemolysis. A second blood specimen is usually obtained 2 to 3 weeks later to determine the acute and convalescent titer.
- A swab of the drainage from the infected area such as the throat, eye, or urethra may be obtained for immunofluorescence testing to determine the presence of an adenoviral infection. The swab specimen should be labeled and taken immediately to the laboratory for testing.

Nursing Implications

- Obtain a history from the client or family concerning the infected area involved. List symptoms the client may have, such as drainage and its color.
- Check with the client concerning contact with other persons who have similarly described symptoms.
- Answer the client or family's questions or refer them to an appropriate health care provider.

ADRENOCORTICOTROPIC HORMONE (ACTH) (PLASMA)

CORTICOTROPIN, CORTICOTROPIN-RELEASING FACTOR (CRF)

Reference Values

7 AM to 10 AM: 8–80 pg/ml; ACTH is highest in early morning
4 PM: 5–30 pg/ml
10 PM to midnight: Less than 10 pg/ml; lowest levels occur at bedtime

Description.   Adrenocorticotropic hormone (ACTH) is stored and released from the anterior pituitary gland (adenohypophysis) under the influence of corticotropin-releasing factor (CRF) from the hypothalamus and plasma cortisol from the adrenal cortex. The negative feedback mechanism controls ACTH releases: when plasma cortisol is low, ACTH is released; when plasma cortisol is high, ACTH release is inhibited. Stress caused by surgery, infections, and physical or emotional trauma increases the ACTH level. ACTH level follows a diurnal pattern, peaks in the early morning or early arising, and ebbs in the late evening or bedtime.

A plasma ACTH is performed to determine whether a decreased plasma cortisol is due to adrenal cortex hypofunction or pituitary hypofunction. Two tests, ACTH suppression and ACTH stimulation, may be ordered to identify the origin of the clinical problem, either the adrenal cortex or the pituitary.

ACTH Suppression Test.   For the ACTH suppression test, a synthetic potent cortisol, dexamethasone (Decadron), is given to suppress the production of ACTH. If an extremely high dose is needed for ACTH suppression, the cause is of pituitary origin, such as pituitary tumor, producing an excess of ACTH secretion. If the plasma cortisol continues to be high with ACTH suppression, the cause could be adrenal cortex hyperfunction (Cushing's syndrome). Suppressing pituitary release of ACTH will not affect a hyperactive adrenal gland.

ACTH Stimulation.   For the ACTH stimulation test, ACTH (cosyntropin) is administered, and the plasma cortisol level should double in 1 h. If the plasma cortisol level remains the same or is lower, adrenal gland insufficiency (Addison's disease) is the cause.

To check for pituitary hypofunction, the drug *metyrapone (Meto pirone)* is given to block the production of cortisol, thus causing an increased ACTH secretion. If the ACTH level does not increase, the problem is pituitary insufficiency.

Purposes
- To determine if a decreased plasma cortisol is due to adrenal cortex hypofunction or pituitary hypofunction

- To evaluate the ACTH suppression test results for health problem of pituitary origin
- To check for adrenal or pituitary hypofunction
- To utilize the ACTH stimulation test to determine the presence of adrenal gland insufficiency

Clinical Problems

Decreased level: Adrenocortical hyperplasia, cancer of the adrenal gland, hypopituitarism

Drugs that may decrease ACTH value: Steroids (cortisone, prednisone, dexamethasone), estrogen, amphetamines, alcohol

Increased level: Stress (trauma, physical or emotional), Addison's disease (adrenal hypofunction), pituitary neoplasm, surgery, pyrogens, pregnancy

Drugs that may increase ACTH value: Metyrapone, vasopressin, insulin

Procedure

- Food and fluid may be restricted. A low-carbohydrate diet may be requested for 24 h prior to the test.
- Collect 5 to 7 ml of venous blood in a lavender-top plastic tube. Pack the tube in ice immediately and send to the laboratory. Blood should not come in contact with glass. Additional testing may be needed since a single plasma value may be misleading.
- If adrenal hypofunction is suspected, blood sample is taken at the peak time (early morning). When adrenal hyperfunction is suspected, blood sample is usually taken at low time (evening).
- Note on the laboratory label the time the blood specimen was drawn. If the test is to be repeated the next morning, the blood sample should be drawn at the same time as the first specimen.
- Restrict activity and stress (if possible) for 8 to 12 h before the test. When possible, restrict drugs such as cortisone until after the test with health care provider's permission.

Factors Affecting Laboratory Results

- Stress and physical activity

Nursing Implications

- Obtain a history of the client's clinical symptoms and drug regimen. Steroids increase the ACTH secretion.
- Relate elevated plasma ACTH levels to plasma cortisol if ordered. With an adrenal gland insufficiency or a pituitary tumor, the ACTH secretions will be increased.

Client Teaching

- Explain to the client having the ACTH suppression test with dexamethasone or ACTH stimulation with ACTH or metyrapone that drugs are used to confirm the cause of the hormonal imbalance.
- Be supportive to the client and the family. Allow time for the client to ventilate his/her fears.

AIDS VIRUS (*SEE* HUMAN IMMUNODEFICIENCY VIRUS [HIV])

ALANINE AMINOTRANSFERASE (ALT) (SERUM)

SERUM GLUTAMIC PYRUVIC TRANSAMINASE (SGPT)

Reference Values

Adult: 10–35 units/l; 4–36 units/l at 37°C (SI units)
Male: Levels may be slightly higher
Child: Infant: could be twice as high as adult; child: similar to adult
Elderly: Slightly higher than adult

Description.   ALT/SGPT, an enzyme found primarily in the liver cells, is effective in diagnosing hepatocellular destruction. Serum ALT level could elevate before jaundice is present. With jaundice and the serum ALT greater than 300 units, the cause is most likely due to a liver disorder and not a hemolytic disorder.

Purpose

- To detect the presence of a liver disorder

Clinical Problems

Increased level: **Highest increase:** acute (viral) hepatitis, severe hepatotoxicity causing necrosis of liver (drug or chemical toxicity); **slight or moderate increase:** cirrhosis, cancer of the liver, congestive heart failure, acute alcohol intoxication; **marginal increase:** acute myocardial infarction (AMI)

Drugs that may increase ALT value: Antibiotics, narcotics, methyldopa (Aldomet), guanethidine, digitalis preparations, indomethacin (Indocin), salicylates, rifampin, flurazepam (Dalmane), propranolol (Inderal), oral contraceptives, lead, heparin

Procedure

- No food or fluid restriction is required.
- Collect 3 to 5 ml of venous blood in a red-top tube. Avoid hemolysis. RBCs have high concentration of ALT.
- Drugs that can cause false-positive levels should be listed on the laboratory slip along with the date and time last given.

Nursing Implications

Elevated Levels

- Relate the client's serum ALT/SGPT to clinical problems and drugs that can cause false-positive levels.
- Check for signs of jaundice. ALT levels rise several days before jaundice begins if it is related to liver damage.
- Be supportive to the client if jaundice is present and isolation technique is enforced.

ALBUMIN (SERUM)

Reference Values

Adult: 3.5–5.0 g/dl; 52% to 68% of total protein
Child: Newborn: 2.9–5.4 g/dl; infant: 4.4–5.4 g/dl; child: 4.0–5.8 g/dl

Description.   Albumin, a component of proteins, makes up more than half of plasma proteins. Albumin is synthesized by the liver. It increases osmotic pressure (oncotic pressure), which is necessary for maintaining vascular fluid (vessels). A decrease in serum albumin will cause fluid to shift from the vessels to the tissues, resulting in edema.

The *A/G ratio* is a calculation of the distribution of two major protein fractions, albumin and globulin. The reference value of A/G ratio is greater than 1.0, which is the albumin value divided by globulin value (albumin ÷ globulin). A high ratio value is considered insignificant; a low ratio value occurs in liver and renal diseases. Protein electrophoresis is more accurate and has replaced the A/G ratio calculation.

Purpose
- To detect an albumin deficit

Clinical Problems
Decreased level: Cirrhosis of the liver, acute liver failure, severe burns, severe malnutrition, preeclampsia, renal disorders, certain malignancies, ulcerative colitis, prolonged immobilization, protein-losing enteropathies, malabsorption
Drugs that may decrease albumin value: Penicillin, sulfonamides, aspirin, ascorbic acid
Increased level: Dehydration, severe vomiting, severe diarrhea
Drug that may increase albumin value: Heparin

Procedure
- No food or fluid restriction is required.
- Collect 3 to 5 ml of venous blood in a red-top tube.

Nursing Implications
- Check for peripheral edema and ascites when serum albumin is low.
- Assess skin integrity if pitted edema or anasarca is present. Use measures to avoid skin breakdown.

Client Teaching
- Suggest that the client includes foods rich in protein if the serum albumin value is decreased and the client does not have cirrhosis.

ALCOHOL (ETHYL OR ETHANOL) (SERUM OR PLASMA)

Reference Values

00.0%—normal, no alcohol; less than 0.05% or 50 mg/dl—no significant alcohol influence; 0.05%–0.10% or 50–100 mg/dl—alcohol influence is present; 0.10%–0.15% or 100–150 mg/dl—reaction time affected; greater than 0.15% or 150 mg/dl—indicative of alcohol intoxication; greater than 0.25% or 250 mg/dl—severe alcohol intoxication; greater than 0.30% or 300 mg/dl—comatose; greater than 0.40% or 400 mg/dl—fatal.

Description.   Ethyl alcohol (ethanol) in the blood is a frequently requested laboratory test for medical and legal reasons. In most states, an alcohol level greater than 0.1% or 100 mg/dl is considered by law to be proof of alcohol intoxication. However, some states consider 0.08% or 80 mg/dl as proof of alcohol intoxication. On an empty stomach, plasma alcohol peaks in 40 to 70 min.

Serum/plasma alcohol may be used as a screening test on an unconscious client. Nurses should check for any legal ramifications (state laws) in reference to drawing blood for plasma alcohol level.

Purpose

- To detect the percent of alcohol in the bloodstream and for DUI (driving under the influence)

Clinical Problems

Increased level: Moderate to severe alcohol intoxication, chronic alcohol consumption, cirrhosis of the liver, malnutrition, folic acid deficiency, acute pancreatitis, gastritis, hypoglycemia, hyperuricemia

Procedure

- Obtain a consent form if required by law.
- Cleanse the venipuncture area with benzalkonium, and then wipe the solution off with a sterile swab. Do not use alcohol to cleanse the area.

- Collect 3 to 5 ml of venous blood in a red-top tube. A green-, lavender-, or blue-top tube can be used. Avoid hemolysis.
- Write on the specimen and laboratory slip the date and time the blood specimen was drawn. The signatures of the collector and a witness should be included on the tube.

Factors Affecting Laboratory Results
- Cleansing the venipuncture site with alcohol or tincture

Nursing Implications
Elevated level: (Greater than 0.10% or Greater than 100 mg/dl)
- Follow legal ramifications in your state for drawing plasma alcohol level.
- Provide safety measures, such as side rails, to prevent physical harm to the client when the serum alcohol level is greatly increased.

Client Teaching
- Instruct the client not to consume alcoholic beverages when taking sedatives, hypnotics, narcotics, tranquilizers (Valium, Librium), anti-convulsants (Dilantin), and anticoagulants (Coumadin).
- Listen to client's concerns.

ALDOLASE (ALD) (SERUM)

Reference Values
Adult: Less than 6 units/l, 22–59 milliunits/l at 37°C (SI units), 3–8 units/dl (Sibley-Lehninger)
Child: Infant: 12–24 units/dl child: 6–16 units/dl

Description.   Aldolase is an enzyme present in many types of cells, particularly in the skeletal and cardiac muscles. This enzyme test is used to monitor skeletal muscle disease such as muscular dystrophy, dermatomyositis, and trichinosis. Aldolase is not elevated in neural origin diseases such as multiple sclerosis and myasthenia gravis.

Serum aldolase is helpful in diagnosing early cases of Duchenne's muscular dystrophy. It is not as effective in diagnosing myocardial infarction (MI). In progressive muscular dystrophy, the serum aldolase may be 10 or more times the normal value.

Purpose
- To aid in the diagnosis of skeletal muscle disease, such as muscular dystrophy

Clinical Problems
Decreased level: Late muscular dystrophy
Drugs that may decrease aldolase value: Large doses of phenothiazides
Increased level: Early and progressive muscular dystrophy, trichinosis, dermatomyositis, acute myocardial infarction (AMI), acute hepatitis, cancer of the gastrointestinal tract, leukemia
Drugs that may increase aldolase value: Alcohol, cortisone, narcotics, aminocaproic acid, insecticides, clofibrate, and intramuscular injections

Procedure
- No food or fluid restriction is required.
- Collect 3 to 5 ml of venous blood in a red-top tube. Unhemolyzed serum must be used when measuring for aldolase.

Nursing Implications
- Check serum aldolase results, and plan the nursing care according to the symptoms present and psychological needs.
- Assist the client with activities of daily living (ADL) as needed. Promote maximum independence.
- List on the laboratory slip any drugs the client is receiving that can elevate the serum aldolase level.
- Be supportive of the client and family regarding the client's physical and psychological limitations.

ALDOSTERONE (SERUM AND URINE)

Reference Values
Adult: Serum: Less than 16 ng/dl (fasting), 4–30 ng/dl (sitting position)
   Urine: 6–25 mcg/24 h
Child: (3–11 years): 5–70 ng/dl
Pregnancy: 2 to 3 times higher than adult

Description.   Aldosterone is the most potent of all mineralocorticoids produced by the adrenal cortex. The major function of aldosterone is to regulate sodium, potassium, and water balance. Aldosterone promotes sodium reabsorption from the distal tubules of the kidney, and potassium and hydrogen excretion. Twenty-five percent of this hormone secretion is influenced by the adrenocorticotropic hormone (ACTH), and 60% to 75% depends on the renin–angiotensin system. Renin promotes aldosterone secretion, thus causing sodium retention, which results in water retention.

A decreased renin level inhibits the conversion of angiotensinogen to angiotensin. Without angiotensin, aldosterone secretion is markedly reduced.

Serum aldosterone is not the most reliable test, because there can be fluctuations caused by various influences. A 24-h urine test is considered more reliable than a random serum aldosterone collection. The urine and serum aldosterone levels are increased by hyponatremia, a low-salt diet, and hyperkalemia. Also, hypernatremia, a high-salt diet, and hypokalemia decrease the serum aldosterone levels.

Purposes
- To detect deficit or excess of aldosterone
- To compare serum and urine aldosterone levels with other laboratory tests for determining overhydration with elevated sodium level and adrenal hypo- or hyperfunction

Clinical Problems
Decreased level—serum and urine: Overhydration with elevated serum sodium level, severe hypernatremia, high-sodium diet, adrenal cortical

hypofunction (Addison's disease), diabetes mellitus, glucose infusion, licorice

Increased level—serum: Dehydration, hyponatremia, low-sodium diet, essential hypertension, adrenal cortical hyperfunction, cancer of the adrenal gland, cirrhosis of the liver, emphysema, severe congestive heart failure (CHF)

Drugs that may increase serum aldosterone value: Diuretics, hydralazine (Apresoline), diazoxide (Hyperstat), nitroprusside, oral contraceptives

Urine: Tumors of the adrenal cortex or primary aldosteronism, same as serum aldosterone

Drugs that may increase urine aldosterone value: Diuretics, lithium, oral contraceptives

Procedure

Serum

- Food and fluids are not restricted, but excess salt may interfere with test result. Normal salt intake is suggested.
- Collect 5 ml of venous blood in a red- or green-top tube.
- The client should be in a supine position for at least 1 h before the blood is drawn.
- Record the date and time on the specimen. Aldosterone levels exhibit circadian rhythm, with peak levels occurring in the morning and lower levels in the afternoon.

Urine

- Collect a 24-h urine specimen in a large container with a preservative such as a boric acid tablet.
- Have the client void and discard urine before beginning the test.
- Label the container with the exact date and time of urine collection (e.g., 7/5/09, 7 AM to 7/6/09, 7:02 AM).

Nursing Implications

- Compare the serum aldosterone and the 24-h urine aldosterone results if both have been ordered.
- Assess the client for signs and symptoms of overhydration due to excess aldosterone secretion and water retention (e.g., constant, irritating cough, dyspnea, vein engorgement, chest rales).

- Assess the client for signs and symptoms of dehydration that may also result from elevated serum aldosterone level. Sodium reabsorption may be greater than excess water retention.
- Monitor vital signs. Report vital sign changes that may indicate dehydration or overhydration.
- Check at regular intervals to determine whether the urine collection is being properly obtained.

Client Teaching

- Instruct the client not to increase or decrease salt intake before the aldosterone tests. Normal salt intake should be encouraged for accurate test results.
- Instruct the client to remain in a supine position for at least 1 h before blood is drawn to prevent false test results. The position of the client when blood was drawn should be noted on the laboratory slip.
- Instruct the client how to collect the 24-h urine specimen. All urine should be saved after the initial urine specimen is discarded. Toilet paper or feces should not be in the urine.

ALKALINE PHOSPHATASE (ALP) WITH ISOENZYME (SERUM)

Reference Values

Adult: 42–136 units/l; ALP^1: 20–130 units/l; ALP^2: 20–120 units/l
Child: Infant and child (0–12 years): 40–115 units/l; older child (13–18 years): 50–230 units/l
Elderly: Slightly higher than adult

Description. ALP is an enzyme produced mainly in the liver and bone and is also produced in the intestine, the kidney, and the placenta. This test is useful for determining liver and bone diseases.

To differentiate between liver and bone disorders, other enzyme tests should be performed (i.e., LAP, GGTP, and/or 5′N). ALP isoenzymes, ALP^1 (liver origin) and ALP^2 (bone origin), are helpful in distinguishing between liver and bone disease.

Purposes
- To determine the presence of a liver or a bone disorder
- To compare ALP results with other laboratory tests for confirmation of liver or bone disorder

Clinical Problems
Decreased level: Hypothyroidism, malnutrition, scurvy (vitamin C deficit), hypophosphatasia, pernicious anemia, placental insufficiency

Drugs that decrease ALP values: Fluoride, oxalate, propranolol (Inderal)

Increased level: Obstructive biliary disease (jaundice); cancer of the liver, hepatocellular cirrhosis; hepatitis; leukemia; cancer of the bone, breast, and prostate; Paget's disease (osteitis deformans); healing fractures; multiple myeloma; osteomalacia; gastrointestinal ulcerative disease; late pregnancy; hyperthyroidism; hyperparathyroidism; rheumatoid arthritis; congestive heart failure (CHF)

Drugs that may increase ALP value: Antibiotics, colchicine, methyldopa (Aldomet), allopurinol, phenothiazines, indomethacin (Indocin), procainamide, some oral contraceptives, tolbutamide, isoniazid (INH), IV albumin

Procedure
- No food or fluid restrictions are required. For ALP isoenzymes, fasting overnight may be indicated.
- Collect 3 to 5 ml of venous blood in a red-top tube. Avoid hemolysis.
- Withhold drugs that can elevate ALP level for 8 to 24 h with health care provider's permission.
- List client's age and drugs that may affect test results on laboratory slip.

Factors Affecting Laboratory Results
- Age of the client (youth and old age) and late pregnancy to 3 weeks postpartum can cause elevated level.

Nursing Implications
- Know factors that can elevate serum ALP levels (e.g., drugs, IV albumin [can elevate serum ALP 5 to 10 times its normal value]); age of

client (child or elderly); late pregnancy to 3 weeks postpartum; and blood drawn 2 to 4 h after fatty meal.
- Record pertinent information from procedure on laboratory slip.

Client Teaching
- Assess for clinical signs and symptoms of liver disease or bone disease.
- Inform client that other enzyme tests may be ordered to verify diagnosis.

ALPHA₁ ANTITRYPSIN (α₁AT) (SERUM)

ALPHA-1-TRYPSIN INHIBITOR
Reference Values
Adult: 78–200 mg/dl, 0.78–2.0 g/l
Child: Newborn: 145–270 mg/dl; infant: similar to adult range

Description.   Antitrypsin (α_1AT), a protein produced by the liver, inhibits proteolytic enzymes that are released by the lung. A deficiency of homozygous antitrypsin (heredity linked) permits proteolytic enzymes to damage lung tissue, thus causing emphysema.

An elevated serum α_1 AT level might be present in inflammatory conditions.

Purposes
- To determine if COPD is caused by a deficiency of alpha₁ antitrypsin protein
- To detect an α_1 AT deficiency

Clinical Problems
Decreased level: Chronic obstructive lung disease (pulmonary emphysema), severe liver damage, malnutrition, severe protein-losing disorders (e.g., nephrotic syndrome)
Increased level: Acute and chronic inflammatory conditions, infections (selected), necrosis, late pregnancy, exercise (returns to normal in 1 day)
Drugs that may increase α_1 AT value: Oral contraceptives

Procedure

- Restrict food and fluids, except for water, for 8 h.
- Collect 3 to 5 ml of venous blood in red-top tube.
- Hold oral contraceptives for 24 h before the test, with the health care provider's permission. Any oral contraceptive taken should be listed on the laboratory slip.

Factors Affecting Laboratory Results

- Oral intake of food before the test can cause an inaccurate result if the client has an elevated serum cholesterol or serum triglyceride level.

Nursing Implications

- List the name of the oral contraceptive and date last taken on the laboratory slip.

Decreased level
Client Teaching

- Explain to the client that the test is ordered to determine an antitrypsin (protein) deficiency that can cause a lung disorder. A nonsmoker with an α_1AT deficiency can have emphysema. Antitrypsin inhibits proteolytic enzymes from destroying lung tissue; with a lack of this protein, the alveoli are damaged.
- Instruct the client with an α_1AT deficit to use preventive methods in protecting lungs (i.e., avoid persons with upper respiratory infection [URI], seek medical care when having a respiratory infection).
- Encourage the client to stop smoking and to avoid areas having high air pollution. Air pollution can cause respiratory inflammation and promote chronic obstructive lung disease.

Increased level

- Check the serum α_1AT level 2 to 3 days after extensive surgery. Inflammation can markedly increase the serum level. A baseline serum level may be ordered before surgery for several reasons (e.g., for determining lung disease and the effects of surgery).
- Report to the health care provider if the serum α_1AT remains elevated 2 weeks after surgery.
- Note that serum α_1AT can be markedly elevated during late pregnancy.

ALPHA FETOPROTEIN (AFP) (SERUM)

Reference Values
Nonpregnancy: Less than 15 ng/ml
Pregnancy

Serum		Amniotic Fluid	
Weeks of Gestation	*ng/ml*	*Weeks of Gestation*	*mcg/ml*
8–12	0–39	14	11.0–32.0
13	6–31	15	5.5–31.0
14	7–50	16	5.7–31.5
15	7–60	17	3.8–32.5
16	10–72	18	3.6–28.0
17	11–90	19	3.7–24.5
18	14–94	20	2.2–15.0
19	24–112	21	3.8–18.0
20	31–122		
21	19–124		

Description.   Serum AFP, a screening test, is usually done between 16 and 20 weeks of gestation to detect the probability of twins, infant of low birth weight, or serious birth defects, such as open neural tube defect. If a high serum AFP level occurs, the test should be repeated. Ultrasound and amniocentesis may be performed to diagnose neural tube defect in the fetus.

Purpose
- To identify the probability of neural tube defects, fetal death, or other anomalies in pregnancy (see Clinical Problems)

Clinical Problems
Increased Level
Nonpregnant: Cirrhosis of the liver (not liver metastasis), germ cell tumor of gonads, such as testicular cancer

Pregnant: Neural tube defects (spina bifida, anencephaly), fetal death, other anomalies (duodenal atresia, tetralogy of Fallot, hydrocephalus, trisomy 13, encephalocele)

Procedure
- No food or fluid restriction is required.
- Collect 5 to 7 ml of venous blood in a red-top tube. Avoid hemolysis.

Factors Affecting Laboratory Results
- Fetal blood contamination could cause an elevated amniotic AFP level.
- Inaccurate recording of gestation week could affect results.
- Multiple pregnancy or fetal death could cause false-positive test.

Nursing Implications
- Explain that the test is for screening purposes. If the test is positive, genetic counseling might be necessary.
- Be supportive to the client and family.

ALZHEIMER'S DISEASE MARKERS (SEE AMYLOID BETA PROTEIN PRECURSOR [CSF])

AMINO ACID (URINE)

Reference Values
Normal values are age dependent: 200 mg/24 h

Description. This test screens for elevated levels of amino acid in the urine (aminoaciduria), which can indicate inborn errors of metabolism. With abnormal metabolism, there can be an excess in one or more amino acids in the plasma and urine. The test is performed when genetic abnormalities are suspected. The amino acid screening test is positive when there is an increase in amino acid or its metabolites in the urine.

Aminoaciduria disease can include phenylketonuria, maple syrup urine disease, cystinuria, and tyrosinemia. Further testing would be needed to confirm the metabolic disorder.

Purposes
- To screen for renal aminoacidurias
- To detect inborn errors of metabolism

Clinical Problems
Increased level: Mental retardation, retarded growth, cystinuria, severe brain damage, oasthouse urine disease, phenylketonuria, tyrosinosis, ketosis
Drugs that may increase urine amino acid: Penicillins, valproic acid

Procedure
- There is no food or fluid restriction.
- Collect a clean random urine specimen. A 24-h urine specimen may be requested.
- Pack the specimen in ice and send immediately to the laboratory. Refrigeration can be used.

Factors Affecting Laboratory Results
- Lack of protein ingestion in 48 h
- Failure to ice or refrigerate the specimen

Nursing Implications
- Obtain a history of health problems that may relate to the abnormal metabolism disorder.
- Check the drug history, notify the health care provider if the client is taking a penicillin derivative.
- Allow the client and family time to express their concerns.

AMINOGLYCOSIDES (SERUM)

AMIKACIN (AMIKIN), GENTAMICIN (GARAMYCIN), KANAMYCIN (KANTREX), NETILMICIN (NETROMYCIN), TOBRAMYCIN (NEBCIN)

Reference Values
Adult and Child

THERAPEUTIC RANGE

Drug Name	Peak	Trough	Toxic Level
Amikacin	15–30 mcg/ml	Less than 10 mcg/ml	Greater than 35 mcg/ml
Gentamicin	6–12 mcg/ml	Less than 2 mcg/ml	Greater than 12 mcg/ml
Kanamycin	15–30 mcg/ml	1–4 mcg/ml	Greater than 35 mcg/ml
Netilmicin	0.5–10 mcg/ml	Less than 4 mcg/ml	Greater than 16 mcg/ml
Tobramycin	5–10 mcg/ml	Less than 2 mcg/ml	Greater than 12 mcg/ml

Description.   Aminoglycosides are broad-spectrum antibiotics that are effective against Gram-negative microorganisms. These agents are not well absorbed from the GI tract and so are given parenterally. Peak action after intramuscular (IM) injection is 0.5 to 1.5 h, and after 30 min IV infusion is 0.5 h. Half-life is about 2 h. Aminoglycosides cross the placental barrier but do not cross the blood–brain barrier. They are excreted mostly unchanged by the kidneys.

Ototoxicity and nephrotoxicity can result from overdose of an aminoglycoside or from long-term administration. Renal function tests (e.g., creatinine, creatinine clearance, and urinalysis) should be assessed periodically (recommended creatinine levels every 2 to 3 days) while the client is receiving these agents. If clients with renal insufficiency receive any of these drugs, dosage should be adjusted (decreased). Drug half-life is usually 24 to 96 h in clients having renal damage.

Purpose
- To assess clients receiving aminoglycosides for therapeutic effect and possible toxic effect by monitoring urinary output, blood urea nitrogen (BUN), and serum creatinine levels

Clinical Problems

Increased levels: Overdose of aminoglycoside, renal insufficiency or failure

Drugs that may increase aminoglycoside value: Diuretics, cephalosporins (increase chance of nephrotoxicity)

Procedure

- No food or fluid restriction is required.
- Collect 3 to 5 ml of venous blood in a red-top tube.
- Collect specimen during steady state, usually 24 to 36 h after drug was started.
- Record on the laboratory requisition slip drug dose, route (IM or IV), and last time the drug was administered. Specific drug levels may need to be checked concurrently with aminoglycoside levels.

Nursing Implications

- Check serum aminoglycoside (amikacin, gentamicin, kanamycin, netilmicin, tobramycin) results, and report nontherapeutic levels to the health care provider immediately.
- Assess intake and output. Notify the health care provider if urine output has greatly decreased. This could be a sign of aminoglycoside toxicity.
- Suggest renal function tests for clients receiving long-term aminoglycoside therapy, especially for those with renal insufficiency.
- Recognize that diuretics and cephalosporins coadministered with an aminoglycoside could enhance the risk of nephrotoxicity.
- Assess hearing status of the client. Any hearing impairment (e.g., loss of high tone) while the client is receiving an aminoglycoside could indicate ototoxicity.
- Observe for signs and symptoms of nephrotoxicity (e.g., proteinuria, elevated creatinine, elevated BUN, decreased creatinine clearance test).
- Observe for signs and symptoms of ototoxicity (e.g., nausea and vomiting with motion, dizziness, headache, tinnitus, decrease in ability to hear high-pitched tones).

AMMONIA (PLASMA)

Reference Values
Adult: 15–45 mcg/dl, 11–35 µmol/l (SI units)
Child: Newborn: 64–107 mcg/dl; child: 29–70 mcg/dl; 29–70 µmol/l (SI units)

Description.   Ammonia, a by-product of protein metabolism, is converted in the liver to urea. The kidneys excrete urea. With severe liver disorder or when blood flow to the liver is altered, the plasma ammonia level is elevated. Although elevated plasma ammonia is correlated with hepatic failure, other conditions that interfere with liver function (CHF, acidosis) can cause a temporary ammonia elevation.

Purpose
* To detect liver disorder from the inability of the liver to convert ammonia to urea

Clinical Problems
Decreased level: Renal failure, malignant hypertension, essential hypertension
Drugs that may decrease ammonia value: Antibiotics (neomycin, kanamycin, tetracycline), monoamine oxidase inhibitors, diphenhydramine (Benadryl), potassium salts, sodium salts
Increased level: Hepatic failure, hepatic encephalopathy or coma, portacaval anastomosis, Reye's syndrome, erythroblastosis fetalis, cor pulmonale, severe congestive heart failure, high-protein diet with liver failure, acidosis, exercise, hyperalimentation
Drugs that may increase ammonia value: Ammonia chloride, diuretics (thiazides, furosemide [Lasix], ethacrynic acid [Edecrin], acetazolamide [Diamox]), ion exchange resin, isoniazid (INH)

Procedure
* No food or fluid restriction is required unless indicated by laboratory. Smoking should be avoided before the test.

- Collect 5 ml of venous blood in a green-top (heparinized) tube. Deliver blood specimen in packed ice immediately to laboratory. Ammonia levels increase rapidly after blood is drawn.
- Minimize use of tourniquet for drawing blood.
- List drugs client is taking that could affect test results.

Factors Affecting Laboratory Results
- A high- or low-protein diet can cause false test result.
- Exercise might increase the plasma ammonia level.

Nursing Implications
Increased Level
- Identify clinical problems and drugs that can increase the plasma ammonia level.
- Notify the laboratory personnel promptly when a plasma ammonia level is drawn so that it can be analyzed immediately to avoid false results.
- Recognize that exercise may be a cause of an elevated plasma ammonia level.
- Observe for signs and symptoms of hepatic failure, especially when the plasma ammonia is elevated (i.e., behavioral and personality changes, lethargy, confusion, flapping tremors of the extremities, twitching, and, later, coma).
- Know various treatments used in decreasing the plasma ammonia level, such as low-protein diet, antibiotics (neomycin) to destroy intestinal bacteria that increase ammonia production, enemas, cathartics (magnesium sulfate) to prevent ammonia formation, and sodium glutamate and L-arginine in IV dextrose solution to stimulate urea formation.

AMYLASE (SERUM AND URINE)

Reference Values
Serum: Adult: 60–160 Somogyi units/dl, 30–170 units/l (SI units)
Pregnancy: slightly increased

Child: usually not done
Elderly: could be slightly higher than adult
Serum isoenzymes: S (salivary) type: 45%–70%
P (pancreatic) type: 30%–55%
Values may differ with method used
Urine: Adult: 4–37 units/12 h

Description.   Amylase is an enzyme that is derived from the pancreas, salivary gland, and liver. In acute pancreatitis, serum amylase is increased to twice its normal level. Its level begins to increase 2 to 12 h after onset, peaks in 20 to 30 h, and returns to normal in 2 to 4 days. An increased serum amylase can occur after abdominal surgery involving the gallbladder (stones or biliary duct) and stomach (partial gastrectomy).

There are two major amylase isoenzymes, P and S types. P-type elevation may occur more frequently in acute pancreatitis. Elevated S type can be due to ovarian and bronchogenic tumors.

The urine amylase level is helpful in determining the significance of a normal or slightly elevated serum amylase, especially when the client has symptoms of pancreatitis. Urine amylase can remain elevated up to 2 weeks after acute pancreatitis.

Purpose
* To assist in the diagnosis of acute pancreatitis and other health problems (see Clinical Problems)

Clinical Problems
Decreased level: IV D$_5$W, advanced chronic pancreatitis, acute and subacute necrosis of the liver, chronic alcoholism, toxic hepatitis, severe burns, severe thyrotoxicosis
Drugs that may decrease amylase value: Glucose, citrates, fluorides, oxalates
Increased level: Acute pancreatitis, chronic pancreatitis (acute onset), partial gastrectomy, peptic ulcer perforation, obstruction of pancreatic duct, acute cholecystitis, cancer of the pancreas, diabetic acidosis, diabetes mellitus, acute alcoholic intoxication, mumps, renal failure, benign prostatic hypertrophy, burns, pregnancy

Drugs that may increase amylase value: Narcotics, ethyl alcohol (large amounts), ACTH, guanethidine, thiazide diuretics, salicylates, tetracycline

Procedure
Serum
- Restrict food for 1 to 2 h before the blood sample is drawn. If the client has eaten or has received a narcotic 2 h before the test, the serum results could be invalid.
- Obtain 3 to 5 ml of venous blood in a red-top tube.
- List on the laboratory slip drugs that could cause false amylase levels.

Urine
- Have client void and discard urine. Collect a 2-h urine specimen.
- Urine specimen should be refrigerated or kept on ice. No preservative is needed.

Factors Affecting Laboratory Results
- IV fluids with glucose can result in false-negative levels.

Nursing Implications
Decreased Level—Serum and Urine
- Determine when the client has ingested food or sweetened fluids. Blood should not be drawn until 2 h after eating, since sugar can decrease the serum amylase level.
- Know that D_5W IV can decrease the serum amylase level, causing a false-negative result.
- Check urinary output for 8 and 24 h. A decreased urine output could result in a decreased urine amylase.

Client Teaching
- Encourage the client to drink water during the test unless water intake is restricted for medical reasons.
- Explain to the client the importance of collecting urine at a specified time, using a urinal or bedpan and saving all urine.

Increased Level—Serum and Urine
- Check serum amylase levels for several days after abdominal surgery. Surgery of the stomach or gallbladder might cause trauma to the pancreas and excess amylase to be released.

- Report symptoms of severe pain when pancreatitis is suspected. The physician may want to draw a serum amylase level before a narcotic is given. An elevated level may indicate an acute pancreatitis.
- Check the serum amylase level and compare with the urine amylase level. A low serum amylase level and an increased urine amylase level could indicate that the acute problem is no longer present.
- Report elevated serum amylase results occurring beyond 3 days. If the serum amylase levels remain elevated beyond 3 days, pancreatic cell destruction could still be occurring.

AMYLOID BETA PROTEIN PRECURSOR (CSF)

ALZHEIMER'S DISEASE MARKER

Reference Values
Adult Normal: 450 units/1 cerebrospinal fluid (CSF)

Description.   A CSF test that can aid in diagnosing Alzheimer's disease is amyloid beta protein precursor test. It is found that the amyloid beta protein is present in the senile plaques within the brain. Amyloid can also be found in the meningeal blood vessels of clients with Alzheimer's disease. It is believed that this type of protein may have neurotoxic effects on the brain cells. Small amounts of amyloid can be found in the CSF of most healthy persons; however, a higher value occurs in the CSF of clients with Alzheimer's, and a somewhat slightly higher value than normal may occur in an aged client with senile dementia.

Purpose
- To aid in the diagnosing of Alzheimer's disease

Clinical Problems
Increased level: Alzheimer's disease, senile dementia

Procedure
- A consent form should be signed.
- There is no food or fluid restriction.

- The bladder should be emptied.
- The client's position for the procedure is lying on his/her side in a "fetal" or a sitting position.
- The client should remain relaxed and still during the procedure. Taking deep breaths may help the client to relax.
- Collect at least 2 ml of CSF and place the fluid specimen in a sterile tube.

Factors Affecting Laboratory Results
- Blood in the spinal fluid can cause false test results.

Nursing Implications
Client Teaching
- Explain to the client and family the test procedure. A family member may wish to be with the client during the test procedure.
- Answer the client or family member's questions, and if unknown, refer the questions to the appropriate health professional.

Post-test
- Place client in a reclining position for 8 to 12 h; the client can turn side to side. The client's head should not be raised to avoid "spinal" headache, which could occur from the leaking of spinal fluid at the needle insertion site.
- Report any numbness or tingling in the extremities.
- Encourage the client to increase fluid intake for the next 24 h.

ANGIOTENSIN-CONVERTING ENZYME (ACE) (SERUM)

ANGIOTENSIN-1-CONVERTING ENZYME

Reference Values
Adult greater than 20 years: 8–67 units/l
Child and adult less than 20 years: Not performed because they normally have elevated ACE levels

Description.   Angiotensin-converting enzyme (ACE) is found primarily in the lung epithelial cells and some in blood vessels and renal cells. The purpose of ACE is to regulate arterial blood pressure by converting angiotensin I to the vasoconstrictor angiotensin II, which increases blood pressure and stimulates the adrenal cortex to release aldosterone (sodium-retaining hormone). However, this test has little value for diagnosing hypertension.

High serum ACE levels are found primarily with active pulmonary sarcoidosis. Seventy percent to 90% of clients with active sarcoidosis have elevated serum ACE levels. Other conditions that have elevated ACE levels include Gaucher's disease (disorder of fat metabolism), leprosy, alcoholic cirrhosis, active histoplasmosis, tuberculosis, pulmonary embolism, hyperthyroidism, and Hodgkin's disease.

Purposes
- To assist in diagnosing various health problems such as pulmonary sarcoidosis related to elevated serum ACE level
- To compare the results of serum ACE level with other laboratory tests for diagnosing health problem

Clinical Problems
Decreased level: Therapy for sarcoidosis, diabetes mellitus, hypothyroidism, respiratory distress syndrome, severe illness, starvation
Drugs that may decrease ACE value: Steroids (prednisone, cortisone), captopril, enalapril
Increased level: Sarcoidosis, Gaucher's disease, leprosy, alcoholic cirrhosis, histoplasmosis, tuberculosis, pulmonary embolism, hyperthyroidism, Hodgkin's disease, myeloma, non-Hodgkin's lymphoma, idiopathic pulmonary fibrosis, scleroderma, diabetes mellitus, asbestosis

Procedure
- Restrict food and fluids for 12 h prior to the test.
- Collect 7 ml of venous blood in a red-top or green-top tube. Check with the laboratory concerning which tube—for clotted blood (red-top) or heparinized (green-top). Avoid hemolysis. Deliver the blood sample immediately to the laboratory.
- Record the client's age on the laboratory slip.

Nursing Implications

- Check blood pressure. This test is not used to determine the cause of hypertension; however, ACE indirectly contributes to an increase in blood pressure.
- Report if the client is taking steroids to the health care provider and on the laboratory slip.
- Record the age of the client on the laboratory slip. Rarely is this test ordered for clients under 20 years of age as there could be a false-positive test result.

Client Teaching

- Instruct the client not to eat or drink for 12 h prior to the test; this would most likely be NPO after dinner.
- Answer questions or concerns the client may have or refer him/her to other health care providers.

ANION GAP

Reference Values

Adult: 10–17 mEq/l (values differ from 7 to 20 mEq/l)

Description.   Anion gap is the difference between the electrolytes, measured cations (sodium and potassium), and measured anions (chloride and bicarbonate [HCO_3]) to determine the unmeasured cations and anions in the serum. These unmeasured ions are phosphates, sulfates, lactates, ketone bodies, and other organic acids that contribute to metabolic acid–base imbalances (metabolic acidosis or alkalosis).

The formula used to determine the anion gap is: Anion gap = (sodium + potassium) – (chloride + [HCO_3] [bicarbonate]).

An elevated anion gap greater than 17 mEq/l is indicative of metabolic acidosis; a decreased anion gap less than 10 mEq/l is indicative of metabolic alkalosis.

Purpose

- To determine the presence of acidosis

Clinical Problems
Decreased level: High electrolyte values such as sodium, calcium, magnesium, multiple myeloma, nephrosis
Drugs that may decrease the anion gap: Diuretics, lithium, chlorpropamide
Increased level: Lactic acidosis, ketoacidosis, starvation, severe salicylate intoxication, renal failure, severe dehydration, paint thinner ingestion
Drugs that may increase the anion gap: Penicillin and carbenicillin in high doses, salicylates, diuretics (thiazides and loop diuretics), methanol ingestion, paraldehyde
Normal level occurring in metabolic acidosis: Diarrhea, renal tubular acidosis, hyperalimentation, ureterosigmoidostomy, small bowel fistula, pancreatic drainage

Procedure
- No food or fluid restriction is required.
- Obtain serum electrolyte values: sodium (Na), potassium (K), chloride (C), and CO_2 (bicarbonate determinant). If electrolytes are not available, collect 7 to 10 ml of venous blood in a red-top tube.

Nursing Implications
- Calculate anion gap from recently obtained electrolyte values of sodium, potassium, chloride, and serum CO_2. Use the formula given in Description.
- Observe for signs and symptoms of metabolic acidosis such as rapid, vigorous breathing (Kussmaul's breathing), flushed skin, increased pulse rate.

ANTHRAX (*SEE* BIOTERRORISM INFECTIONS)

ANTIBIOTIC SUSCEPTIBILITY (SENSITIVITY) TEST

CULTURE AND SENSITIVITY (C & S) TEST

Reference Values
Adult: Organism is sensitive, intermediate, or resistant to the antibiotic disks
Child: Same as adult

Description.   It is important to identify not only the organism responsible for the infection but also the antibiotic(s) that will inhibit the growth of the bacteria. The health care provider orders a C & S test when a wound infection, urinary tract infection (UTI), or other types of infected secretions are suspected. The choice of antibiotic depends on the pathogenic organism and its susceptibility to the antibiotics.

Purpose
- To check the effectiveness of selected antibiotics to a specific bacterium from a culture

Clinical Problems
Resistant (R):   Antibiotic is noneffective against the organism
Intermediate (I):   Bacterial growth retardation is inconclusive
Sensitive (S):   Antibiotic is effective against the organism

Procedure (See Cultures—Procedure)
- The specimen for C & S should be taken to the laboratory within 30 min of collection or refrigerated.
- It usually takes 24 h for bacterial growth and 48 h for the test results.

Nursing Implications
- Collect specimen for C & S before preventive antibiotic therapy is started. Antibiotic therapy started before specimen collection could cause an inaccurate result.
- Record on the laboratory slip the antibiotic(s) the client is receiving, the dosages, and how long the antibiotic(s) has (have) been taken.
- Check laboratory report for C & S result. If the client is receiving an antibiotic and the report shows the organism is resistant to that antibiotic, notify the health care provider.

Client Teaching
- Inform the client that the culture test results will be available in 48 h.

ANTICARDIOLIPIN ANTIBODIES (ACA) (SERUM)

ANTIPHOSPHOLIPID ANTIBODIES (APA); CARDIOLIPIN ANTIBODIES (aCl); IgG CARDIOLIPIN ANTIBODIES AND IgM CARDIOLIPIN ANTIBODIES

Reference Value

Negative

Description. Anticardiolipin antibodies (ACA) are autoantibodies found in some clients with systemic lupus erythematosus (SLE). They occur in 45% of clients with SLE and less than 7% of clients without SLE. These antibodies were originally found in clients with SLE and were called *lupus anticoagulants* (LA). Later it was determined that these antibodies did not act as anticoagulants and that they were found in health problems other than lupus. ACA and LA are members of the antiphospholipid antibodies (APA) family of immunoglobulins active against phospholipids. ACA may also be present in clients having thrombocytopenia, spontaneous or recurrent thrombosis, and fetal loss.

Purposes
- To aid in the diagnosis of SLE, especially in clients who have thrombocytopenia and repeated fetal loss
- To detect ACA syndrome in clients with other health problems

Clinical Problems
Increased level: SLE, thrombocytopenia, thrombosis, fetal loss, infection, severe hemorrhage (rate), malignancy, acquired immunodeficiency syndrome (AIDS)
Drugs that can increase ACA level: Chlorpromazine, procainamide, quinidine, penicillin, various antibiotics, phenytoin

Procedure
- There is no food or fluid restriction.

• Collect 3 to 5 ml of venous blood in a red-top tube. Avoid hemolysis; send the specimen immediately to the laboratory.

Factors Affecting Laboratory Results
• Hemolysis of the blood specimen may cause a false test result.

Nursing Implications
• Obtain a history of the client's health problem with current symptoms.
• Observe for signs and symptoms of SLE (e.g., fatigue, fever, rash butterfly over the nose, leukopenia).

Client Teaching
• Instruct the client to have daily rest periods, which help to decrease symptoms.
• Explain to the client the purpose of oral anticoagulant or platelet inhibitor therapy for thrombocytopenia or recurrent thrombosis if these treatments are ordered.
• Listen to the client's concerns; answer questions or refer them to another health care provider.

ANTIDEPRESSANTS (TRICYCLICS) (SERUM)

AMITRIPTYLINE, DESIPRAMINE, DOXEPIN, IMIPRAMINE, NORTRIPTYLINE

Reference Values
Adult

Drug Name	Therapeutic Range (ng/ml)	Toxic Level (ng/ml)
Amitriptyline HCI (Elavil)	75–225	Greater than 500
Desipramine HCI (Norpramin)	125–300	Greater than 500
Doxepin HCI (Sinequan)	150–300	Greater than 500
Imipramine HCI (Tofranil)	150–300	Greater than 500
Nortriptyline HCI (Aventyl)	75–150	Greater than 300

Description.   Antidepressants are used primarily for unipolar or endogenous depression, which is characterized by loss of interest in work or home, inability to complete tasks, and deep depression. There are three groups of antidepressants: tricyclic antidepressants (TCAs), second-generation antidepressants (newest group), and monoamine oxidase (MAO) inhibitors. A common side effect of tricyclic antidepressants is anticholinergic symptoms. With second-generation antidepressants, extrapyramidal symptoms (EPS) are common. Clients taking MAO inhibitors should avoid foods rich in tyramine (cheese, cream, chocolate, bananas, beer, red wines). Hypertensive crisis could occur when taking foods rich in tyramine and MAO inhibitors.

Purposes

- To regulate tricyclic drug level for obtaining a therapeutic drug level
- To monitor tricyclic drug dose
- To avoid toxic drug level

Clinical Problems

Decreased level: Mild, reactive, unipolar, and/or atypical depression
Drugs that may decrease antidepressant level: Barbiturates, chloral hydrate
Increased level: Toxic tricyclic antidepressant
Drugs that may increase antidepressant level: Hydrocortisone, neuroleptics, cimetidine, oral contraceptives

Procedure

- No food or fluid restriction is required.
- Collect 7 ml of venous blood in a red-top tube. Deliver blood container immediately to the laboratory.
- Obtain blood specimen 2 h before the next drug dose.

Nursing Implications

- Assess client's history related to depression.
- Record drugs that the client presently is taking. CNS depressants and alcohol, if taken with antidepressants, could cause respiratory depression and hypotension.
- Monitor vital signs and urinary output. Report abnormal findings.

- Check serum tricyclic level of the drug client is taking. Report if the level is NOT within therapeutic range.
- Assess client's compliance to drug therapy. Report changes.

Client Teaching
- Discuss the importance of drug compliance with the client. This is important to maintain a therapeutic drug level and possibly to avoid toxic level if the drug is taken in excess.
- Discuss possible side effects, such as dry mouth, blurred vision, fatigue, urinary retention, postural hypotension, and GI disturbances, and report any of these to the health care provider.
- Discuss foods to avoid if the client is taking an MAO inhibitor (see Description).

ANTIDIURETIC HORMONE (ADH) (PLASMA)

VASOPRESSOR

Reference Values
Adult: 1–5 pg/ml; 1–5 ng/l

Description.   Antidiuretic hormone (ADH) is produced by the hypothalamus and stored in the posterior pituitary gland (neurohypophysis). Primary function of ADH is for water reabsorption from the distal renal tubules in response to the serum osmolality. Antidiuretic means "against diuresis." There is more ADH secreted from the posterior pituitary gland when the serum osmolality is increased, greater than 295 mOsm/kg (concentrated body fluids); thus, more water is reabsorbed, which dilutes the body fluid. When the serum osmolality is decreased, less than 280 mOsm/kg, less ADH is secreted, and thus more water is excreted via kidneys.

Syndrome (secretion) of inappropriate ADH (SIADH) is an excess secretion of ADH that is not influenced by the serum osmolality level. SIADH causes excess water retention. Stress, surgery, pain, and certain drugs (narcotics, anesthetics) contribute to SIADH.

Purposes
- To detect a deficit or excess in ADH secretion
- To identify the presence of body fluid deficit or excess

Clinical Problems
Decreased level: Diabetes insipidus, psychogenic polydipsia, nephrotic syndrome
Drugs that may decrease ADH value: Alcohol, lithium, demeclocycline, phenytoin (Dilantin)
Increased level: SIADH, brain tumor, cancer (ectopic ADH), pulmonary tuberculosis, pain, intermittent positive pressure breathing (IPPB), surgery, pneumonia
Drugs that may increase ADH value: Anesthetics, narcotics, estrogens, oxytocin, antineoplastic (anticancer) drugs, thiazides, antipsychotics, tricyclic antidepressants

Procedure
- Restrict food and fluids for 12 h. Avoid strenuous exercise for 12 h. Stress should be decreased or avoided.
- Collect 5 to 7 ml of venous blood in a lavender-top plastic tube or plastic syringe. Glass container can cause degradation of the antidiuretic hormone. If blood is drawn in glass, prechill the glass and separate immediately.
- Deliver the blood specimen immediately (within 10 min) to the laboratory.

Factors Affecting Laboratory Results
- Blood specimen taken at night or from a client in standing position can cause the ADH to be elevated.

Nursing Implications
- Report drugs the client is taking that can affect test results. These drugs should be withheld 12 h prior to the test.

- Record in the client's chart and on the laboratory slip if the client is having undue stress or pain. This could increase the ADH secretion (SIADH) and plasma level.
- Take the blood specimen immediately to the laboratory. The serum should be separated from the clot within 10 min.
- Listen to client's concerns.

ANTIGLOMERULAR BASEMENT MEMBRANE ANTIBODY (ANTI-GBM, AGBM) (SERUM)

GLOMERULAR BASEMENT MEMBRANE ANTIBODY

Reference Values

Negative or none detected

Description.   This test is performed to detect circulating glomerular basement membrane (GBM) antibodies that can damage the glomerular basement membranes in the glomeruli. Beta-hemolytic *Streptococcus* can cause an antibody response in the renal glomeruli.

Glomerulonephritis, caused by anti-GBM, is usually severe and rapidly progressive. Pulmonary hemorrhage often occurs due to cross-reactivity of anti-GBM with pulmonary vascular basement membrane.

Purpose

- To detect GBM antibodies that could cause or is causing renal disease

Clinical Problems

Positive result: Anti-GBM nephritis, tubulointerstitial nephritis, pulmonary capillary basement membranes

Procedure

- No food or fluid restriction is required.
- Collect 5 to 7 ml of venous blood in a red-top tube. Test should be run immediately, and if not, the blood should be frozen.
- Tissue from kidney biopsy might be the specimen. Tissue should be frozen after collection.

Nursing Implications
- Obtain a history of a streptococcal throat infection.
- Monitor urine output. As the glomeruli are damaged, oliguria usually occurs.
- Assess for signs and symptoms of renal (glomerular) disease (i.e., edema of the extremities, shortness of breath, proteinuria, hematuria, increased blood pressure, elevated serum BUN and creatinine, decreased urine output).

Client Teaching
- Instruct the client to follow a medical regimen of diet, drugs, and rest.

ANTIMITOCHONDRIAL ANTIBODY (AMA) (SERUM)

Reference Values
Negative: At a 1:5 to 1:10 dilution
Intermediate level: 1:20 to 1:80 dilution
Strongly suggestive of primary biliary cirrhosis: greater than 1:80
Positive for primary biliary cirrhosis: greater than 1:160

Description.   The antimitochondrial antibody (AMA) test is used to differentiate between primary biliary cirrhosis and other liver disease. Eighty percent to 90% of clients with primary biliary cirrhosis have a positive titer for AMAs. A positive test result would usually rule out extrahepatic biliary obstruction and acute infectious hepatitis. To confirm biliary cirrhosis, other liver tests should be performed, such as ALT, GGT, alkaline phosphatase, serum bilirubin.

This test is usually performed in conjunction with anti–smooth muscle antibodies (ASMA) test. ASMA titer is elevated with biliary cirrhosis and chronic active hepatitis. Like AMA, ASMA is seldom elevated with extrahepatic biliary obstruction. The antibodies may also be associated with autoimmune disease.

Purposes
- To aid in the diagnosis of biliary cirrhosis
- To determine liver function

- To differentiate between biliary cirrhosis and extrahepatic disease (liver biopsy may be needed)

Clinical Problems

Positive titer: Primary biliary cirrhosis, chronic hepatitis, autoimmune disorders (i.e., systemic erythematosus [SLE], rheumatoid arthritis, pernicious anemia)

Procedure

- NPO for 8 h prior to the test. Food and fluids may not need to be restricted; check with the laboratory.
- Collect 3 to 5 ml of venous blood in a red- or a gray-top tube. Avoid hemolysis. Take blood specimen immediately to the laboratory.

Nursing Implications

- Assess for the presence of jaundice.
- Check other liver tests and compare test results.
- Check with the laboratory as to whether NPO is necessary.

Client Teaching

- Listen to client's concern. Answer appropriate questions.
- Tell the client that if a hematoma occurs to apply warm wet compresses or soaks. Clients with hepatic disease have an increased bleeding tendency.

ANTIMYOCARDIAL ANTIBODY (SERUM)

Reference Values

Negative: None detected
Positive: Titer levels

Description.   Antimyocardial antibody develops due to a specific antigen in the heart muscle that can cause autoimmune damage to the heart. This antibody may be detected in the blood prior to or soon after heart disease. The antibody may be present after cardiac surgery, myocardial infarction, streptococcal infection, and rheumatic fever. This test may be used to monitor therapeutic response to treatment.

Purpose
- To identify the presence of antimyocardial antibody as the cause of the cardiac condition

Clinical Problems
Increased titer: Myocardial infarction, myocarditis, pericarditis, following cardiac surgery, acute rheumatic fever, chronic rheumatic diseases, streptococcal infections, idiopathic cardiomyopathy, endomyocardial fibrosis, thoracic injury, systemic lupus erythematosus (SLE)

Procedure
- No food or fluid restriction is required.
- Collect 3 to 5 ml of venous blood in a red-top tube. Send to the laboratory immediately.

Nursing Implications
- Obtain a history of heart disease.
- Check cardiac enzyme levels, CPK, AST, LDH, and if elevated, heart disease is likely.
- Observe for signs and symptoms of heart disease, such as chest pain, dyspnea, diaphoresis, and indigestion.
- Listen to client's concerns.

ANTINUCLEAR ANTIBODIES (ANA) (SERUM)

Reference Values
Adult: Negative

Description.   The ANA test is a screening test for diagnosing systemic lupus erythematosus (SLE) and other collagen diseases. The total ANA can also be positive in scleroderma, rheumatoid arthritis, cirrhosis, leukemia, infectious mononucleosis, and malignancy. It is normally present (95%) in lupus nephritis.

Purpose
- To compare ANA with other laboratory tests for diagnosing SLE or other collagen disease

Clinical Problems
Increased level: (Greater than 1:20) SLE, progressive systemic sclerosis, scleroderma, rheumatoid arthritis, leukemia, cirrhosis of the liver, infectious mononucleosis, myasthenia gravis, malignancy

Drugs that may increase ANA value: Antibiotics (penicillin, tetracycline, streptomycin), antihypertensives (hydralazine [Apresoline], methyldopa [Aldomet]), isoniazid (INH), diuretics (acetazolamide [Diamox], thiazides [hydrochlorothiazide/HydroDIURIL]), phenytoin (Dilantin), oral contraceptives, antiarrhythmics (procainamide [Pronestyl], quinidine), trimethadione (Tridione), chlorpromazine (Thorazine)

Procedure
- No food or fluid restriction is required.
- Collect 3 to 5 ml of venous blood in a red-top tube. Take to the laboratory immediately, since serum needs to be separate from cells.
- Withhold drugs the client is receiving that can cause a false-positive titer before test with health care provider's permission. If given, list the drugs on the laboratory slip.

Nursing Implications
- Relate clinical problems and drugs to positive ANA results. With SLE, the ANA titer may fluctuate according to the severity of the disease.
- Compare test result with other tests for lupus.
- Assess for signs and symptoms of SLE (e.g., skin rash over the cheeks and nose, joint pain).

Client Teaching
- Promote rest during an acute phase.

ANTIPARIETAL CELL ANTIBODY (APCA) (BLOOD)

PARIETAL CELL ANTIBODY

Reference Values
Negative: less than 1:120 titer
Positive: 1:180 titer

Description.   Parietal cells in the stomach secrete hydrochloric acid (HCl), which is needed for protein catabolism. Parietal cell antibody is frequently caused by an autoimmune response.

Antiparietal cell antibody (APCA) at approximately 80% to 90% is sensitive for detecting pernicious anemia (PA). The APCA titer may decrease during the duration of PA. Also this test helps in differentiating between autoimmune chronic gastritis and that of pernicious anemia. Intrinsic factor (IF) antibodies may also be found in pernicious anemia because of the disruption of the IF production caused by the autoimmune process. PA may have a genetic tendency that is not caused by an autoimmune response.

An elevated APCA may be present in other autoimmune disorders such as myasthenia gravis, Type 1 diabetes mellitus or insulin-dependent diabetes mellitus (IDDM). APCA titer level may increase with age. It should not be the only test used for diagnosing pernicious anemia.

Purposes
- To screen for the presence of pernicious anemia (PA)
- To rule out the occurrence of other autoimmune disorders, for example, myasthenia gravis, Type 1 diabetes mellitus

Clinical Problems
Increased titer level: Pernicious anemia, chronic gastritis, gastric ulcer, Type 1 diabetes mellitus, gastric cancer, myasthenia gravis, thyroid disease

Procedure
- There is no food or fluid restriction.
- Collect 7 to 10 ml of venous blood in a red- or gray-top tube.

Nursing Implications

- Obtain a history from the client related to the present health complaint. Clinical manifestations of pernicious anemia may include weakness, orthopnea, burning sensation of the tongue, dyspnea, lightheadedness, sensitivity to temperature changes.

Client Teaching

- Encourage the client to have a balanced diet high in protein, vitamins, and iron. Foods rich in fish, red meat, eggs, and milk help to increase the daily Vitamin B_{12} intake.
- Inform the client other tests may be necessary to confirm the diagnosis (especially if pernicious anemia is suggestive).

ANTISCLERODERMA ANTIBODY (Scl-70) (SERUM)

ANTIBODIES TO Scl-70 ANTIGEN

Reference Values
Negative: Borderline: 20–25 units
Positive: Greater than 25 units

Description.   Antiscleroderma antibodies occur in 40% to 70% of clients with advanced or diffused cutaneous scleroderma, interstitial pulmonary fibrosis, and peripheral vascular disease. The presence of antibodies to Scl-70 antigen is seldom present in other rheumatic disorders, such as systemic lupus erythematosus (SLE) and rheumatoid arthritis.

A negative test result does not indicate the absence of sclerodermal disease. Scleroderma is considered an autoimmune collagen disorder.

Purpose

- To assist in the diagnosis of scleroderma

Clinical Problems
Increased levels: Scleroderma, CREST syndrome, progressive systemic sclerosis

Drugs that may increase Scl-70 levels: Aspirin, diphenhydramine (Benadryl), isoniazid, methyldopa, ethosuximide, penicillin, tetracycline, streptomycin

Procedure
- There is no food or fluid restriction.
- Collect 5 ml of venous blood in a red-top tube.

Factors Affecting Laboratory Results
- See drug list that can cause a false-positive test result.

Nursing Implications
- Obtain a history of health problems. Record if the client has any physical symptoms such as a rash. There can be localized or systemic forms of scleroderma.

Client Teaching
- Explain to the client that other tests may be requested by the health care provider.
- If the client is diagnosed with systemic scleroderma, inform the client that most systemic forms of scleroderma progress very slowly.
- Tell the client to dress warmly, including gloves, because cold weather may increase discomfort and pain.

ANTI–SMOOTH MUSCLE ANTIBODY (ASMA, ASTHMA) (SERUM)

Reference Values
Negative: Less than 1:20 titer
Positive: Greater than 1:20 titer

Description. Anti–smooth muscle antibody (ASMA, ASTHMA) is associated primarily with autoimmune chronic active hepatitis (CAH). With CAH, the titer level is usually greater than 1:160. The titer elevation of ASTHMA occurs in more than 70% of clients with CAH, and most of the clients are females. CAH is frequently referred to as an autoimmune disease. Clients with primary biliary cirrhosis may have a slight titer elevation. Lower titer levels may be present in other conditions, such as cancer, viral infections, and acute viral hepatitis. The antimitochondrial antibody (AMA) test and antinuclear antibody (ANA) test may be prescribed with the ASTHMA test to differentiate the cause of the liver disorder. An elevated AMA titer is more prevalent with biliary cirrhosis, whereas ASTHMA and ANA elevations occur with chronic active hepatitis, which is referred to as lupoid hepatitis. With CAH, the ASTHMA is usually higher than the ANA.

Purpose
- To assist with the diagnosis of CAH

Clinical Problems
Increased levels: *High titers:* Chronic active hepatitis. *Low titers:* Primary biliary cirrhosis, cancer of the liver, infectious mononucleosis, multiple sclerosis (MS), rheumatoid arthritis, acute viral hepatitis, intrinsic asthma

Procedure
- There is no food or fluid restriction.
- Collect 5 to 7 ml of venous blood in a red-top tube.
- Apply pressure to the venipuncture site to decrease bleeding. Clients with liver dysfunction tend to bleed more readily.

Nursing Implications
- Obtain a history from the client related to the health problem. Jaundice may be present.
- Record drugs that the client is taking that may be a contributing cause of CAH.

Client Teaching
- Explain to the client that other laboratory tests may be performed, for example, ANA, AMA, bilirubin, and a liver biopsy may be requested to ensure the diagnosis.

- If steroids are prescribed for CAH, explain how the steroid drug should be taken, such as with food. If steroid drugs are discontinued, the daily dose should be tapered over a period of days to avoid adverse effects.
- Listen to the client's concerns. Refer questions to other health professionals as needed.

ANTISPERM ANTIBODY TEST (SEMEN, BLOOD/SERUM)

ANTISPERMATOZOAL ANTIBODY

Reference Values
Male: Negative for sperm agglutinating antibody
Negative: 0%–15%
Moderately positive: 50%
Strongly positive: 100%

Description. Infertility can result from antisperm antibody production. When the sperm is blocked in the efferent testicular ducts, the formation of autoantibodies to sperm occurs in the blood. Antisperm antibodies may occur in approximately 50% of men following a vasectomy. Most of these men are infertile after repair of the ducts postvasectomy.

Using the enzyme-linked immunoabsorbent assay (ELISA), IgA and IgG antisperm antibodies can be identified. The IgA antisperm antibodies are associated with poor sperm motility. The IgG antisperm antibodies are associated with poor fusion of the sperm and ovum. By testing the sperm in the males and the cervical mucus in the female, the presence of antisperm antibodies can be identified, and the cause of infertility may be determined.

Purposes
- To determine the cause of infertility
- To identify the presence of antisperm antibodies

Clinical Problems
Increased presence of antisperm antibodies: Infertility, blocked efferent ducts in the testes, post vasectomy

Procedure
- No food or fluid restriction is required.

Blood/Serum
- Collect 7 ml of venous blood in a red- or red/gray-top tube.

Semen Specimen
- Inform the male not to have an ejaculation for 3 days before the test.
- Instruct the male to collect a fresh semen specimen in a clean plastic container.
- Instruct the male not to use a condom or lubricant when collecting the specimen.
- If the semen specimen is collected at home, he should take the specimen to the laboratory within 1–2 h. The specimen should be kept warm during the transportation. Check with the laboratory; their procedure may differ.

Vaginal Mucus Specimen
- Collect approximately 1 ml of cervical specimen in a plastic vial. The specimen should be immediately frozen.

Factors Affecting Laboratory Results
- Intercourse occurring before semen collection
- Use of lubricants with semen collection
- Heavy coffee consumption and smoking may decrease sperm motility

Nursing Implications
- Obtain a history of the problems concerning infertility.
- Obtain a history of drugs the clients are taking.
- Provide privacy to the male when collection of the semen occurs on site.

Client Teaching

- Instruct the male on how to collect the semen specimen.
- Instruct the female of how the cervical specimen is obtained.
- Explain to the couple when the test results would be available.
- Permit the couple to ventilate concerns and questions about the test and possible results.
- Encourage the couple to seek genetic counseling if appropriate.

ANTISTREPTOLYSIN O (ASO) (SERUM)

Reference Values

Upper limit of normal varies with age, season, and geographic area.

Adult: Less than 100 international units/ml

Child: Newborn: similar to mother's; 2–5 years: less than 100 international units/ml; 12–19 years: less than 200 international units/ml

Description.   The beta-hemolytic streptococcus secretes an enzyme known as streptolysin O that acts as an antigen and stimulates the immune system to develop antistreptolysin O (ASO) antibodies. A high serum ASO could indicate an acute rheumatic fever or acute glomerulonephritis. The ASO antibodies appear 1 to 2 weeks after an acute streptococcal infection, peak 3 to 4 weeks later, and could remain elevated for months. A fourfold increase in titer between acute and convalescent phase is suggestive of a recent group A streptococcal infection.

Purposes

- To identify clients who are susceptible to specific autoimmune disorders (e.g., collagen disease)
- To aid in determining the effect of beta-hemolytic streptococcus in secreting the enzyme streptolysin O

Clinical Problems

Drugs that may decrease ASO value: Antibiotic therapy

Elevated level: Acute rheumatic fever, acute glomerulonephritis, streptococcal upper respiratory infections, rheumatoid arthritis (mildly elevated), hyperglobulinemia with liver disease, collagen disease (mildly elevated)

Procedure

* No food or fluid restriction is required.
* Collect 3 to 5 ml of venous blood in a red-top tube. Avoid hemolysis of blood specimen.
* Repeated ASO testing (once or twice a week) is advisable to determine the highest level of increase.

Factors Affecting Laboratory Results

* An increased level may occur in healthy persons (carriers).

Nursing Implications

* Check serum ASO levels when the client is complaining of joint pain in the extremities.
* Note that antibiotic therapy could decrease antibody response.
* Check the urinary output when the serum ASO is elevated. A urinary output of less than 600 ml/24 h may be associated with acute glomerulonephritis.

APOLIPOPROTEINS (APO) (PLASMA/SERUM)

APOLIPOPROTEIN A-1 (APO A-1), APOLIPOPROTEIN B (APO B), APOLIPOPROTEIN E (APO E), LIPOPROTEIN (A) (LP[A])

Reference Values

Apo-A-1:
Young adult: Male: 80–155 mg/dl; 0.80–1.55 g/l (SI units)
                              Female: 80–186 mg/dl; 0.80–1.86 g/l (SI units)
Middle-aged adult: Male: 100–165 mg/dl; 1.00–1.65 g/l (SI units)
                                         Female: 93–200 mg/dl; 0.93–2.00 g/l (SI units)
Elderly: Male: 85–166 mg/dl; 0.85–1.66 g/l (SI units)
                      Female: 120–215 mg/dl; 1.2–2.15 g/l (SI units)
Child: Male: 67–150 mg/dl; 0.67–1.50 g/l (SI units)

Female: 60–150 mg/dl; 0.60–1.50 g/l (SI units)

Adolescent: Male: 88–148 mg/dl; 0.88–1.48 g/l (SI units)

Female: 83–150 mg/dl; 0.83–1.50 g/l (SI units)

Apo B:

Adult/elderly: Male: 50–170 mg/dl; 0.50–1.70 g/l (SI units)

Female: 46–155 mg/dl; 0.46–1.55 g/l (SI units)

Five to 17 years old: Male: 46–139 mg/dl; 0.46–1.39 g/l (SI units)

Female: 41–96 mg/dl; 0.41–0.96 g/l (SI units)

Newborn–1-year-old: 11–31 mg/dl; 0.11–0.31 g/l (SI units)

Ratio: Apo A-1/Apo B:

Male: 0.82–2.20

Female: 0.75–3.20

Description.   *Apolipoproteins* are protein components of lipoproteins. They are used to determine risks of atherogenic disease.

Apolipoprotein A-1 (Apo A-1) is a major component of high-density lipoprotein (HLD). As HLD increases Apo-A-1 also increases. Apo A-1 helps to transport peripheral cholesterol to the liver for excretion. It is the "good" apolipoprotein that does not contribute to coronary artery disease or stroke.

Apolipoprotein B (Apo B) is the major component of low-density lipoprotein (LDL) composing about 75% of the protein. Apo B exists in two forms, Apo B-100 and Apo B-48. Apo B-100 has very low-density lipoproteins (VLDL) as well as LDL. Apo B-100 is produced in the liver and Apo B-48 is produced in the small intestine. Apo B-100 is a better indicator of coronary artery disease than LDL. The reference values for African-Americans for apolipoproteins may be 5%–10% higher than that for Caucasians. Also the ratio of Apo A-1 and Apo B is thought to help in identifying atherosclerosis.

Apo B-48, the second Apo B, is of intestinal origin and found in chylomicrons. This Apo B transports lipids that have been digested in the intestines to the bloodstream.

Ratio of Apo A-1 to Apo B is thought to be more useful in identifying atherosclerosis heart disease than LDL or VLDL alone. A decrease in Apo A-1 and an increase in Apo B-100 suggest an increased risk of coronary artery disease.

Apolipoprotein E (Apo E) has a role in the clearance of Apo B-containing lipoproteins including VLDL and chylomicrons. A deficit in Apo E usually produces an increase in Apo B lipoproteins. Apo E has three alleles, E-2, E-3, and E-4. It has been stated that E-4 contributes to coronary artery disease (CAD) and to Alzheimer's disease. There has been some evidence with Apo E-4 allele in that there is the development of plaques and neurofibrillary tangles, and loss of brain tissue volume associated with Alzheimer's disease.

Lipoprotein (a) (Lp[a]) is another lipoprotein referred to as little "a" lipoprotein. The two polypeptide components of Lp(a) are Apo A-1 (dissolves fibrin clots) and Apo B-100. An increase in Lp(a) inhibits fibrin in microthrombi, thus causing atherosclerotic damage to the arterial walls. Increased levels of Lp(a) usually occurs with familial hypercholesterolemia and renal failure, and in women it is associated with a decrease in estrogen levels.

Purposes
- To aid in the diagnosis of coronary artery disease
- To identify the presence of atherosclerotic disease

Clinical Problems
Apo A-1:
Decreased level: CAD, ischemic coronary artery disease, MI, stroke, renal disease, chronic renal failure, nephrotic syndrome, smoking
Drugs that may decrease Apo A-1 value: Androgens, beta-adrenergic blockers, diuretics, progestins, and Synthroid
Increased level: Familial hyperalphalipoproteinemia
Drugs that may increase Apo A-1 value: Anticonvulsants, estrogen, hormonal replacement therapy, statins, niacin, furosemide (Lasix), ethyl alcohol. *Others:* weight reduction
Apo B:
Decreased level: Chronic anemia, Tangier disease, alpha lipoprotein deficiency, joint inflammation, chronic pulmonary disease, Reye's syndrome, malnutrition. *Others:* weight reduction.
Drugs that may decrease Apo B value: Synthroid, captopril, niacin, statin drugs

Increased level: CAD, hyperlipoproteinemia, diabetes mellitus, MI, Cushing's syndrome, familial lipidemia, nephronic syndrome, pregnancy, hepatic disease

Drugs that may increase Apo B value: Beta adrenergic blockers, corticosteroids, oral contraceptives, alcohol abuse, androgens

Apo E-4:

Increased level: CAD, Alzheimer's disease

Lp(a):

Decreased level: Chronic hepatocellular disease, malnutrition

Increased level: CAD, diabetes mellitus, familial hypercholesterolemia, estrogen deficit, chronic renal failure

Procedure
- Restrict food and fluids for 12 h before the test.
- Collect 7 ml of venous blood in a red- or lavender-top tube.
- A ratio of Apo A-1 to Apo B-100 may be ordered to predict CAD.
- Avoid smoking before the test.

Factors Affecting Laboratory Results
- Smoking may decrease Apo levels
- Food ingested before the test
- Drugs; see drugs that decrease or increase levels in Clinical Problems section
- Acute illness can increase Apo B levels
- Diet high in fat and carbohydrate (CHO) can increase Apo B levels

Nursing Implications
- Obtain a history of client's health problems.
- Relate apolipoprotein levels with cholesterol HDL and LDL.
- List drugs client is taking that may affect test results.

Client Teaching
- Explain to the client not to eat for 12 h before the test. Fluid (water) and medications are not restricted unless indicated by the health care provider.

- Encourage overweight clients with increased Apo B to reduce weight. A nutritionist may be suggested.
- Instruct client to decrease foods high in saturated fats and cholesterol.
- Encourage client to exercise if approved by the health care provider.
- Explain that high alcohol consumption can affect test results.
- Encourage client to stop or decrease smoking; this can affect test results.

ARTERIAL BLOOD GASES (ABGs) (ARTERIAL BLOOD)*

BLOOD GASES

Reference Values

Adult: pH: 7.35–7.45; $PaCO_2$: 35–45 mm Hg; PaO_2: 75–100 mm Hg; SaO_2: greater than 95%; SvO_2: greater than 70%; HCO_3: 24–28 mEq/l; base excesses (BE): +2 to −2 mEq/l

Child: pH: 7.36–7.44. Other measurements are same as adult

Description.   Arterial blood gases (ABGs) are usually ordered to assess disturbances of acid–base (A-B) balance caused by a respiratory disorder and/or a metabolic disorder. The basic components of ABGs include the pH, $PaCO_2$, PaO_2, SO_2, HCO_3, and BE.

pH: The pH, the negative logarithm of the hydrogen ion concentration, determines the acidity or alkalinity of body fluids. A pH less than 7.35 indicates acidosis, either respiratory or metabolic acidosis. A pH greater than 7.45 indicates alkalosis, either respiratory or metabolic alkalosis.

PaCO₂: The partial pressure of carbon dioxide ($PaCO_2$) reflects the adequacy of alveolar ventilation. When there is alveolar damage, carbon dioxide (CO_2) cannot escape. Carbon dioxide combines with water to form carbonic acid ($H_2O + CO_2 = H_2CO_3$), causing an acidotic state. When the client has alveolar hypoventilation, the $PaCO_2$ is elevated, and respiratory acidosis results. Chronic obstructive lung disease is a major cause of

---

*Updated by Ellen B. Boyda, RN, MSN, NP

respiratory acidosis. When the client has alveolar hyperventilation (blowing off CO_2 by rapid deep breathing), the $PaCO_2$ is decreased, and respiratory alkalosis results.

PaO_2:   The partial pressure of oxygen (PaO_2) determines the amount of oxygen available to bind with hemoglobin. The pH affects the combining power of oxygen and hemoglobin, and with a low pH, there will be less oxygen in the hemoglobin. The PaO_2 is decreased in respiratory diseases, such as emphysema, pneumonia, and pulmonary edema; in the presence of abnormal hemoglobin (CO Hb, Meth Hb, Sulfa Hb); and in polycythemia.

SO_2:   The oxygen saturation (SO_2) is the percentage of oxygen in the blood that combines with hemoglobin. It is measured indirectly by calculation of the PaO_2 and pH or measured directly by co-oximetry. The combination of oxygen saturation, partial pressure of oxygen, and hemoglobin indicates tissue oxygenation.

HCO_3 and BE: Bicarbonate ion (HCO_3) is an alkaline substance that comprises over half of the total buffer base in the blood. When there is a deficit of bicarbonate and other bases or an increase in nonvolatile acid such as lactic acid, metabolic acidosis occurs. If a bicarbonate excess is present, then metabolic alkalosis results. The bicarbonate plays a very important role in maintaining a pH of 7.35 to 7.45 on an ongoing basis and also in compensation for an acidotic or alkalotic state.

The base excess (BE) value is frequently checked with the HCO_3 value. A base excess of less than -2 is acidosis and greater than $+2$ is alkalosis.

Acid-Base Imbalances: To determine the type of A-B imbalance, the pH, $PaCO_2$, HCO_3, and BE are checked. The $PaCO_2$ is a respiratory determinant, and the HCO_3 and BE are metabolic determinants. The $PaCO_2$, HCO_3, and BE values are compared to the pH. A pH of less than 7.35 is acidosis and one of greater than 7.45 is alkalosis.

1. If the pH is less than 7.35, the $PaCO_2$ is greater than 45 mm Hg, and the HCO_3 and BE are normal, the A-B imbalance is respiratory acidosis.
2. If the pH is greater than 7.45, the $PaCO_2$ is less than 35 mm Hg, and the HCO_3 and BE are normal, the A-B imbalance is respiratory alkalosis.
3. If the pH is less than 7.35, the $PaCO_2$ is normal, the HCO_3 and BE are less than 24 mEq/l and less than -2, the A-B imbalance is metabolic acidosis.

4. If the pH is greater than 7.45, the $PaCO_2$ is normal, the HCO_3 and BE are greater than 28 mEq/l and greater than +2, the A-B imbalance is metabolic alkalosis.

Acid-Base (A-B)

Imbalance	pH	PaCO₂	HCO₃	BE
Respiratory acidosis	↓	↑	N	N
Respiratory alkalosis	↑	↓	N	N
Metabolic acidosis	↓	N	↓	↓
Metabolic alkalosis	↑	N	↑	↑

Key: ↑ = increase; ↓ = decrease; N = normal

Purposes

* To detect metabolic acidosis or alkalosis, or respiratory acidosis or alkalosis
* To monitor blood gases during an acute illness and evaluate need for medical intervention

Clinical Problems

Respiratory Acidosis (pH less than 7.35; $PaCO_2$ greater than 45 mm Hg): Chronic obstructive lung disease (emphysema, chronic bronchitis, severe asthma), acute respiratory distress syndrome (ARDS) obesity, drug overdose, severe head injury, Guillain-Barré syndrome, anesthesia, pneumonia, severe sleep apnea. *Drug Influence:* Narcotics, sedatives

Respiratory Alkalosis (pH greater than 7.45; $PaCO_2$ less than 35 mm Hg): Salicylate toxicity (early phase), anxiety, hysteria, tetany, strenuous exercise (swimming, running), severe pain, fever, hyperthyroidism, delirium tremens, pulmonary embolism, pregnancy

Metabolic Acidosis (pH less than 7.35; HCO_3 less than 24 mEq/l): Diabetic ketoacidosis, severe diarrhea, starvation/malnutrition, shock, burns, kidney failure, acute myocardial infarction

Metabolic Alkalosis (pH greater than 7.45; HCO_3 greater than 28 mEq/l): Severe vomiting, gastric suction, peptic ulcer, potassium loss (as in diuretic therapy), excess administration of bicarbonate, hepatic failure, cystic fibrosis. *Drug Influence:* Sodium bicarbonate, sodium oxalate, potassium oxalate

Procedure
- There is no food or fluid restriction.
- If the client is receiving anticoagulant therapy or taking aspirin or has a clotting problem, the laboratory, nurse, or pulmonary technician drawing the blood should be notified.
- Collect 1–5 ml of arterial blood in a heparinized needle and syringe, remove the needle, make sure there is no air in the syringe, and apply an airtight cap over the tip of the syringe.
- Place the syringe with arterial blood in an ice-water bag (to minimize the metabolic activity of the sample) and deliver it immediately to the laboratory. Ice water is colder than ice.
- Indicate on the laboratory slip whether the client is receiving oxygen and the flow rate, type of O_2 administration device (e.g., cannula, mask), and the client's current temperature.
- Apply pressure to the puncture site for 5 min, longer for persons on anticoagulants or streptokinase therapy.

Factors Affecting Laboratory Results
- Improper handling of the blood sample, such as not using ice water, exposure of specimen to air, and not expelling all the heparin out of the collection syringe, causes inaccurate results.
- Hemolysis of the blood sample causes false results.
- Narcotics and sedatives can contribute to the respiratory acidotic state, and sodium bicarbonate could cause metabolic alkalosis.
- Inaccurate results can occur as a result of suctioning, changes in O_2 therapy, and ventilator use; exposure to carbon monoxide or nitrate; and blood transfusion.

Nursing Implications
Respiratory Acidosis
- Assess for signs and symptoms of respiratory acidosis, such as dyspnea, headache, disorientation, and increased $PaCO_2$ (greater than 45 mm Hg).
- Perform chest clapping to break up bronchial and alveolar secretions when applicable. Carbon dioxide can be trapped in the lungs because of excess secretions and mucous plugs.

- Administer oxygen at a low concentration (2 to 3 l/min) when emphysema is present.
- Check for metabolic compensatory mechanism with respiratory acidosis—HCO_3 would be elevated, greater than 28 mEq/l.

Client Teaching

- Teach the client breathing exercises to enhance CO_2 excretion from the lungs.
- Instruct the client on how to properly use the incentive spirometer device or mininebulizer if ordered.
- Demonstrate the postural drainage procedure, if not contraindicated, by lowering the head of the bed or having the client lie over the side of the bed. Secretions are mobilized and excreted by gravity.

Respiratory Alkalosis

- Relate a low $PaCO_2$ value to clinical problems associated with tachypnea (rapid respiratory rate). Anxiety, hysteria, nervousness, and strenuous physical exertion can cause tachypnea. With rapid breathing, an excess of CO_2 is lost.
- Assess for signs and symptoms of respiratory alkalosis, such as tachypnea, dizziness, tingling of fingers, tetany spasms, and a $PaCO_2$ less than 35 mm Hg.
- Adjustments may need to be made if client is receiving mechanical ventilation.

Client Teaching

- Instruct the client to breathe slowly and deeply. Breathing into a paper bag will help to decrease hyperventilation.

Metabolic Acidosis

- Relate decreased values of HCO_3 and BE to metabolic acidosis. When there is tissue breakdown from shock, malnutrition, severe diarrhea and such, acid metabolites (e.g., lactic acid) are released. Another cause of metabolic acidosis is the presence of ketone bodies (fatty acid) from diabetic ketoacidosis.
- Assess for signs and symptoms of metabolic acidosis, such as rapid, vigorous breathing (Kussmaul's breathing), flushed skin, restlessness,

decreased bicarbonate (HCO_3) value of less than 24 mEq/l, and decreased BE less than -2.

- Check for respiratory compensatory mechanism with metabolic acidosis: $PaCO_2$ would be decreased to less than 35 mm Hg. The lung compensates by blowing off CO_2 through hyperventilation to decrease carbonic acid in the blood, thereby decreasing the acidotic state.

Metabolic Alkalosis

- Relate elevated HCO_3 and BE values to metabolic alkalosis. With severe vomiting and gastric suction, hydrogen and chloride (hydrochloric acid) are lost, causing an alkalotic state. Drugs containing sodium bicarbonate taken in excess or over a long period of time could cause metabolic alkalosis.
- Assess for signs and symptoms of metabolic alkalosis, such as shallow breathing, vomiting, elevated HCO_3 value of greater than 28 mEq/l, and elevated BE value of greater than $+2$.
- Stop nasogastric drainage or decrease amount of vomiting as necessary.

Client Teaching

- Instruct the client not to ingest large quantities of antacids containing base substances like bicarbonate. An alkalotic state could result.

ASCORBIC ACID (VITAMIN C) (PLASMA AND SERUM)

Reference Values

Adult: 0.6–2.0 mg/dl (plasma), 34–114 umol/l (SI units, plasma), 0.2–2.0 mg/dl (serum), 12–114 umol/l (SI units, serum)
Child: 0.6–1.6 mg/dl (plasma)

Description. Ascorbic acid (vitamin C) is a water-soluble vitamin found in fresh fruits and vegetables. Deficiencies of vitamin C still occur, but the severe deficiency known as scurvy is rare.

Vitamin C is important for the formation of collagen substances and certain amino acids, in wound healing, and in withstanding the stresses of injury and infection. Because vitamin C is vitally important to the body's defense mechanisms in dealing with stress caused by injury and disease, the client's ascorbic acid level should be known. This test can also be used to determine whether the ascorbic acid therapy is adequate. Excess ingestion of vitamin C is not considered toxic, as is excess ingestion of vitamins A and D, because excess vitamin C is water soluble and is excreted in the urine.

Purpose
- To determine if the ascorbic acid therapy is adequate

Clinical Problems
Decreased level: Scurvy, low vitamin C diet, malabsorption, pregnancy, infections, cancer, severe burns
Causes of false-negative readings: Test for occult blood in stool, serum triglycerides
Increased level: Excess vitamin C ingestion
Causes of false-positive readings: Clinitest, serum creatinine, serum uric acid, serum bilirubin, serum ALT and AST, blood glucose, serum cholesterol

Procedure
- There is no food or fluid restriction.
- Collect 5 to 7 ml of venous blood in a gray-top tube (plasma) or a red-top tube (serum).

Factors Affecting Laboratory Results
- High doses of ascorbic acid can cause inaccurate results.

Nursing Implications
- Recognize the functions of ascorbic acid in maintaining the state of wellness. Ascorbic acid has been taken by persons in large doses (less than 1 g) to prevent colds. This has not been medically proved effective.
- Answer the client's questions concerning the importance of vitamin C. It helps with the healing process.

Decreased Level

- Relate vitamin C deficit to certain clinical problems (e.g., infections, burns). Vitamin C is lost during severe infections and burns.

Client Teaching

- Teach the client to eat food rich in vitamin C (e.g., oranges, grapefruits, strawberries, cantaloupe, pineapple, broccoli, cabbage, spinach, kale, turnips). Approximately 23% of the population has an ascorbic acid deficit in the body.

Increased Level

- Record on the client's chart habitual use of high doses of vitamin C. High doses of ascorbic acid can cause false-positive laboratory results.

ASPARTATE AMINOTRANSFERASE (AST) (SERUM)

SERUM GLUTAMIC OXALOACETIC TRANSAMINASE (SGOT)

Reference Values

Adult: *Average range:* 8–38 units/l; (Frankel), 4–36 international units/l, 16–60 units/ml at 30°C (Karmen), 8–33 units/l at 37°C (SI units). Female values may be slightly lower than those in men. Exercise tends to increase serum levels.

Child: Newborns: four times the normal level; child: similar to adults

Elderly: Slightly higher than adults

Description.   AST/SGOT is an enzyme found mainly in the heart muscle and liver; it is found in moderate amounts in the skeletal muscle, the kidneys, and the pancreas. High levels of serum AST are found following an acute myocardial infarction (AMI) and liver damage. After severe chest pain due to AMI, serum AST level rises in 6 to 10 h and peaks in 24 to 48 h. If there is no additional infarction, the AST level returns to normal in 4 to 6 days. Other cardiac enzyme tests are used in diagnosing an AMI (e.g., CPK, LDH).

In liver disease the serum level increases by ten times or more and remains elevated for a longer period of time. Serum levels of AST and ALT are frequently compared.

Purposes

- To detect an elevation of serum AST, an enzyme that is mainly in the heart muscle and liver and that increases during an acute myocardial infarction and liver damage
- To compare AST results with CPK and LDH for diagnosing an acute myocardial infarction

Clinical Problems

Decreased level: Pregnancy, diabetic ketoacidosis, beriberi

Increased level: Acute myocardial infarction (AMI), encephalitis, liver necrosis, musculoskeletal disease and trauma, acute pancreatitis, cancer of the liver, severe angina pectoris, strenuous exercise, acute pulmonary embolism, eclampsia, CHF

Drugs that may increase AST value: Antibiotics, narcotics, vitamins (folic acid, pyridoxine, vitamin A), antihypertensives (methyldopa [Aldomet], guanethidine), theophylline, digitalis preparations, cortisone, flurazepam (Dalmane), indomethacin (Indocin), isoniazid (INH), rifampin, oral contraceptives, salicylates, intramuscular (IM) injections

Procedure

- No food or fluid restriction is required.
- Collect 3 to 5 ml of venous blood in a red-top tube. Avoid hemolysis of blood specimen. Draw blood before drugs are given.
- List on the laboratory slip drugs that can cause false-positive levels with date and time last given.

Factors Affecting Laboratory Results

- IM injections could cause increased serum AST levels.

Nursing Implications

- Alleviate anxiety by explaining purpose of the test. Be supportive to the client and family.
- Hold drugs causing an elevated serum AST for 24 h prior to the blood test, with the health care provider's permission.
- Do not administer IM injections before the blood test. IM injections can increase the serum AST level. A few medications (e.g., morphine) can be given IV without affecting the serum level.

- Assess the client for signs and symptoms of AMI (e.g., chest and arm pain, dyspnea, diaphoresis).
- Compare serum AST and serum ALT levels to determine if liver damage could be responsible for the abnormal values.

Client Teaching
- Instruct the client to report symptoms of chest and/or arm pain, nausea, and/or diaphoresis immediately—day or night.

ATRIAL NATRIURETIC HORMONE (ANH) (PLASMA)

ATRIAL NATRIURETIC FACTOR (ANF), ATRIAL NATRIURETIC PEPTIDES (ANP)

Reference Values
20–77 pg/ml; 20–77 ng/l (SI units)

Description.   Atrial natriuretic hormone (ANH) is secreted from the atria of the heart. It is released during expansion of the atrium, produces vasodilation, and increases glomerular filtration rate. ANH reduces renal reabsorption of sodium, blocks renin release by the kidney, and blocks aldosterone secretion from the adrenal glands; thus, it has an antihypertensive effect. With the physiologic effects of ANH, preload, afterload, and blood volume are reduced. An elevated ANH level can be used to detect cardiovascular disease, early asymptomatic left ventricular disorder, and congestive heart failure (CHF). However, with chronic level CHF, the ANH is decreased, while with acute congestive heart failure, the ANH level is elevated.

Purposes
- To detect cardiovascular disease, particularly CHF
- To detect asymptomatic fluid volume (cardiac) overload

Clinical Problems
Decreased level: Chronic CHF
Drugs that may decrease plasma ANH: Prazosin, urapidil

Increased level: Acute CHF, paroxysmal atrial tachycardia, early cardiovascular disease, subarachnoid hemorrhage

Procedure
- NPO for 8 to 12 h prior to test.
- Withhold cardiac drugs (e.g., beta blockers, calcium blockers, diuretics, vasodilators, and digoxin) until after test.
- Collect 5 ml of venous blood in a lavender-top tube. Ice the tube and take it immediately to the laboratory.

Factors Affecting Laboratory Results
- Cardiac drugs (see Procedure)

Nursing Implications
- Obtain a health and drug history from the client.
- Take vital signs. Compare findings to baseline readings.
- Answer the client's questions. Be supportive of the client.

Client Teaching
- Inform the client that medications that were withheld may be taken following the test.
- Instruct the client to notify his/her health care provider of difficulty in breathing, shortness of breath, chest pain, and/or indigestion.

BETA$_2$ MICROGLOBULIN (B$_2$ M, BMG) (BLOOD, SERUM, URINE)

Reference Values
Blood/Serum: *Adult*: less than 2 mcg/ml, 0.2 mg/dl, 1.0–2.4 mg/l
Elderly: 0.25 mg/dl
Urine: Less than 120 mcg/24 h

Description.   Beta$_2$ microglobulin (B$_2$ M, BMG) is a protein of low molecular weight found on the surface of many cells and is a component of class 1 human leukocyte antigen (HLA), particularly on lymphatic cells. B$_2$ M is filtered by the glomeruli and 95% is reabsorbed by the tubules of the kidneys. With renal disease, both blood and urine specimens are obtained for B$_2$ M to differentiate between glomerular and tubular disease. If the blood level of B$_2$ M is increased and the urine level is decreased, the glomerular renal disease is suspected. If the blood level is low and the urine level is increased, then tubular renal disease is suggested. Blood B$_2$ M increases early with renal transplant rejection.

Other causes of an elevated B$_2$ M include lymphomas, leukemias, many neoplasms, multiple myeloma, and severe chronic inflammatory disease. It is a useful tumor marker to determine the stage of cancerous tumor—its growth rate and the prognosis.

B$_2$ M is increased in AIDS clients especially those with opportunistic infection. It has been combined with CD$_4$ lymphocyte count for determining the probability of an HIV-infected person developing AIDS in the next 3–4 years.

Purposes
- To detect glomerular or tubular renal disease
- To determine the stage of the tumor and prognosis
- To determine the progression of HIV to AIDS

Clinical Problems
Blood
Increased level: Glomerular renal disease; renal transplant rejection; some malignancies—lymphomas, leukemia, multiple myeloma; AIDS; Crohn's diseases; mercury exposure; chronic inflammatory disease
Drugs that may affect test results: Aminoglycoside toxicity

Urine
Increased level: Tubular renal disease, lymphomas, leukemia, multiple myeloma, AIDS, mercury exposure

Procedure
Blood
- Food and fluid are not restricted.
- Collect 5 ml of venous blood in a red- or lavender-top tube.

Urine: 24 h

- Discard the first morning urine specimen.
- Collect all urine for the next 24 h in a large container with a preservative. Keep container refrigerated.
- Have client void at the end of the 24 h.
- Label the urine container with the client's name, date, and the exact time of collection (e.g. 6/3/09, 7:01 AM to 6/4/09, 6:59 AM).
- No toilet paper or feces should be present in the urine collection.

Factors Affecting Test Results

- Radioactive dyes given within a week before the test.
- Acid urine causing B_2M to be unstable.
- Discard urine specimen during the 24-h collection time.

Nursing Implications

- Obtain a history of health problems.
- Determine if the client received radioactive dye within a week before the test.

Client Teaching

- Encourage the client to ventilate feelings and concerns by providing a private calm environment.

Urine

- Collect urine specimen in a container with a preservative during the 24 h. Keep urine collection container in a refrigerator or on ice.
- Follow strictly the date and times for the urine collection.

BILIRUBIN (TOTAL, DIRECT, INDIRECT) (SERUM)

Reference Values

Adult: Total: 0.1–1.2 mg/dl, 1.7–20.5 μmol/l (SI units)

Direct (conjugated): 0.1–0.3 mg/dl, 1.7–5.1 μmol/l (SI units)

Indirect (unconjugated): 0.1–1.0 mg/dl, 1.7–17.1 μmol/l (SI units)

Child: Total: newborn: 1–12 mg/dl, 17.1–205 μmol/l (SI units); child: 0.2–0.8 mg/dl

Description.   Bilirubin is formed from the breakdown of hemoglobin by the reticuloendothelial system and is carried in the plasma to the liver, where it is conjugated (directly) and excreted in the bile. There are two forms of bilirubin in the body: the conjugated, or direct reacting (soluble); and the unconjugated, or indirect reacting (protein bound). If the total bilirubin is within normal range, direct and indirect bilirubin levels do not need to be analyzed. If one value of bilirubin is reported, it represents the total bilirubin. Jaundice is frequently present when serum bilirubin (total) is greater than 3 mg/dl. Total serum bilirubin in newborns can be as high as 12 mg/dl; the panic level is greater than 15 mg/dl.

Increased direct or conjugated bilirubin is usually the result of obstructive jaundice, either extrahepatic (from stones or tumor) or intrahepatic (damaged liver cells). Indirect or unconjugated bilirubin is associated with increased destruction of RBCs (hemolysis).

Transcutaneous bilirubin test is a test to check for the presence of hyperbilirubinemia in newborns. This small device is placed on the newborn's sternum to check the bilirubin level. It is estimated that 60% of newborns and 80% of preterm infants develop jaundice during the first week of life and with preterm infants, most jaundice is noted while these infants are receiving nursing care. In many of these cases, the nurse will check the bilirubin level. It has been recommended by the American Academy of Pediatrics (AAP) that newborns be tested for hyperbilirubinemia by using the transcutaneous bilimeter (Draeger Medical's Minolta JM 103 model). By using this method, the results of the bilirubin are obtained in 7 seconds. With the serum bilirubin test for newborns, the blood is taken from the heel of the infant and the sample is sent to the laboratory. The serum method can cause discomfort to the infant. It has been determined that the transcutaneous test is as accurate as the serum test and is less traumatic to the infant. At present this form of test to determine bilirubin values is not universally used.

Purposes
- To monitor bilirubin levels associated with jaundice
- To suggest the occurrence of liver disorder

Clinical Problems
Decreased Level
Direct: Iron deficiency anemia

Drugs that may decrease bilirubin value: Barbiturates, aspirin (large amounts), penicillin, caffeine

Increased level

Direct: Obstructive jaundice caused by stones or neoplasms, hepatitis, cirrhosis of the liver, infectious mononucleosis, liver cancer, Wilson's disease

Indirect: Erythroblastosis fetalis, sickle cell anemia, transfusion reaction, hemolytic anemias, pernicious anemia, malaria, septicemia, CHF, decompensated cirrhosis

Drugs that may increase bilirubin value: Antibiotics, sulfonamides; diuretics; isoniazid (INH); diazepam (Valium); narcotics; barbiturates; flurazepam (Dalmane); indomethacin (Indocin); methyldopa (Aldomet); procainamide (Pronestyl); steroids; oral contraceptives; tolbutamide (Orinase); vitamins A, C, and K

Procedure

- Restrict food and fluids, except for water.
- Collect 3 to 5 ml of venous blood in a red-top tube. Avoid hemolysis.
- List drugs client is taking that may affect test results.
- Protect the blood specimen from sunlight and artificial light, as light will reduce the bilirubin content. Blood should be sent to the laboratory immediately so that separation of serum from the cells can be performed.
- There is no laboratory test for indirect bilirubin. Indirect bilirubin is calculated by subtracting direct bilirubin from total bilirubin: Total bilirubin − direct bilirubin = indirect bilirubin.

Factors Affecting Laboratory Results

- A high-fat dinner prior to the test may affect bilirubin levels.
- Carrots and yams may increase the serum bilirubin level.

Nursing Implications

- Check the serum bilirubin (total), and if it is elevated, check the direct bilirubin level. To obtain the indirect bilirubin level, subtract the direct bilirubin from the total bilirubin. An elevated direct bilirubin level is usually due to a liver problem, and an elevated indirect bilirubin level is most likely due to a hemolytic problem.

- Check the sclera of the eyes and the inner aspects of the arm for jaundice.
- Be supportive to client and family. Answer questions and refer unknown answers to other professionals.

Client Teaching
- Instruct the client not to eat carrots, yams, or foods high in fat the night before.

BILIRUBIN (URINE)

Reference Values
Adult: Negative, 0.02 mg/dl

Description.   Bilirubin is not normally present in urine; however, a very small quantity may be present without being detected by routine test methods. Bilirubin is formed from the breakdown of hemoglobin; it is conjugated in the liver and is excreted as bile. Conjugated, or direct, bilirubin is water soluble and is excreted in the urine when there is an increased serum level.

Bilirubinuria (bilirubin in urine) has a characteristic color of dark amber. It is an indicator of liver damage or biliary obstruction such as stones. Bilirubinuria can be tested by the floor nurse using a dipstick such as bili-Labstix or tablet (Ictotest-Ames). The more accurate testing is Ictotest (tablet). Values of serum bilirubin should be compared with urine bilirubin to diagnose the cause of the jaundice. If serum bilirubin is elevated (hyperbilirubinemia) and the urine bilirubin is negative, unconjugated (fat-soluble) hyperbilirubinemia is probable. Conjugated (water-soluble) hyperbilirubinemia is excreted in the urine.

Purpose
- To compare urine bilirubin level with serum bilirubin and other liver enzyme tests to detect liver disorder

Clinical Problems
Increased level: Obstructive biliary disease, liver disease (hepatitis, toxic agents), CHF with jaundice, cancer of the liver (secondary)

Drugs that may increase urine bilirubin: Phenothiazines, chlorprothixene (Taractan), phenazopyridine (Pyridium), chlorzoxazone (Paraflex)

Procedure
- No food or fluid restriction is required.
- Use either bili-Labstix or Ictotest reagent tablets for the bilirubinuria test. The bili-Labstix is dipped in urine and, after 20 s, is compared to a color chart on the bottle.
- With the Ictotest, place 5 drops of urine on the asbestos-cellulose test mat. Place the reagent tablet on the mat and add 2 drops of water. If the test is positive for bilirubin, the mat color will turn blue or purple. Pink or red color indicates a negative test result.
- Urine bilirubin test should be performed within 1 h. Keep urine away from ultraviolet light.

Nursing Implications
- Compare the urine bilirubin result with the serum bilirubin test (direct and total). If the serum bilirubin (direct) is elevated and the urine bilirubin is positive (bilirubinuria), the cause of the jaundice is most likely conjugated hyperbilirubinemia.
- Check the color of the urine. If it is dark amber in color, shake the urine specimen and note whether a yellow foam appears.
- Record the results of the bili-Labstix and the urine color on the client's chart.
- Notify the health care provider of amber urine with yellow foam and test results.

BIOTERRORISM INFECTIOUS PRODUCTS TESTS

ANTHRAX (*BACILLUS ANTHRACIS*), BOTULISM (*CLOSTRIDIUM BOTULINUM*), SMALLPOX (VARIOLA VIRUS [DNA VIRUS])

Reference Values
Negative: The organism being tested

Description.   There are many products used in bioterrorism; however, three of them, anthrax, botulism, and smallpox, are presented because these seem to be the most common infectious agents used in bioterrorism. Use of any of these agents in bioterrorism should be reported to the Department of Public Health and the Centers for Disease Control and Prevention (CDC).

Anthrax

Anthrax is caused by the *Bacillus anthracis,* which is a spore-forming Gram-positive bacillus. The spores of this organism can be transmitted via inhalation, through gastrointestinal (GI) tract, and cutaneously (skin) from infected animals and their products, or through intentional release for bioterrorist attack. Inhalation of the spores is the most serious transmission of Anthrax and frequently is fatal. For suspected GI anthrax, culture of the blood, gastric secretions, food, and feces is recommended. If cutaneous (skin) anthrax is suspected, a culture of the skin vesicle is done. Immunization is suggested for clients working directly with animals and their products, and also for clients who can be contaminated with anthrax in direct warfare.

Common symptoms of anthrax include fever, fatigue, skin lesions, and/or respiratory failure. If pulmonary anthrax is present, the symptoms would include fever, dyspnea, chest pain, coughing, and cyanosis due to a lack of oxygen. Treatment for anthrax is through repeated doses of antibiotics.

Botulism

Botulism is caused by *Clostridium botulinum,* which is a spore-forming anaerobic bacteria/toxin. The botulinum toxin is transmitted mainly via the GI tract and the lungs. However, the organism can pass from the person's infected wound into the bloodstream. This organism is found in the soil and in undercooked food exposed to room temperature for a long period. It may be used as a bioterrorism agent.

Symptoms may begin 6 to 12 h following consumption of contaminated food and the symptoms mostly include dysphagia, blurred vision, muscle weakness, and flaccid paralysis. The organism is not contagious. Treatment is given using equine antitoxin to decrease nerve damage.

Smallpox

Smallpox is caused by variola virus, a DNA virus. It has been controlled with the smallpox vaccination. The concern today is that it could be used as a bioterrorism weapon.

There are two types of the variola virus; variola major, which is the most severe form of smallpox and is the most common type, and variola minor, which is less severe and not as common. With the variola major, the fever is very high and the rash is more extensive.

The early symptoms of smallpox are fever, body aches, and malaise. Rash usually appears first in the mouth and then on the skin. Then it becomes a vesicular rash with fluid. Persons who are at risk for a bioterrorism attack of smallpox should be vaccinated.

Purposes

- To test for the organism/toxin that could cause anthrax, botulism, or smallpox
- To notify the Department of Public Health and CDC of the suspected bioterrorism agent

Clinical Problems

Anthrax: *Bacillus anthracis*
Botulism: *Clostridium botulinum*
Smallpox: variola virus; DNA virus

Procedure
Anthrax

- No food or fluid restriction is required.
- Obtain a culture of blood, sputum, stool, and/or fluid from the skin vesicle. Use two sterile cotton swabs to obtain the fluid from the vesicle that has been opened. The blood and sputum specimens are used for testing pulmonary anthrax.
- Take precautions as outlined by the institution when taking specimens.

Botulism

- No food or fluid restriction is required.

- Obtain gastric secretions, vomitus, and/or stool specimen when GI botulism is suspected.
- Collect 10 ml of venous blood in a red-top tube. Thirty milliliters of blood may be requested.
- Refrigerate all specimens.

Smallpox
- No food or fluid restriction is required.
- Collect vesicle fluid using sterile cotton swab(s). Remove the scab if present to obtain a culture of the vesicle fluid; however, the scab may be used for testing.
- An electron microscope can identify the brick-shaped virions of smallpox.

Factors Affecting Laboratory Results
- Insufficient amount of collected specimen
- Contamination of specimen with other organisms
- Not keeping the specimen iced or refrigerated as indicated

Nursing Implications
- Obtain a history related to his/her contact with the infectious agent.
- Notify appropriate health officials if a bioterrorism agent is suspected. Further testing and isolation of the client may be necessary until the agent is identified.
- Use guidelines for client care prepared by the health department, CDC, and/or the institution. Take precautions as necessary.
- Report and document the signs and symptoms experienced by the client.
- Administer medications and treatment as prescribed.

Client Teaching
- Explain to the client the types of medications and treatment he/she is to receive. If the client is being isolated, explain to the client and family the purpose of isolation.
- Answer the client and family's questions or refer the questions to the appropriate health professionals.
- Be supportive to the client and family.

BLEEDING TIME (BLOOD)

Reference Values
Adult: Ivy method: 3–7 min; Duke method: 1–3 min (seldom performed)

Description.   Two methods, Ivy and Duke, are used to determine whether bleeding time is normal or prolonged. Bleeding time is lengthened in thrombocytopenia (decreased platelet count [less than 50,000]). The test is frequently performed when there is a history of bleeding (easy bruising), familial bleeding, or preoperative screening. The Ivy technique, in which the forearm is used for the incision, is the most popular method. Aspirins and anti-inflammatory medications can prolong the bleeding time.

Purpose
- To check bleeding time for various health problems

Clinical Problems
Prolonged time: Thrombocytopenic purpura, platelet function abnormality, vascular abnormalities, severe liver disease, disseminated intravascular coagulation (DIC), aplastic anemia, factor deficiencies (V, VII, XI), Christmas disease, hemophilia, leukemia

Drugs that may increase bleeding time: Salicylates (aspirins, others), warfarin (Coumadin), dextran, streptokinase (fibrinolytic agent)

Procedure
Ivy Method
- Test should NOT be performed while taking anticoagulant or aspirin. Client should withhold these medications 3 to 7 days prior to test, with health care provider's permission. Aspirin therapy will prolong bleeding time.
- Cleanse the volar surface of the forearm (below the antecubital space) with alcohol and allow it to dry. Inflate the blood pressure cuff to 40 mm Hg, and leave it inflated during the test. Puncture the skin 2.5 mm deep on the forearm; start timing with a stopwatch. Blot

blood drops carefully every 30 seconds until bleeding ceases. The time required for bleeding to stop is recorded.

Duke method
- The area used is the earlobe.
- No food or fluid restriction is required.

Nursing Implications
- Explain the procedure step by step.
- Allow time for the client to ask questions.
- Obtain a drug history of the last time (date) the client took aspirin or anticoagulants. Aspirin prevents platelet aggregation, and bleeding can be prolonged by taking only one aspirin tablet (5 grains or 325 mg) 3 days prior to test. A history of taking cold medications should be recorded, since many cold remedies contain salicylates.

Client Teaching
- Instruct the client not to take aspirin and over-the-counter cold remedies for 3 days before the test. Notify the health care provider or laboratory, or both, if client has taken aspirin compounds.

BLOOD UREA NITROGEN (BUN) (SERUM)

Reference Values
Adult: 5–25 mg/dl
Child: Infant: 5–15 mg/dl; child: 5–20 mg/dl
Elderly: Could be slightly higher than adult
Urea nitrogen/creatinine ratio: 10:1–20:1; averages: 15:1

Description.   Urea is an end product of protein metabolism. An elevated BUN level could be an indication of dehydration, prerenal failure, or renal failure or gastrointestinal bleeding, or both. Dehydration from vomiting, diarrhea, inadequate fluid intake, or all three is a common cause of an elevated BUN (up to 35 mg/dl). With dehydration, the serum creatinine level would most likely be normal or high normal. Once the client is hydrated (if dehydrated), the BUN should return to normal; if it does not, prerenal or renal failure should be suspected. Digested blood from gastrointestinal bleeding is a source of protein and can cause the BUN to elevate. A low BUN value usually indicates overhydration (hypervolemia).

Urea nitrogen/creatinine ratio may be affected due to liver function, dietary protein intake, and muscle mass. A decreased ratio can occur from acute renal tubular necrosis, malnutrition, low-protein diet, or overhydration. The ratio may be increased due to reduced renal perfusion, obstructive uropathy, shock, GI bleeding, dehydration, and high protein intake.

Purpose
- To detect renal disorder or dehydration associated with increased BUN levels

Clinical Problems
Decreased level: Overhydration (hypervolemia); severe liver damage, low-protein diet, malnutrition (negative nitrogen balance), IV glucose fluids, pregnancy
Drugs that may decrease BUN value: Phenothiazines
Increased level: Dehydration, high protein intake, prerenal failure (low blood supply), renal insufficiency/failure, kidney diseases (glomerulonephritis, pyelonephritis, acute nephritis), gastrointestinal bleeding, sepsis, AMI, diabetes mellitus, licorice (excessive ingestion)
Drugs that may increase BUN value: Diuretics, antibiotics, methyldopa (Aldomet), guanethidine (Ismelin), sulfonamides, propranolol (Inderal), morphine, lithium carbonate, salicylates

Procedure
- No food or fluid restriction is required. Test results may be more accurate if the patient is NPO for 8 h.
- Collect 3 to 7 ml of venous blood in a red-top tube.

Factors Affecting Laboratory Results
- Hydration status of the client should be known. Dehydration or overhydration may cause false results.

Nursing Implications

- Compare serum BUN and serum creatinine results. If both BUN and creatinine levels are elevated, kidney disease should be highly suspected.
- Check vital signs every 8 h and urinary output in 8 and 24 h for decreased urinary output due to dehydration or renal disease.
- Assess for signs and symptoms of dehydration (e.g., poor skin turgor, increased pulse rate and respiration, dry mucous membrane, decrease in urine output [less than 25 ml/h]).
- Observe for signs and symptoms of overhydration due to renal disorder (glomerulonephritis), such as dyspnea, neck vein engorgement, peripheral edema, puffy eyelids, and weight gain.
- Assess client's dietary intake.

Client Teaching

- Encourage client to increase fluid intake when BUN is 26 to 35 mg/dl, with health care provider's permission, to help correct dehydration status.

BLOOD UREA NITROGEN (BUN)/CREATININE RATIO (SERUM)

UREA NITROGEN/CREATININE RATIO

Reference Values
Adult: 10:1 to 20:1 (BUN:creatinine); average: 15:1

Description.   The BUN:creatinine ratio is a test primarily for determining renal function. BUN level can increase due to dehydration or a high-protein diet as well as renal dysfunction. The creatinine level does not increase with dehydration but definitely increases with renal dysfunction. This ratio test is more sensitive to the relationship of BUN to creatinine than separate tests of BUN and creatinine. However, liver function, dietary protein intake, and muscle mass may affect test result.

A decreased ratio can occur from acute renal tubular necrosis and low protein intake. The ratio may be increased due to reduced renal perfusion, glomerular disease, obstructive uropathy, or high protein intake.

Purpose
- To determine renal function

Clinical Problems
Decreased ratio: Acute renal tubular necrosis, low protein intake, malnutrition, pregnancy, liver disease, hemodialysis (urea loss), prolonged IV fluid therapy, ketosis
Drug that may decrease ratio: Phenacemide
Increased ratio: Overproduction or lowered excretion of urea nitrogen, reduced renal perfusion (dehydration, heart failure), glomerular disease, tissue or muscle destruction, high protein intake, obstructive uropathy, azotemia, shock, hypotension, GI bleeding
Drugs that may increase ratio: Tetracycline, corticosteroids

Procedure
- No food or fluid restriction is required.
- Collect 3 to 7 ml of venous blood in a red-top tube.

Nursing Diagnoses
- Altered patterns of urinary elimination related to a decreased or elevated BUN:creatinine ratio secondary to renal disorder
- Ineffective coping related to renal impairment

Nursing Implications
- Assess the client's renal function including urine output, BUN, and serum creatinine level. Urine output should be at least 600 ml/day.
- Assess the client's dietary intake. Record increase or decrease in protein intake.
- Check his or her hydration status. Dehydration may cause increase in the BUN:creatinine ratio.

Client Teaching
- Instruct the client that urine needs to be measured and to urinate in a urinal or bedpan. Inform the health care providers after each voiding so that urine can be measured. Tell the client not to put toilet paper in the urine.

BRAIN NATRIURETIC PEPTIDE (BNP) (PLASMA)

TRIAGE BNP, N-TERMINAL PRO-BRAIN NATRIURETIC PEPTIDE, NT-proBNP

Reference Values

Desired Values: Less than 100 pg/ml; less than 100 ng/l (SI units)
Positive Values: Greater than 100 pg/ml; greater than 100 ng/l (SI units)
Severe heart failure (HF): greater than 400 pg/ml; greater than 400 ng/l (SI units)

Description.   Brain natriuretic peptide or B-type natriuretic peptide (BNP) is a neurohormone secretion primarily in the cardiac ventricles and increases in response to volume expansion and pressure overload. BNP does not exist in the brain, though it was first found in the brain of pigs, but exists in the cardiac ventricular muscle. It is the second type of the natriuretic peptide group; atrial natriuretic peptide (ANP), being the first, exists in the cardiac atrial muscle. The BNP test has been approved by the Food and Drug Administration (FDA) to aid in the diagnosis of HF. Heart failure is difficult to diagnose among persons with lung disease and among those who are obese or elderly; thus, BNP is ordered to determine heart failure. Also BNP is considered a more sensitive test than ANP for diagnosing HF.

Triage BNP and N-terminal proBNP are tests that measure the level of brain natriuretic peptide BNP. BNP is more highly elevated in clients with HF than those with a lung disease. Frequently, the BNP is higher than 100 pg/ml in women who are 65 years old or older. An 80-year-old woman's BNP may be 160 pg/ml; however, with HF, the BNP is markedly higher and can be greater than 400 pg/ml. This test does not replace other clinical findings and tests for diagnosing HF, but if HF is suspected, BNP is helpful in confirming the diagnosis. If the BNP is within normal range for a client having difficulty in breathing, the client's condition is most likely noncardiac dyspnea.

Purpose

- To aid in the diagnosis of heart failure

Clinical Problems

Increased level: Heart failure (HF), left ventricular hypertrophy, myocarditis, early rejection of heart transplants, prolonged systemic hypertension, acute myocardial infarction (AMI), Cushing's syndrome, renal failure

Procedure

- No food or fluid restriction is required.
- Collect 5 ml of venous blood in a red-top tube.

Factors Affecting Laboratory Results

- None known

Nursing Implications

- Assess the client for signs and symptoms of HF (e.g., dyspnea, coughing, edema).
- Obtain a history of previous health problems such as heart failure.

Client Teaching

- Tell the client to report difficulty in breathing, swelling of the extremities, coughing.
- Inform the client that more than one laboratory test may be needed to diagnose the health problem.
- Instruct the client to keep health/medical appointments, which are usually necessary to decrease or control the problem of HF if diagnosed.
- Instruct the client to take the prescribed medications for HF. Clients may stop taking the medications for HF when they feel better and, unfortunately, HF may reoccur.

BREAST CANCER GENETIC TESTING (BRCA-1, BRCA-2) (BLOOD)

Reference Values

Adult: Negative findings of genetic mutation of BRCA-1 and BRCA-2

Description. Predisposition to breast and ovarian cancers can be determined by the mutations in BRCA-1 and BRCA-2. Approximately 22% of families susceptible to breast cancer have inherited the BRCA-1 gene, and another 20% of families have the BRCA-2 gene. The genetic defect is an autosomal dominant gene. The BRCA-1 and BRCA-2 can be passed on to children by the female and by the male. Males who carry the BRCA-1 and BRCA-2 genes are susceptible to breast cancer, and they have a higher risk for developing prostate or colon cancer. However, genetic testing is ordered mostly for women who are at risk of breast or ovarian cancer.

Women who carry the BRCA gene have a strong family history of breast cancer and have a 50% risk of developing breast cancer by age 50, a 70% to 90% risk by the age of 70. If the woman already has breast cancer, she would have a 65% chance for developing breast cancer in the other breast during her lifetime.

BRCA genetic testing can also indicate if the woman is susceptible to ovarian cancer. Only 2% of women develop ovarian cancer by the age of 70. However, if the woman has a strong familial history of ovarian cancer and has the BRCA-1 gene, her risk for developing ovarian cancer by the age of 50 is 30%. By the age of 70, her risk for developing ovarian cancer would be 25% to 45%.

Purposes
- To identify clients who are at risk for developing breast cancer
- To identify clients who are at risk for developing ovarian cancer

Clinical Problems
Increased level: Risk for breast cancer, risk for ovarian cancer

Procedure
- Food and fluid are not restricted.
- Collect 5 ml of venous blood in a lavender- or blue-top tube.
- Do not freeze the blood specimen.

Factors Affecting Laboratory Results
- Frozen blood specimen

Nursing Implications

- Obtain a family history of breast or ovarian cancer.

Client Teaching

- Inform the client that BRCA genetic testing may or may not be covered by medical insurance.
- Suggest that the client receive genetic counseling regardless of whether the test is negative or positive.
- Encourage the client to ventilate his/her feelings and concerns in a private environment.

BREAST CANCER TUMOR PROGNOSTIC MARKERS

ESTROGEN RECEPTOR ASSAY (ER ASSAY), DNA PLOIDY, S-PHASE FRACTION, CATHEPSIN D, HER-2/c-erb-B 2/neu ONCOPROTEIN, p53 PROTEIN

Findings: Favorable and unfavorable

ER assay: Favorable: greater than 11% of cell nuclei stained
Unfavorable: less than 10% of cell nuclei stained

DNA ploidy: Favorable: diploid
Unfavorable: aneuploid (rapid cell replication and tumor growth)

S-phase fraction: Favorable: less than 5%
Unfavorable: greater than 5% (higher S-phase fraction)

Cathepsin D: Favorable: less than 10%
Unfavorable: less than 10%

Her-2/c-erb-B 2/neu oncoprotein: Favorable: less than 10% partial staining in cancer cells
Moderately unfavorable: 10% to 20% partial staining in cancer cells
Strongly unfavorable: greater than 20% partial staining in cancer cells

p53 protein: Favorable: less than 10%
Unfavorable: greater than 10%, mutated p53 protein in tumor cells

Description.   Thirty percent of clients whose tumors have been removed and who have no evidence of lymph node involvement will have a recurrence of malignancy. There are new tumor markers that can predict if more extensive therapy is needed.

Estrogen Receptor Assay (ER Assay)

Tumors with a positive ER assay are more responsive to antiestrogen therapy (estrogen deprivation) and/or removal of the ovaries than tumors that have a negative ER assay. On primary breast cancer tumors, ER assay should be performed. Postmenopausal women have breast tumors that are mostly estrogen-positive tumors compared to premenopausal women.

DNA Ploidy

This test determines cell replication. Aneuploid cells (rapidly replicating cells) have a poorer prognosis. Unfortunately 65% of breast cancer cells are aneuploid. Those with a diploid tumor have a more favorable prognosis.

S-phase Fraction

Tumors that have a high S-phase fraction have a poorer survival rate than those with a low S-phase fraction and diploid tumors. More aggressive cancer cells are in the S-phase stage.

Cathepsin D

Clients with an increase in Cathepsin D protein in the breast cancer cells have an unfavorable prognosis. Increased cathepsin D has been associated with metastatic cancer and recurrence of breast cancer.

Her-2/c-erb-B 2/neu Oncoprotein

The presence of a high level of Her-2/c-erb-B 2/neu oncoprotein in the tumor is associated with poor prognosis. Her-2/c-erb-B 2/neu may be identified in the blood. Clients with Her-2/c-erb-B 2/neu oncoprotein may benefit from trastuzumab (Herceptin), a chemotherapy drug. Herceptin may control the cancer when the client has not responded to other treatments.

p53 Protein

Increase in p53 protein is observed in more aggressive breast cancer. Mutant p53 protein occurs on the surface of cancer cells. Increased levels indicate poor prognosis. This test is frequently done along with lymph node testing.

Purposes

- To determine the prognosis of breast cancer from the biopsy of the tissue or the entire tumor
- To determine if the cancer has reoccurred
- To predict if the cancer has metastasized

Clinical Problems

Increased level: Favorable and unfavorable prognosis of breast cancer, recurrence of breast cancer, breast cancer that has metastasized

Procedure

- Obtain a signed consent form.
- No food or fluid restriction is required with a needle biopsy. With an incision, NPO may be required.
- Cleanse the breast area.
- Obtain a sample of the breast tumor tissue. A needle biopsy of the tumor may be used to aspirate tissue and fluid.
- Place the sample tumor tissue in formalin.
- The container with the tissue is marked with the client's name and date. Indicate on the container the location of the tissue.
- The tissue may be frozen. Check with the laboratory.
- Apply a dressing to the incisional site.

Factors Affecting Laboratory Results

- Inadequate amount of tissue specimen
- Improper preservative agent in the container

Nursing Implications

- Check that the consent form is signed.
- Obtain a familial history of breast cancer.
- Obtain from the client the location of the lump. The mammogram is usually available.
- Indicate which breast, right or left, and mark the location of the lesion.
- Obtain vital signs.

Client Teaching

- Permit client to express her concerns with the procedure and the probability of having breast cancer. Emotional support may be needed. Allow her to vent her feelings.
- Monitor vital signs.
- Instruct the client to report excessive bleeding or redness at the incisional area.
- Inform the client to take analgesics and antibiotics if ordered. Tell the client that if antibiotics are ordered, all of the tablets/capsules should be taken as prescribed.
- Inform the client that the test results should be available in 1 week.
- Instruct the client about how and when to clean the incisional area.
- Tell the client to call for a follow-up appointment.

CALCITONIN (hCT) (SERUM)

Reference Values

Adult: Male: Less than 40 pg/ml or ng/l; female: less than 25 pg/ml or ng/l
Child: Less than 70 pg/ml; less than 70 ng/l (SI units)
Newborn: Usually higher than in adult

Description.   Calcitonin is a potent hormone secreted by the thyroid gland to maintain serum calcium and phosphorus levels. This hormone inhibits calcium reabsorption in the bone and promotes calcium excretion by the kidneys, thus lowering the serum calcium level. Calcitonin acts as an antagonist to the parathyroid hormone (PTH) and vitamin D.

Excess calcitonin secretion occurs in medullary carcinoma of the thyroid gland. Serum has higher values than plasma. A serum calcitonin value between 500 and 2,000 pg/ml most likely indicates thyroid medullary carcinoma; a value greater than 2,000 pg/ml is a definite indicator of thyroid medullary carcinoma.

When the serum calcitonin level is slightly to moderately elevated (100–500 pg/ml), a calcitonin stimulation test may be conducted to diagnose thyroid medullary carcinoma. This test consists of either a calcium infusion or a 10-s pentagastrin infusion with measurement of serum calcitonin before and after the infusion. Positive test result is a rapid rise over the baseline result.

Purpose
- To aid in the diagnosis of thyroid medullary carcinoma or parathyroid hyperplasia or adenoma

Clinical Problems
Increased level: Thyroid medullary carcinoma, carcinoma of the lung or breast, chronic renal failure, parathyroid hyperplasma or adenoma, pernicious anemia, Zollinger–Ellison syndrome, acute or chronic thyroiditis, islet cell tumors, pheochromocytoma

Drugs that may increase calcitonin value: Calcium infusion, epinephrine, estrogens, glucagon, pentagastrin, oral contraceptives

Procedure
- Restrict food and fluids after midnight. A small amount of water may be given if needed.
- Collect 5 to 7 ml of venous blood in a green- or lavender-top tube or in a chilled red-top tube. Avoid hemolysis. Send blood specimen immediately to the laboratory for analysis or freeze to avoid deterioration.

Nursing Implication
- Obtain a health history that may suggest thyroid medullary carcinoma as indicated by a markedly elevated serum calcitonin value. If a slightly elevated serum calcitonin value is present, the nurse may collaborate with the health care provider regarding a calcitonin stimulation test.

CALCIUM (Ca) (SERUM AND URINE)

QUANTITATIVE (24-H URINE COLLECTION)

Reference Values
Adult: Serum: 4.5–5.5 mEq/l, 9–11 mg/dl, 2.3–2.8 mmol/l (SI units).
    Ionized Ca: 4.25–5.25 mg/dl, 2.2–2.5 mEq/l, 1.1–1.24 mmol/l

Urine: 24 h: low-calcium diet less than 150 mg/24 h, less than 3.75 mmol/24 h (SI units); average-calcium diet 100–250 mg/24 h, 2.5–6.25 mmol/24 h; high-calcium diet 250–300 mg/24 h, 6.25–7.50 mmol/24 h

Child: Serum: newborn: 3.7–7.0 mEq/l, 7.4–14.0 mg/dl; infant: 5.0–6.0 mEq/l, 10–12 mg/dl; child: 4.5–5.8 mEq/l, 9–11.5 mg/dl

Description.   Approximately 50% of the calcium is ionized, and only ionized calcium can be used by the body; however, in most laboratories the total serum calcium level determination does not differentiate between ionized and nonionized calcium. In acidosis, more calcium is ionized, regardless of the serum level, and in alkalosis, most of the calcium is protein bound and cannot be ionized. Calcium imbalances require immediate attention, for serum calcium deficit (hypocalcemia) can cause tetany symptoms, unless acidosis is present, and serum calcium excess (hypercalcemia) can cause cardiac dysrhythmias.

A 24-h urine specimen for calciuria is useful for determining parathyroid gland disorders. In hyperparathyroidism, hyperthyroidism, and osteolytic disorders, the urinary calcium excretion is usually increased; it is decreased in hypoparathyroidism.

Purposes
- To check for serum calcium excess or deficit
- To monitor calcium levels
- To detect calcium imbalance

Clinical Problems
Serum
Decreased level: Malabsorption of calcium from the gastrointestinal tract, lack of calcium and vitamin D intake, hypoparathyroidism, chronic renal failure caused by phosphorus retention, laxative abuse, extensive infections, burns, pancreatitis, alcoholism, diarrhea, pregnancy
Drugs that may decrease calcium value: Cortisone preparations, antibiotics (gentamicin, methicillin), magnesium products (antacids), excessive use of laxative, heparin, insulin, mithramycin, acetazolamide (Diamox)
Increased level: Hyperparathyroidism; malignant neoplasm of the bone, lung, breast, bladder, or kidney; hypervitaminosis D, multiple myeloma,

prolonged immobilization, multiple fractures, renal calculi, exercise, milk-alkali syndrome

Drugs that may increase calcium value: Thiazide diuretics, alkaline antacids, estrogen preparation, calcium salts, vitamin D

Procedure
Serum
- No food or fluid restriction is required, unless SMA_{12} or electrolytes are ordered. Many laboratories prefer that breakfast be withheld until after blood specimen is drawn.
- Collect 3 to 5 ml of venous blood in a red-top tube.

Urine
- Label the bottle for a 24-h urine collection with the exact date and time of the urine collection. Preservatives are required by some laboratories; however, the urine specimen may be refrigerated or kept on ice.
- Indicate on the laboratory slip the client's calcium intake (limited, average, or high).

Nursing Implications
Decreased Level
- Observe for signs and symptoms of tetany due to hypocalcemia (e.g., muscular twitching and tremors, spasms of the larynx, paresthesia facial spasms, and spasmodic contractions).
- Check serum calcium values and report abnormal results to the physician, especially if tetany symptoms are present.
- Assess for positive Chvostek's and Trousseau's signs of hypocalcemia.
- Observe for symptoms of tetany when the client is receiving massive transfusions of citrated blood. Citrates prevent calcium ionization. The serum calcium level may not be affected.
- Monitor the pulse regularly if the client is receiving a digitalis preparation and calcium supplements. Calcium excess enhances the action of digitalis and can cause digitalis toxicity (nausea, vomiting, anorexia, bradycardia).
- Administer IV fluids with 10% calcium gluconate slowly. Calcium should be administered in D_5W and not in a saline solution, as

sodium promotes calcium loss. Calcium should not be added to solutions containing bicarbonate, since rapid precipitation will occur.

Client Teaching

* Instruct the client to avoid overuse of antacids and to prevent the chronic laxative habit, which could lower calcium level.
* Encourage the client to consume foods high in calcium and protein needed to enhance calcium absorption.
* Teach the client with hypocalcemia to avoid hyperventilation and crossing his or her legs, which could cause tetany symptoms.

Increased Level

* Observe for signs and symptoms of hypercalcemia (e.g., lethargy, headaches, weakness, muscle flaccidity, heart block, anorexia, nausea, and vomiting).
* Promote active and passive exercises for bedridden clients. This will prevent calcium loss from the bone.
* Identify symptoms of digitalis toxicity when the client has an elevated serum calcium and is receiving a digitalis preparation.
* Notify the health care provider if the client is receiving a thiazide diuretic, for this will inhibit calcium excretion and promote hypercalcemia.

Client Teaching

* Instruct clients to avoid foods high in calcium, to be ambulatory when possible, and to increase oral fluid intake.

CANCER TUMOR MARKERS (CA 15-3, CA 19-9, CA 27.29, CA 50, CA 125) (SERUM)

CANCER ANTIGEN 15-3, CA 19-9, CA 27.29, CA 50, CA 125

Reference Values

CA 15-3:   Less than 30 units/ml; less than 30 kU/l (SI units)
CA 19-9:   Less than 37 units/ml; less than 37 kU/l (SI units)
CA 27.29:   Less than 37 units/ml; less than 37 kU/l (SI units)
CA 50:   Less than 17 units/ml; less than 17 kU/l (SI units)
CA 125:   Less than 35 units/ml; less than 35 kU/l (SI units)

Description.   Tumor markers is a term used to refer to molecules that can be detected in a blood sample. Common clinical uses of tumor markers are for cancer detection; these markers are frequently used to screen and diagnose the presence of possible cancer, to monitor the response to cancer treatment, and to determine the reoccurrence of cancer. Some of these cancer tumor markers are specific to a type of cancer, for example, CA 15-3 for breast cancer. A single test value should not be the only method used to determine if cancer is or is not occurring. Several tumor markers taken, which could be over a period of time, are more useful for diagnostic and monitoring purposes.

CA 15-3 is a marker for identifying breast cancer and monitoring clients' response to treatment. It is a more sensitive test for breast cancer than CEA (carcinoembryonic antigen). Greater than 80% of clients with metastatic breast cancer have an elevated CA 15-3 level. Elevated CA 15-3 may also occur with ovarian, lung, pancreatic, colon, and prostatic cancers.

CA 19-9 is a cancer antigen used in the diagnosis of pancreatic, hepatobiliary, gastric, and colorectal cancers. It is also useful in monitoring the success of treatment and for detecting reoccurrence of the cancer.

CA 27.29 is a tumor marker to detect breast cancer reoccurrence in clients with stage II or III. This test is not approved for screening of breast cancer.

CA 50 is found in clients with gastrointestinal tumors and biliary tract tumors. It tends to be a more sensitive marker when the disease progresses and not when the disease regresses. CA 50 can also be used in diagnosing pancreatic cancer.

CA 125 is mostly found in nonmucinous epithelial ovarian cancer. Approximately 25% of women with benign ovarian tumors have elevated CA 125. Women with elevation of CA 125, greater than 65 units/ml, are associated with ovarian cancer. CA 125 is useful to monitor the client's response to chemotherapy and to check if the cancer is reoccurring. It may also be increased in cancer of the breast, colon, and lung.

Purposes
- To identify clients with elevated serum cancer markers
- To monitor the effects of treatment for the cancer
- To determine the recurrence of the cancer

Clinical Problems

Decreased level: Effective response to treatment, benign disease

Increased levels:

CA 15-3: Breast cancer (most common); metastatic cancer; ovarian, lung, pancreas, colon, prostate cancers; chronic hepatitis; cirrhosis

CA 19-9: Cancer of the pancreas (most common), colon, liver, gastric; pancreatitis; cholecystitis; cirrhosis

CA 27.29: Breast cancer, reoccurrence of breast cancer, metastatic breast cancer, benign disease

CA 50: Gastrointestinal tumor, biliary tract tumors

CA 125: Ovarian cancer (most common); benign ovarian tumors; uterine tumors; cancer of the pancreas, breast, colon, lung; pregnancy, endometriosis; cirrhosis, pancreatitis

Procedure

- No food or fluid restriction is required.
- Collect 5–7 ml of venous blood in a red-top tube.
- Blood sample should be refrigerated immediately.

Factors Affecting Laboratory Results

- Benign breast and ovarian disease may be associated with an increase in CA 15-3, CA 27.29, CA 125
- Menstruation may cause a slight elevation of CA 125
- Radioisotopes given 30 days before detection of CA 15-3, CA 19-9, CA 50, CA 125
- False-positive increased level of CA 50 may occur with benign liver disease

Nursing Implications

- Explain the test procedure to the client.
- Explain to the client to call the health care provider or physician for the test results.
- Have blood sample refrigerated unless it is immediately tested.

Client Teaching

- Be available for client to express feelings or concerns about a specific cancer tumor marker test.

- Be available to answer questions or have the questions answered by another health care professional.

CANDIDA ANTIBODY TEST (SERUM)

Reference Values
Negative
Positive: Greater than 1:8 titer

Description.   This antibody test is to identify systemic candidiasis most often caused by *Candida albicans,* a yeast infection. Candidiasis frequently occurs in the immunocompromised person, and if untreated, the condition can become life threatening. *Candida* sp infection accounts for approximately 80% of all major systemic fungal infections. It is the fourth most common organism found in bloodstream infections. Nosocomial candidiasis increased about fivefold in the 1980s, which contributes to the prolongation of hospitalization.

Vulvovaginal candidiasis may result from prolonged use of potent broad-spectrum antibiotics (oral or intravenously administered) and glucocorticoid therapy. This type of candidiasis is associated with debilitating diseases, uncontrolled diabetes mellitus, and pregnancy. If untreated, it can lead to systemic candidiasis. Usually candidiasis occurs to the skin and mucous membrane.

Purpose
- To diagnose systemic candidiasis that cannot be determined by culture or by the tissue specimen

Clinical Problems
Increased level: Systemic candidiasis

Procedure
- There is no food or fluid restriction.
- Collect 5 ml of venous blood in a red-top tube. Avoid hemolysis by not shaking the tube.

Factors Affecting Laboratory Results
• Hemolysis of the blood specimen

Nursing Implications
• Obtain a history of the client's health complaint. Determine if the client is immunocompromised because of HIV or a debilitating disease.
• Record the drugs that the client is taking.
• Check vital signs. Report abnormal findings.

Client Teaching
• Instruct the client to remain on the drug treatment regimen for candidiasis. Stopping the therapy could cause a relapse.
• Listen to the client's concerns. Answer questions, and if unknown, refer the client to other health professionals.

CANNABINOID (MARIJUANA) (URINE)

Reference Values
Negative: Less than 50 ng/ml (cutoff concentration)

Description.   Marijuana is a mixture of dried leaves and flowering tops of the plant *Cannabis sativa* L. The agents that produce the hallucinogenic and biological effects of marijuana are called *cannabinoids*. A positive test for cannabinoids indicates the presence of cannabinoid metabolites of which carboxy THC is the major one.

Peak plasma levels of carboxy THC occur within 10 min of inhalation and approximately 1 h after ingestion. Excretion in the urine begins within 72 h after exposure and the length of detection can be 30 to 60 days. With chronic users, carboxy THC may accumulate in the fatty tissues leading to a longer detection time in the urine because it is released from these sites slowly over time.

Purposes
• To evaluate the use of marijuana
• To determine if marijuana toxicity has occurred

Clinical Problems

Increased level: Presence of carboxy THC, use of marijuana, marijuana toxicity

Procedure

- No food or fluid restriction is required.
- Collect 20 ml of urine specimen. Repeat urine collection in 1 or 2 days or more if needed.
- Chain-of-custody documentation may be required if testing is for legal purposes.

Factors Affecting Laboratory Tests

- Early urine specimen collection

Nursing Implications

- Obtain a history of the use of marijuana, when able to obtain information from client or friends.
- Monitor vital signs (VS).
- Have another health professional verify or check urine collection for legal purposes. Complete necessary forms for the urine specimen according to the policy of the health department or institution if needed.

Client Teaching

- Be supportive to the client, family, and friends. Refer test results requested by family to appropriate health professionals.
- Do not express judgment about marijuana use to client or family.

CARBON DIOXIDE (CO$_2$) COMBINING POWER (SERUM OR PLASMA)

CO$_2$ COMBINING POWER

Reference Values

Adult: 22–30 mEq/l, 22–30 mmol/l (SI units)
Panic Range: Less than 15 mEq/l and greater than 45 mEq/l
Child: 20–28 mEq/l

Description.   The serum CO_2 test, usually included with the electrolyte (lyte) test, is performed to determine metabolic acid–base abnormalities. The serum CO_2 acts as a bicarbonate (HCO_3) determinant. When serum CO_2 is low, HCO_3 is lost and acidosis results (metabolic acidosis). With an elevated serum CO_2 excess, HCO_3 is conserved and alkalosis results (metabolic alkalosis).

Purpose
- To check for the presence of metabolic acidosis or alkalosis

Clinical Problems
Decreased level: Metabolic acidosis, diabetic ketoacidosis, starvation, severe diarrhea, dehydration, shock, acute renal failure, salicylate toxicity, exercise

Drugs that may decrease CO_2 value: Thiazide, diuretics, triamterene (Dyrenium), antibiotics (methicillin, tetracycline), nitrofurantoin (Furadantin), paraldehyde

Increased level: Metabolic alkalosis, severe vomiting, gastric suction, peptic ulcer, hypothyroidism, potassium deficit

Drugs that may increase CO_2 value: Barbiturates, steroids, loop diuretics

Procedure
- No food or fluid restriction is required.
- Collect 3 to 5 ml of venous blood in a red- or green-top tube.

Nursing Implications
Decreased Level
- Assess for signs and symptoms of metabolic acidosis when serum CO_2 is decreased, especially when less than 15 mEq/l. Symptoms include deep, vigorous breathing (Kussmaul's breathing) and flushed skin.
- Report clinical findings of metabolic acidosis to the health care provider.

Increased Level
- Assess for signs and symptoms of metabolic alkalosis with vomiting or gastric suction for several days. Signs and symptoms include

shallow breathing, a serum CO_2 greater than 30 mEq/l, and a base excess greater than $+2$.

CARBON MONOXIDE, CARBOXYHEMOGLOBIN (BLOOD)

Reference Values

Adult: Nonsmoker: Less than 2.5% of hemoglobin; smoker: 4%–5% saturation of hemoglobin; heavy smoker: 5%–12% saturation of hemoglobin. Toxic: greater than 15% saturation of hemoglobin

Child: Similar to adult nonsmoker

Description.   Carbon monoxide (CO) combines with hemoglobin to produce carboxyhemoglobin, which can occur 200 times more readily than the combination of oxygen with hemoglobin (oxyhemoglobin). When CO replaces oxygen in the hemoglobin in excess of 25%, CO toxicity occurs.

CO is formed from incomplete combustion of carbon-combining compounds, as in automobile exhaust, fumes from improperly functioning furnaces, and cigarette smoke. Continuous exposure to CO, increasing carboxyhemoglobin by more than 60%, leads to coma and death. The treatment for CO toxicity is to administer a high concentration of oxygen.

Purpose

- To determine the percentage of carbon monoxide in the hemoglobin; if high, it could be fatal

Clinical Problems

Increased level: Smoking and exposure to smoking, automobile exhaust fumes, defective gas-burning appliances

Procedure

- No food or fluid restriction is required.
- Collect 5 to 7 ml of venous blood in a lavender-top tube.

- The most common method of analysis is performed with a CO oximeter, a direct-reading instrument.

Factors Affecting Laboratory Results
- Heavy smoking

Nursing Implications
- Determine from the client's history (obtained from the client, family, or friends) where carbon monoxide inhalation could have occurred.
- Assess for mild to severe carbon monoxide toxicity. Symptoms of mild CO toxicity are headache, weakness, malaise, dizziness, and dyspnea with exertion. Symptoms of moderate to severe toxicity are severe headache, bright red mucous membranes, and cherry-red blood. When carboxyhemoglobin exceeds 40%, the blood's residue is brick red.
- Identify individuals who might be candidates for CO poisoning. Clients who are living 24 h a day in a house with an old heating system in the winter should have a blood CO test performed. This is especially true if those persons have continuous headaches.

CARCINOEMBRYONIC ANTIGEN (CEA) (SERUM OR PLASMA)

Reference Values
Adult: Nonsmokers: Less than 2.5 ng/ml; smokers: Less than 5 ng/ml
Acute inflammatory disorders: Greater than 10 ng/ml
       Neoplasms: Greater than 12 ng/ml

Description.   CEA has been found in the gastrointestinal epithelium of embryos and has been extracted from tumors in the gastrointestinal tract. Originally, the CEA test was used to detect colon cancer, especially adenocarcinoma. Elevated levels might occur during an acute inflammatory disorder. CEA should never be used as the sole criterion for diagnosis of colon and pancreatic cancer.

The primary role of the CEA test is to monitor the treatment of colon and pancreatic carcinoma. If the levels fall after treatment, the cancer is most likely under control. CEA test may also be useful for clinical staging of the carcinoma and for determining if client has had a recurrence or relapse of cancer.

Purposes
* To monitor the treatment for colon or pancreatic carcinoma
* To compare with other laboratory tests for diagnosing an inflammatory condition, or gastrointestinal or pancreatic cancer

Clinical Problems
Increased level: Cancer: gastrointestinal tract (esophagus, stomach, small and large intestine, rectum), pancreas, liver, lung, breast, cervix, prostate, bladder, testes, kidney, leukemia; inflammatory bowel disease; chronic cigarette smoking; ulcerative colitis; cirrhosis of the liver; bacterial pneumonia; pulmonary emphysema; acute pancreatitis; acute renal failure; chronic ischemic heart disease

Procedure
* Heparin should not be administered for 2 days before the test, since it interferes with the results. Check with the health care provider.
* No food or fluid restriction is required.
* Collect 5 to 7 ml of venous blood in a red- or lavender-top tube. Avoid hemolysis.

Factors Affecting Laboratory Results
* Heparin interferes with the result of the CEA test.

Nursing Implications
* Relate clinical problems to elevated CEA levels. CEA levels over 10 ng/ml do not always indicate cancer, nor do levels below 10 ng/ml indicate an absence of cancer. Usually, the CEA is used for management of cancer treatment.

- Be supportive of client and family while awaiting test results. Answer questions or, if unable to, refer the questions to health professionals.
- If heparin is given, note date and time on the laboratory slip.

CARDIOVASCULAR DISEASE (CVD) GENETIC TEST (SERUM, BLOOD)

ANGIOTENSINOGEN (AGT) GENE

Reference Values

Negative: Absence of angiotensinogen (AGT) gene

Description. Many clients with cardiovascular disease (CVD) do not have risk factors for CVD, for example, hypercholesterolemia, high blood pressure (hypertension), diabetes mellitus, and/or obesity. The angiotensinogen (AGT) gene is a strong indicator of CVD. AGT is an autosomal recessive gene, and when the client has a pair of elevated AGT genes, he/she has a greater chance of developing CVD at an early age. These clients have a risk of life-threatening angina pectoris, myocardial infarction (MI), hypertension, and cardiomegaly. With a high risk for CVD, the client should be monitored frequently for signs and symptoms of CVD, for example, chest pain, dyspnea, fluid retention, high blood pressure, elevated lipids, and diabetes mellitus. Treatment might include lipid-lowering drugs, antihypertension drugs, diuretics, and management of diabetes. Genetic counseling may be suggested.

Purposes

- To identify the client who is at risk for CVD, that is, familial history of CVD
- To monitor signs and symptoms of CVD

Clinical Problems

Increased level: Elevated AGT gene, hypercholesterolemia, hypertension, diabetes mellitus, angina pectoris, MI

Procedure
- No food or fluid restriction is required. Some institutions may have a restriction.
- Collect 5–7 ml of venous blood in a red- or lavender-top tube.

Factors Affecting Laboratory Results
- None known

Nursing Implications
- Obtain a history of familial CVD and signs and symptoms of CVD.
- Assess laboratory results, that is, AGT, lipid profile, electrolytes.
- Take baseline vital signs (VS). Monitor VS as indicated.

Client Teaching
- Suggest that the client seek genetic counseling when the AGT levels are elevated.
- Be available to answer questions that the client may have or refer the questions to other health professionals.
- Be supportive of the client during and following testing for genetic CVD.

CAROTENE (SERUM)

Reference Values
Adult: 60–300 mcg/dl, 0.74–3.72 umol/l (SI units); varies with diet
Child: 40–130 mcg/dl

Description.   Carotene is a fat-soluble vitamin found in yellow and green vegetables and fruits. After absorption from the intestine, carotene is stored in the liver and can be converted to vitamin A, according to body needs. When fat absorption is decreased, the serum carotene level is decreased, which is indicative of fat malabsorption syndrome. Causes of serum carotene deficit include poor diet, malabsorption, high fever, and pancreatic insufficiency.

Purpose
- To determine the cause of malabsorption syndrome or liver disease

Clinical Problems
Decreased level: Malabsorption syndrome, pancreatic insufficiency, protein malnutrition, febrile illness, severe liver disease, cystic fibrosis
Increased level: Hyperlipidemia, diabetes mellitus, chronic nephritis, hypothyroidism, diet high in carrots, hypervitaminosis A (slightly elevated), pregnancy, hypocholesterolemia

Procedure
- Collect 7 ml of venous blood in a red-top tube. Protect from light.
- Foods rich in carotene—yellow and green vegetables, vegetable juice, and fruits—should be omitted for 2 to 3 days before the test (check laboratory procedure). If the health care provider wishes to check the serum carotene level for determining the absorption ability, a diet high in carotene will be ordered for several days. Water is permitted.
- NPO, a diet low in carotene, or a diet high in carotene should be recorded on the laboratory slip.

Factors Affecting Laboratory Results
- Mineral oil will interfere with carotene absorption.
- Foods rich in carotene can affect the serum results.

Nursing Implications
Client Teaching
- Explain to the client that diet will be high or low in carotene, depending on the health care provider's clinical assumptions and orders. Drinking water is permitted.
- Explain to the client that the test is to determine whether there is a vitamin (carotene) deficiency.
- Answer the client's questions concerning what foods to avoid or to eat before the test. Vegetables and fruits are rich in carotene.

CATECHOLAMINES (PLASMA AND URINE)

Reference Values

Plasma: Epinephrine: supine: less than 50 pg/ml; sitting: less than 60 pg/ml; standing: less than 90 pg/ml

Norepinephrine: supine: 110–410 pg/ml; sitting: 120–680 pg/ml; standing: 125–700 pg/ml

Dopamine: supine and standing: less than 87 pg/ml

Pheochromocytoma: total catecholamines: greater than 1,000 pg/ml

Urine

Adult: Total: less than 100 mcg/24 h (higher with activity), less than 0.59 μmol/24 h (SI units), 0–14 mcg/dl (random); epinephrine: less than 20 mcg/24 h; norepinephrine: less than 100 mcg/24 h. Values may differ with laboratories

Child: Level less than adult because of weight differences

Description.   The three main catecholamines are epinephrine (adrenaline), norepinephrine, and dopamine, which are hormones secreted by the adrenal medulla. These catecholamines respond to stress, fear, hypoxia, hemorrhage, and strenuous exercise by increasing the blood pressure. Catecholamines can be measured from plasma or by a 24-h urine collection specimen. The 24-h urine catecholamine collection has the advantage of determining the daily secretion of hormones. A single plasma catecholamine level could be misleading due to catecholamine fluctuation, but it is considered 75% effective in diagnosing pheochromocytomas. Urinary catecholamine levels are 3 to 100 times greater than normal in cases of pheochromocytoma. In children, the urine test may be used to diagnose malignant neuroblastoma.

Fractional analysis of catecholamine levels (epinephrine, norepinephrine, dopamine) is helpful for identifying certain adrenal medullary tumors suspected in hypertensive clients. A comparison of plasma catecholamine level with a 24-h urine catecholamine test can aid in diagnosing pheochromocytoma.

Purpose

- To assist in the diagnosis of the health problem related to the abnormal amount of catecholamines in the plasma and urine

Clinical Problems

Decreased level: Norepinephrine: anorexia nervosa, orthostatic hypotension; dopamine: parkinsonism

Increased level: Epinephrine and norepinephrine: pheochromocytoma (continuous elevation with epinephrine); ganglioblastoma, ganglioneuroma, and neuroblastoma (higher elevations with norepinephrine); diabetic ketoacidosis; kidney disease; shock; thyrotoxicosis; acute myocardial infarction (AMI); strenuous exercise; manic-depressive disorder

Drugs that may increase plasma and urine catecholamines: Epinephrine, norepinephrine, bronchodilators, amphetamines, aminophylline, selected beta adrenergics (isoproterenol), antihypertensives, antibiotics, chlorpromazine (Thorazine)

Procedure

Plasma

- Avoid foods rich in amines 2 days prior to test, such as chocolate, cocoa, wine, beer, tea, aged cheese, nuts (especially walnuts), and bananas.
- Avoid selected drugs 2 days prior to the test, such as OTC cold medications that contain sympathomimetics, diuretics, or antihypertensives, with the approval of the health care provider.
- Avoid strenuous exercise and smoking prior to the test.
- Restrict food and fluids 12 h prior to the test.
- An indwelling venous catheter may be inserted for collection of blood samples. Having an IV in place helps to avoid a surge in catecholamine release when a venipuncture is performed during collection of blood sample. The test may require a blood sample while the client is in a supine position and a sample while in standing position. Blood should be collected early in the morning.
- Collect 7 to 10 ml of venous blood in a green- or lavender-top tube. Place the blood sample immediately in an ice bath and take to the laboratory. The laboratory should be notified when the specimen is obtained, because the blood should be spun down and frozen immediately. This blood sample is usually sent to another laboratory.

Urine

- Avoid drugs, coffee, chocolate, bananas, and vanilla for 3 to 7 days before the test. Check with the laboratory. No other food or fluid restriction is necessary.

- Collect urine for 24 h in a large container with a preservative (10 to 15 ml of hydrochloric acid), and keep the bottle refrigerated. The pH of the urine collection should be below 3.0, and if not, more hydrochloric acid may be required.
- Label the large container with the client's name and the dates and exact times of the 24-h urine collection (e.g., 4/15/09, 7:15 AM to 4/16/09, 7:15 AM).

Nursing Implications
- Monitor the client's blood pressure. Report blood pressure that remains elevated and responds poorly to drug therapy.
- Check urine output. Report abnormal decreases in urine output. This may indicate renal insufficiency as well as affect the urine catecholamine test results.
- Ascertain if the client is extremely apprehensive or has given indications of stressful situation(s). Catecholamine levels are increased during stressful conditions.
- Report to the health care provider and record any strenuous activity, severe anxiety, and rising blood pressure readings.

Plasma
- Alert the laboratory of the order for plasma catecholamine. This is necessary so that the test can be processed in the laboratory within 5 min after blood sample is obtained.

Client Teaching
- Explain the procedure for the plasma catecholamine test to the client. Explanations should be given at least 24 h before the test. Writing the procedure for the client may be helpful in relieving anxiety.
- Encourage the client to relax as much as possible prior to the test and not exercise or smoke before the test.
- Listen to the client's concerns. Refer questions to other health care providers as needed.

Urine
- Withhold drugs that can cause false positives for 3 days or more, with physician's permission. Record the drugs that the client must take on the laboratory slip.

Client Teaching

- Explain that all urine should be saved in the refrigerated container. Inform the client that toilet paper and feces should not be put in the urine.
- Explain to the client that there is a strong acid as a preservative in the urine container and not to urinate directly into the container.
- Explain that fasting can increase catecholamine levels. Foods are not restricted except for those listed under Procedure.

CEREBROSPINAL FLUID (CSF)

SPINAL FLUID

Reference Values

	Color	Pressure (mm H$_2$O)	mm^3 WBC	Protein mg/dl	Chloride mEq/l	Glucose mg/dl
Adult	Clear, colorless	75–175	0–8	15–45	118–132	40–80
Child	Clear	50–100	0–8	14–45	120–128	35–75
Premature infant			0–20	<400		
Newborn 1–6 months	Clear		0–15	30–200 30–100	110–122	20–40

Description.   CSF/spinal fluid is obtained by a lumbar puncture (spinal tap) performed in the lumbar sac at L3–4 or at L4–5. First, CSF pressure is measured, then fluid is aspirated and placed in sterile test tubes. Data from the analysis of the spinal fluid is important for diagnosing spinal cord and brain diseases.

Purpose

- To detect color, pressure, WBC, protein, glucose, and presence of bacteria in CSF

Clinical Problems

Increased level: Intracranial pressure (ICP) due to meningitis, subarachnoid hemorrhage, brain tumor, brain abscess, encephalitis, viral infection

Procedure

- No food or fluid restriction is required.
- Collect a sterile lumbar puncture tray, an antiseptic solution, a local anesthetic, sterile gloves, and tape.
- Place the client in a fetal position, with the back bowed, the head flexed on the chest, and the knees drawn up to the abdomen.
- Label the three test tubes 1, 2, and 3.
- The physician checks the spinal fluid pressure, using a manometer attached to the needle, and collects a total of 10 to 12 ml of spinal fluid: 3 ml in tube 1, 3 ml in tube 2, and 3 ml in tube 3. The first tube is most likely contaminated (with blood from the spinal tap) and is usually discarded; the second tube is for cell count, glucose, and protein determination; and the third tube is for microbiologic studies.
- Use aseptic technique in collecting and handling specimen.
- Label the tubes with the client's name, date, and room number. Take the test tubes immediately to the laboratory.

Queckenstedt Procedure.   The Queckenstedt procedure is performed during a lumbar puncture when spinal block is suspected. Temporary pressure is applied to the jugular veins while the CSF pressure is monitored. Normally the CSF pressure will rise when the jugular veins are compressed. In partial or total CSF block, the pressure fails to rise with jugular vein compression, or it takes 15 to 30 seconds for CSF pressure to drop after compression is released.

Factors Affecting Laboratory Results

- Refrigeration may affect the results of the culture.
- A traumatic spinal tap could cause the presence of blood in the fluid specimen, which could be mistaken for a clinical problem.
- Hyperglycemia could increase the CSF glucose level.

- IV fluid containing chloride could invalidate the CSF chloride level determination.

Nursing Implications

- Explain the procedure for the lumbar puncture to the client by giving a step-by-step explanation.
- Collect specimen in numerical order of tubes.
- Check the vital signs before the procedure and afterwards at specified times (e.g., 0.5, 1, 2, and 4 h).
- Assess for changes in the neurologic status after the procedure (e.g., increased temperature, increased blood pressure, irritability, numbness and tingling in the lower extremities, and nonreactive pupils).
- Administer an analgesic as ordered to relieve a headache.
- Be supportive of client before, during, and after procedure.

Client Teaching

- Instruct the client to remain flat in bed in the prone or supine position for 4 to 8 h following the lumbar puncture. Headaches are common because of spinal fluid leaking from the site of the lumbar puncture.

CERULOPLASMIN (Cp) (SERUM)

Reference Values
Adult: 18–45 mg/dl, 180–450 mg/l (SI units)
Child: Infant: less than 23 mg/dl; 1–5 years old: 26–55 mg/dl; greater than 6 years old: same as adult

Description. Ceruloplasmin (Cp) is a copper-containing glycoprotein known as one of the alpha$_2$ globulins in the plasma. Ceruloplasmin is produced in the liver and binds with copper. With decreased serum ceruloplasmin levels, there is increased urinary excretion of copper and increased deposits of copper in the cornea (Kayser-Fleischer rings [green-gold rings]), brain, liver, and kidneys, thus causing damage and destruction to the organs. A deficit of ceruloplasmin or hypoceruloplasmin may result in Wilson's disease, usually seen between the ages of 7 and 15 and in early middle age.

Purpose
- To detect Wilson's disease or liver disorder

Clinical Problems
Decreased level: Wilson's disease (hepatolenticular degeneration), protein malnutrition, nephrotic syndrome, newborns and early infancy
Increased level: Cirrhosis of the liver, hepatitis, pregnancy, Hodgkin's disease, cancer of the bone, stomach, lung, myocardial infarction, rheumatoid arthritis, infections and inflammatory process, exercise, ingestion of excess copper, estrogen therapy, lymphomas, systemic lupus erythematosus (SLE)
Drugs that may increase ceruloplasmin value: Carbamazepine, estrogen products, oral contraceptives, phenytoin, methadone, barbiturates

Procedure
- No food or fluid restriction is required.
- Withhold drugs containing estrogen for 24 h before the blood test, with the health care provider's permission.
- Collect 5 ml of venous blood in a red-top tube.

Factors Affecting Laboratory Results
- Estrogen therapy, pregnancy, or exercise could cause an elevated serum ceruloplasmin level.

Nursing Implications
- Associate a decreased serum ceruloplasmin to Wilson's disease, a genetic problem in which there is excess accumulation of copper in the liver, eye, brain, and kidney.
- Assess for jaundice due to liver disorder from excess copper deposits.
- Check the cornea of the eye for a discolored (green-gold) ring from copper deposits.
- Assess for signs and symptoms of Wilson's disease, such as abnormal muscular rigidity (dystonia), tremors of the fingers, dysarthria, and mental disturbances.

CHLAMYDIA TEST (SERUM AND TISSUE SMEAR OR CULTURE)

Reference Values
Normal titer: Less than 1:16
Positive titer: Greater than 1:64

Description.   *Chlamydia* is a bacterium-like organism and has some features of a virus. There are two species of *Chlamydia: C psittaci,* which can cause psittacosis in birds and humans, and *C trachomatis,* which appears in three types (lymphogranuloma venereum [venereal disease], genital and other infections, and trachoma [eye disorder]).

The occurrence of *C psittaci* organism is more common for persons working in pet stores who may have contact with infected birds such as parakeets, and those working in the poultry industry who may come in contact with infected turkeys. A respiratory infection may result, causing chlamydial pneumonia. Serologic testing or tissue culture may be performed for diagnosis.

The strain of *C trachomatis,* lymphogranuloma venereum (LGV), venereal disease, is transmitted through sexual intercourse. It can occur in both male and female, causing enlargement of the inguinal and pelvic lymph nodes. Pregnant women can pass chlamydia infection to the newborn during birthing. This can cause trachoma ophthalmia neonatorum in the infant, which may lead to blindness later if untreated. Untreated genital infections caused by *C trachomatis* could lead to sterility.

With psittacosis and LGV, the serum titer level is greater than 1:64 (greater than fourfold of the reference value). The titer for genital infection caused by *C trachomatis* is usually between 1:16 and 1:64. Normally, the general population has a titer level less than 1:16. Tissue culture may be used to confirm test results with titer level. Tetracycline or erythromycin are usually the antibiotics used to treat chlamydia, not penicillin.

Purpose
- To identify the presence of a chlamydia infection, *C psittaci* or *C trachomatis*

Clinical Problems

Positive titer: Psittacosis; lymphogranuloma venereum (LGV); genital infections—pelvic inflammatory disease (PID), salpingitis, endometriosis; trachoma ophthalmia neonatorum; chlamydial pneumonia

Negative titer: Antibiotic therapy

Procedure

- No food or fluid restriction is required.
- Collect 3 to 5 ml of venous blood in a red-top tube. Avoid hemolysis.
- Tissue smear or culture may be obtained from the cervix or other areas.

Factors Affecting Laboratory Results

- Antibiotic therapy taken before tests could cause negative test results.

Nursing Implications

- Obtain a history from the client of any contact with birds that may be infected with *C psittaci.* Employees who work in pet shops or the poultry industry may be infected with *C psinaci* and have psittacosis.
- Check for signs and symptoms of psittacosis, which include a non-productive or slightly productive cough, chills, fever, headache, gastrointestinal symptoms, bradycardia, and mental changes.
- Assess if the woman is pregnant and has enlargement of the pelvic or inguinal lymph nodes. Genital infection from *Chlamydia* could be passed to the infant during the vaginal birthing process. Prenatal screening of pregnant women for chlamydial infection is being considered. Symptoms can be vague. The incidence of chlamydial infection in infants is 28 out of 1,000 live births.
- Withhold antibiotic drug, with physician's approval, until after the specimen has been obtained.

Client Teaching

- Encourage the client with *C trachomatis* infection to give name(s) of sexual partner(s). Certain antibiotic therapies can eliminate the organism and prevent passing the infection to others. The sexual partner(s) may also need treatment.

- Explain to the mother with a chlamydial infection that the infant should be checked.
- Inform clients with titer less than 1:16 that an acute chlamydial infection is unlikely.
- Listen to the client's concerns. Respond or refer questions to other health care providers.

CHLORIDE (CI) (SERUM)

Reference Values
Adult: 95–105 mEq/l, 95–105 mmol/l (SI units)
Child: Newborn: 94–112 mEq/l; infant: 95–110 mEq/l; child: 98–105 mEq/l

Description.   Chloride, an anion found mostly in the extracellular fluid, plays an important role in maintaining body water balance, osmolality of body fluids (with sodium), and acid–base balance. Most of the chloride ingested is combined with sodium (sodium chloride [NaCl], or salt).

Purpose
- To check chloride level in relation to potassium, sodium, acid–base balance

Clinical Problems
Decreased level: Vomiting, gastric suction, diarrhea, low serum potassium or sodium (or both), low-sodium diet, continuous IV D$_5$W, gastroenteritis, colitis, adrenal gland insufficiency, heat exhaustion, acute infections, burns, excessive diaphoresis, metabolic alkalosis, chronic respiratory acidosis, HF
Drugs that may decrease chloride value: Thiazide and loop diuretics, bicarbonates
Increased level: Dehydration, high serum sodium level, adrenal gland hyperfunction, multiple myeloma, head injury, eclampsia, cardiac decompensation, excessive IV saline (0.9% NaCl), kidney dysfunction, metabolic acidosis

Drugs that may increase chloride value: Ammonium chloride, cortisone preparations, ion exchange resins, prolonged use of triamterene (Dyrenium), acetazolamide (Diamox)

Procedure
- No food or fluid restriction is required.
- Collect 3 to 5 ml of venous blood in a red- or green-top tube.

Nursing Implications
Decreased Level
- Assess for signs and symptoms of hypochloremia (e.g., hyperexcitability of the nervous system and muscles, tetany, slow and shallow breathing, and hypotension).
- Inform the health care provider when the client is receiving IV D_5W continuously. A chloride deficit could occur.
- Check the serum potassium and sodium levels. Chloride is frequently lost with sodium and potassium.
- Observe for symptoms of overhydration when the client is receiving several liters of normal saline for sodium and chloride replacement. Sodium holds water. Symptoms of overhydration include a constant, irritating cough; dyspnea; neck-and-hand vein engorgement; and chest rales.

Client Teaching
- Encourage the client with deficit to drink fluids containing sodium and chloride (e.g., broth, tomato juice, *no* plain water).

Increased Level
- Assess for signs and symptoms of hyperchloremia (similar to acidosis: i.e., weakness; lethargy; and deep, rapid, vigorous breathing).
- Monitor daily weights and intake and output to determine whether fluid retention is present because of sodium and chloride excess.
- Notify the health care provider if the client is receiving IV fluids containing normal saline and has an elevated serum chloride level. Check for symptoms of overhydration.

Client Teaching
- Instruct the client to avoid drinking or eating salty foods and to use salt substitute.
- Instruct the client to read labels of salt substitutes, since many contain calcium chloride and potassium chloride.

CHOLESTEROL (SERUM)

Reference Values (See also Lipoproteins)
Adult: Desirable level: less than 200 mg/dl; moderate risk: 200–240 mg/dl; high risk: greater than 240 mg/dl. Pregnancy: high risk levels but returns to prepregnancy values 1 month after delivery
Child: Infant: 90–130 mg/dl; child 2–19 years; desirable level: 130–170 mg/dl; moderate risk: 171–184 mg/dl; high risk: greater than 185 mg/dl

Description.   Cholesterol is a blood lipid synthesized by the liver. Cholesterol is used by the body to form bile salts for fat digestion and for the formation of hormones by the adrenal glands, ovaries, and testes. Thyroid and estrogen hormones decrease the concentration of cholesterol. Approximately one third of American people have serum cholesterol levels below 200 mg/dl.

Purposes
- To check client's cholesterol level
- To monitor cholesterol levels

Clinical Problems
Decreased level: Hyperthyroidism, starvation, malabsorption
Drugs that may decrease cholesterol value: Thyroxine, estrogens, aspirin, antibiotics (tetracycline and neomycin), nicotinic acid, heparin, colchicine
Increased level: Hypercholesterolemia; AMI; atherosclerosis; hypothyroidism; uncontrolled diabetes mellitus; biliary cirrhosis; pancreatectomy; pregnancy (third trimester); heavy stress periods; type II, III, V hyperlipoproteinemia; high-cholesterol diet; nephrotic syndrome

Drugs that may increase cholesterol value: Oral contraceptives, epineph-rine, phenothiazines, vitamins A and D, sulfonamides, phenytoin (Dilantin)

Procedure
- Restrict food and fluids for 12 h prior to test. List food and drugs taken prior to laboratory test on the laboratory slip.
- Instruct client to have a low-fat meal the night prior to the test.
- Collect 3 to 5 ml of venous blood in a red-top tube. Avoid hemolysis.

Factors Affecting Laboratory Results
- A high-cholesterol diet before the test could cause an elevated serum cholesterol level.
- Severe hypoxia could increase the serum cholesterol level.

Nursing Implications
Client Teaching
- Instruct the client with hypercholesterolemia to decrease the intake of foods rich in cholesterol (e.g., bacon, eggs, fatty meats, seafood, chocolate, and coconut).
- Encourage client to lose weight if overweight and has hypercholes-terolemia. If obese, losing weight can decrease serum cholesterol level.
- Answer questions regarding cholesterol and the blood test.
- Explain to the client and family what is considered a normal serum cholesterol level and the effects of an elevated cholesterol level.

COAGULATION FACTORS (PLASMA) (*SEE FACTOR ASSAY*)

COLD AGGLUTININS (SERUM)

COLD HEMAGGLUTININ

Reference Values
Adult: Normal: 1:8 antibody titer (elderly may have higher levels); greater than 1:16 significantly increased; greater than 1:32 definitely positive
Child: Similar to adult

Description. Cold agglutinins (CAs) are antibodies that agglutinate RBCs at temperatures between 0°C and 10°C. Elevated titers (greater than 1:32) are usually found in clients with primary atypical pneumonia or with other clinical problems, such as influenza and pulmonary embolism. The CAs test is often done during the acute and convalescent phases of illness.

Purposes
- To determine the presence of an increased antibody titer significant for atypical pneumonia, influenza, or leukemia
- To compare test results with other laboratory tests

Clinical Problems
Increased level: Primary atypical pneumonia, influenza, cirrhosis, lymphatic leukemia, multiple myeloma, pulmonary embolism, acquired hemolytic anemias, malaria, infectious mononucleosis, viral infections (Epstein-Barr [EB] virus [mononucleosis] and cytomegalovirus), tuberculosis (TB)

Procedure
- No food or fluid restriction is required.
- Collect 5 to 7 ml of venous blood in a red-top tube. Keep specimen warm. Take to laboratory immediately.
- The laboratory may rewarm the blood sample for 30 min before the serum is separated from the cells.

Factors Affecting Laboratory Results
- Antibiotic therapy may cause inaccurate results.
- Elevated cold agglutinins may interfere with type- and cross-matching.

Nursing Implications
- Answer the client's questions concerning the significance of the test.
- Assess for signs and symptoms of viral infection (e.g., elevated temperature).

- Notify the health care provider of a recurrence of an acute inflammation. The health care provider may wish to order a serum C-reactive protein (CRP) test.
- Check the results of the serum CRP level. If the titer is decreasing, the client is responding to treatment, and/or the acute phase is declining.
- Compare CRP with erythrocyte sedimentation rate (ESR). The serum CRP level will elevate and return to normal faster than the ESR level.

COMPLEMENT: TOTAL (SERUM)

Reference Values
Adult: 75–160 units/ml; 75–160 kU/l (SI units)

Description.   Total complement plays an important role in the immunologic enzyme system reacting to an antigen–antibody response. The complements make up about 10% of the serum globulins. The complement system has over 20 components, with 9 major components numbered C1 to C9. C3 and C4 are the most abundant complements and are discussed separately in the text. The total complement may be referred to as total hemolytic complement or CH_{50}. CH_{50} assesses the function of the complement system. When the complement system is stimulated, it increases phagocytosis, lysis, or destruction of bacteria, and produces an inflammatory response to infection.

Most assays for CH_{50} are most sensitive to changes in C2, C4, and C5. Assay should be used as a screen for overall complement function and not as a quantitative measure of C1 activation during the course of disease states.

Purposes
- To identify the effects of the immunologic enzyme system regarding the presence of inflammatory condition(s) or tissue rejection
- To compare serum complement tests with serum immunoglobulins to determine the cause of the health problem

Clinical Problems
Decreased level: Allograft rejection, hypogammaglobulinemia, acute poststreptococcal glomerulonephritis, acute serum sickness, systemic

lupus erythematosus (SLE), lupus nephritis, hepatitis, subacute bacterial endocarditis, hemolytic anemia, rheumatic fever, multiple myeloma, advanced cirrhosis

Increased level: Acute rheumatic fever, rheumatoid arthritis, acute myocardial infarction (AMI), ulcerative colitis, diabetes mellitus, thyroiditis, Wegener's granulomatosis, obstructive jaundice

Procedure

- No food or fluid restriction is required.
- Collect 3 to 5 ml of venous blood in a red-top tube. Avoid hemolysis. Allow to clot at room temperature. Spin at 4°C. Transfer serum and freeze immediately. This test may be sent to a large reference laboratory.

Nursing Implications

- Obtain a history from the client of an infectious process or abnormal response to infection. Complement deficiency may occur to those persons susceptible to infection and with certain autoimmune diseases.
- Assess the client's vital signs and urine output. Report abnormal findings.
- Compare total complement results with serum immunoglobulins. Complement results give information about the client's immune system.

COMPLEMENT C3 AND C4 TEST (SERUM)

C3 AND C4 COMPONENT OF THE COMPLEMENT SYSTEM

Reference Values

Adult: C3: *Male:* 80–180 mg/dl. *Female:* 76–120 mg/dl; C4: 15–45 mg/dl, 150–450 mg/l (SI units)

Elderly: Slightly higher than adult

Description. The complement system (a group of 11 proteins) is activated when the antibodies are combined with antigens. C3 is the most abundant component of the complement system and contributes about 70% of the total protein. Increased C3 levels occur in inflammatory disorders. A decrease in C3 and C4 is commonly found in diseases such as systemic lupus erythematosus (SLE), glomerulonephritis, and renal transplant rejection.

Purposes
- To assist in the detection of acute inflammatory disease (e.g., rheumatoid arthritis) and other health problems (see Clinical Problems)
- To compare test results with other laboratory tests to determine health problem

Clinical Problems
Decreased level: SLE (C4 decreased time is longer than C3), glomerulonephritis, lupus nephritis, acute renal transplant rejection, protein malnutrition, anemias (pernicious, folic acid), multiple sclerosis (slightly lower), cirrhosis of the liver

Increased level: Acute inflammatory disease, acute rheumatic fever, rheumatoid arthritis, early SLE, AMI, ulcerative colitis, cancer

Procedure
- No food or fluid restriction is required.
- Collect 3 to 5 ml of venous blood in a red-top tube; take to the laboratory *immediately*. C3 is unstable at room temperature.

Nursing Implications
- Compare the serum C3 value with other laboratory studies that are ordered and related to the specific health problem.
- Compare the serum C3 and C4 results.
- Be supportive of client and family.

COOMBS' DIRECT (BLOOD—RBC)

DIRECT ANTIGLOBULIN TEST

Reference Values
Adult: Negative
Child: Negative

Description.   The direct (antiglobulin) Coombs' test detects antibodies other than the ABO group, which attach to RBCs.

The RBCs are tested and if sensitized will agglutinate. A positive Coombs' test reveals antibodies present on RBCs, but the test does not identify the antibody responsible.

Purpose
* To detect antibodies on red blood cells

Clinical Problems
Positive (+1 to +4):   Erythroblastosis fetalis, hemolytic anemia (autoimmune or drugs), transfusion hemolytic reactions (blood incompatibility), leukemias, SLE

Drugs that may increase Coombs' direct: Antibiotics (cephalosporins [Keflin], penicillin, tetracycline, streptomycin), aminopyrine (Pyradone), phenytoin (Dilantin), chlorpromazine (Thorazine), sulfonamides, antiarrhythmics (quinidine, procainamide [Pronestyl]), L-dopa, methyldopa (Aldomet), antituberculins (isoniazid [INH], rifampin)

Procedure
* No food or fluid restriction is required.
* Collect 5 to 7 ml of venous blood in a lavender-top tube. A red-top tube could be used. Avoid hemolysis. Venous blood from the umbilical cord of a newborn may be used.

Nursing Implications
* Report previous transfusion reactions.
* Observe for signs and symptoms of blood transfusion reactions (e.g., chills, fever [slight temperature elevation], and rash).

COOMBS' INDIRECT (SERUM)

ANTIBODY SCREEN TEST

Reference Values
Adult: Negative
Child: Negative

Description.   The indirect Coombs' test detects free circulating antibodies in the serum. This screening test will check for antibodies in recipient's and donor's serum prior to transfusions to avoid a transfusion reaction. It does not directly identify the specific antibody. It is done as part of crossmatch blood test.

Purpose
- To check recipient's and donor's blood for antibodies prior to blood transfusion

Clinical Problems
Positive (+1 to +4):   Incompatible crossmatched blood, specific antibody (previous transfusion), anti-Rh antibodies, acquired hemolytic anemia
Drugs that may increase Coombs' indirect: Same as for direct Coombs' test

Procedure
- No food or fluid restriction is required.
- Collect 5 or 7 ml of venous blood in a red-top tube.

Nursing Implications
- Obtain a history of previous transfusions, and report any previous transfusion reactions.
- Observe for transfusion reactions.
- List drugs that can cause false-positive test results on the laboratory slip.

COPPER (Cu) (SERUM AND URINE)

Reference Values
Serum: Male: 70–140 mcg/dl, 11–22 μmol/l (SI units); female: 80–155 mcg/dl, 12.6–24.3 μmol/l (SI units); pregnancy: 140–300 mcg/dl
   Child: newborn: 20–70 mcg/dl; child: 30–190 mcg/dl; adolescent: 90–240 mcg/dl

Urine: Adult and child: 0–60 mcg/24 h, 0.095 μmol/24 h
Wilson's disease: greater than 100 mcg/24 h

Description.   Copper (Cu) is required for hemoglobin synthesis and activation of respiratory enzymes. Approximately 90% of the copper is bound to alpha$_2$ globulin, referred to as ceruloplasmin, which is the means of copper transportation in the body. In hepatolenticular disease (Wilson's disease), the serum copper level is less than 20 mcg/dl, and the urinary copper level is greater than 100 g/24 h. There is a decrease in copper metabolism with Wilson's disease, and excess copper is deposited in the brain (basal ganglia) and liver, causing degenerative changes. Wilson's disease is more likely to be found in the Italian and Sicilian populations and in the Eastern European Jewish people.

Serum copper and serum ceruloplasmin tests are frequently ordered together and compared. Both show decreased serum levels with Wilson's disease, and the urine copper level is elevated.

Purposes
- To aid in the diagnosis of Wilson's disease (hepatolenticular disease)
- To screen infants and children with familial history of Wilson's disease

Clinical Problems
Serum
Decreased level: Wilson's disease, protein malnutrition, chronic ischemic heart disease
Increased level: Cancer (bone, stomach, large intestine, liver, lung), Hodgkin's disease, leukemias, hypo/hyperthyroidism, anemias (pernicious and iron deficiency), rheumatoid arthritis, systemic lupus erythematosus, pregnancy, cirrhosis of the liver
Drugs that may increase copper level: Oral contraceptives

Urine
Increased level: Wilson's disease, biliary cirrhosis, rheumatic arthritis, nephrotic syndromes

Procedure
A serum and a urine specimen may be requested simultaneously.

Serum
- No food or fluid restriction.
- Collect 5 ml of venous blood in a royal blue-top tube (used for trace metal).

Urine
- Discard the first morning urine specimen and then begin a 24-h urine collection in a container specified for this test.

Factors Affecting Laboratory Results
- Blood sample inserted into a siliconized stopper may cause a false reading.

Nursing Implications
- Assess for signs and symptoms of Wilson's disease (e.g., rigidity, dysarthria, dysphagia, incoordination, and tremors).
- Check for a Kayser-Fleischer ring (dark ring) around the cornea. This is a copper deposit that the body has not been able to metabolize.
- Compare the serum copper level with the urine copper level and the serum ceruloplasmin level if ordered. With Wilson's disease, the serum copper and ceruloplasmin levels would be decreased and the urine copper level would be increased.

Client Teaching
- Explain to the client with Wilson's disease that foods rich in copper, such as organ meats, shellfish, mushrooms, whole-grain cereals, bran, nuts, and chocolate, should be avoided. Canned foods should be omitted. A low-copper diet and D-penicillamine promote copper excretion.

CORTISOL (PLASMA)

Reference Values
Adult: 8 AM–10 AM: 5–23 mcg/dl, 138–635 nmol/l (SI units). 4 PM–6 PM: 3–13 mcg/dl, 83–359 nmol/l (SI units)
Child: 8 AM–10 AM: 15–25 mcg/dl; 4 PM–6 PM: 5–10 mcg/dl

Description.   Cortisol is a potent glucocorticoid released from the adrenal cortex in response to adrenocorticotropic hormone (ACTH) stimulation. Levels of plasma cortisol are higher in the morning and lower in the afternoon. When there is adrenal or pituitary dysfunction, the diurnal variation in cortisol function ceases.

Purposes
- To determine the occurrence of an elevated or decreased plasma cortisol level
- To associate a decreased cortisol level with an adrenocortical hypofunction

Clinical Problems
Decreased level: Adrenocortical hypofunction (Addison's disease), anterior pituitary hypofunction, respiratory distress syndrome (low-birth-weight newborns), hypothyroidism
Drugs that may decrease cortisol value: Androgens, phenytoin (Dilantin)
Increased level: Adrenocortical hyperfunction (Cushing's syndrome), cancer of the adrenal gland, stress, pregnancy, AMI, diabetic acidosis, hyperthyroidism, pain, fever
Drugs that may increase cortisol value: Oral contraceptives, estrogens, spironolactone (Aldactone), triparanol

Procedure
- Have client rest in bed for 2 h before blood is drawn.
- Draw blood before meals.
- Collect 5 to 7 ml of venous blood in a green-top (heparinized) tube.
- If the client has taken estrogen or oral contraceptives in the last 6 weeks, the drug(s) should be listed on the laboratory slip. Recommendation: stop medication 2 months before test with the health care provider's approval.

Factors Affecting Laboratory Results
- Physical activity prior to the test might decrease the cortisol level.
- Obesity can cause an elevated serum level.

Nursing Implications

- Obtain a history of drugs taken prior to test. List drugs, especially oral contraceptives and estrogen, on the laboratory slip and inform the health care provider.

Client Teaching

- Instruct the client to rest for 2 h prior to the test.
- Instruct client to be NPO 2 h before test, both AM and PM.

Decreased Level

- Observe for signs and symptoms of Addison's disease. Symptoms are anorexia, vomiting, abdominal pain, fatigue, dizziness, trembling, and diaphoresis.

Increased Level

- Observe for signs and symptoms of Cushing's syndrome. Symptoms are fat deposits in the face (moon face), neck, and back of chest; irritability; mood swings; bleeding (gastrointestinal or under skin); muscle wasting; weakness.

C-PEPTIDE (SERUM)

CONNECTING PEPTIDE INSULIN, PRO-INSULIN C-PEPTIDE

Reference Values
Adult: Fasting: 0.8 to 1.8 ng/ml; 0.27 to 0.63 nmol/l (SI units)

Description.   C-Peptide is an inactive amino acid formed during the conversion of pro-insulin to insulin in the beta cells of the pancreas. The C-peptide levels can indicate the beta cell activity in the production of insulin. Normally, C-peptide levels correlate with the insulin levels because both are released from the beta cells of the pancreas in similar amounts. C-Peptide has a long half-life compared to insulin, so C-peptide levels can be increased in blood circulation.

The C-peptide levels can indicate the presence of insulin antibodies in a diabetic client receiving (exogenous) insulin. When exogenous insulin increases the serum insulin levels, C-peptide levels remain unaffected or decreased. The C-peptide levels are high with insulinoma.

Purposes
- To identify excess insulin administration in the diabetic or nondiabetic patient; insulin level is increased and the C-peptide level is decreased
- To assist in the diagnosis of insulin antibodies
- To assist in the diagnosis of insulinoma
- To evaluate the insulin reserve in insulin-dependent diabetic patient or Type 1 diabetes mellitus
- To detect the cause of hypoglycemia

Clinical Problems
Decreased level: Type 1 diabetes mellitus, pancreatectomy
Drugs that may decrease C-peptide levels: Atenolol, calcitonin, rosiglitazone, troglitazone
Increased level: Insulinoma, Type 2 diabetes mellitus, beta cell transplants, renal failure
Drugs that may increase C-peptide levels: Sulfonylurea and glyburide (oral hypoglycemic drug groups); cortisone drugs, for example, prednisone, betamethasone; oral contraceptives; estrogen drugs; chloroquine; terbutaline

Procedure
- Nothing by mouth (NPO), except some water, 8–10 h before the test
- Collect 5–7 ml of venous blood in a red-top tube. Insulin specimen should be placed on ice

Factors Affecting Laboratory Results
- Hemolysis of the blood sample
- Liver dysfunction can cause an increased C-peptide level
- Renal failure can cause an increased C-peptide level
- For drugs, see Decreased and Increased Levels, Clinical Problems
- Radioisotope testing before the blood is drawn for C-peptide

Nursing Implications

- Obtain a history of client's health problems related to diabetes mellitus, for example, symptoms related to hypoglycemia.
- Obtain a list of medications the client is taking.

Client Teaching

- Explain to the client that he/she should adhere to the American Diabetic Association diet. Have a nutritionist speak to the client.
- Explain to the client the importance of insulin regulation, diet, and weight control.
- Listen to the client's concerns. Answer questions or refer them to other health professionals.

C-REACTIVE PROTEIN (CRP) (SERUM) AND N HIGH SENSITIVITY CRP (hs CRP)

Reference Values

Adult: Not usually present: *Qualitative:* greater than 1.2 titer, *Positive:* Quantitative: 20 mg/dl
Child: Not usually present.

N High Sensitivity CRP (hs CRP)
Adult: Less than 0.175 mg/l

Description.   C-Reactive protein (CRP) is produced in the liver in response to tissue injury and inflammation. It appears in the blood 6 to 10 h after an acute inflammatory process and tissue destruction. Also it peaks within 48 to 72 h. Serum CRP is also found in many body fluids, such as pleural, peritoneal, and synovial fluids.

This type of protein is needed to fight injury and infection. Inflammation can cause the protein to become an inflammatory protein. Many references believe that the inflammatory protein is an important factor in cardiovascular disease.

Chronic infection, fat cells, hypertension, smoking, cardiovascular and peripheral disease, stroke, and rheumatoid arthritis can produce these inflammatory proteins, which weaken the fatty plaques and cause them to erupt. The pieces of plaques become clots that lead to decreased blood flow and even heart attacks. Higher levels of inflammatory proteins in the blood indicate a higher potential for atherosclerosis.

N High Sensitivity CRP (hs CRP).   This test is a highly sensitive test for detecting the risk of cardiovascular and peripheral vascular diseases. It is frequently combined with cholesterol screening. Approximately one third of the population who has had a heart attack have normal cholesterol levels and normal blood pressure. A positive hs CRP test may indicate that the client is at a high risk for coronary artery disease (CAD). This test can detect an inflammatory process occurring that is caused by the build-up of plaque (atherosclerosis) in the arterial system, particularly coronary arteries. Positive serum hs CRP values are much lower than the standard serum CRP, which makes it a more valuable test for predicting coronary heart disease.

Purposes
- To associate an increased CRP titer with an acute inflammatory process
- To detect the risk of coronary heart disease (hs CRP)
- To compare test results with other laboratory tests, such as ESR, anti-streptolysin O

Clinical Problems
Increased level: Chronic infections, cardiovascular and peripheral diseases, acute myocardial infarction (AMI), inflammatory bowel disease, rheumatoid arthritis, rheumatic fever, systemic lupus erythematosus, bacterial infections, late pregnancy, intrauterine contraceptive devices, cancer with metastasis
Drugs that may increase the CRP or hs CRP levels: Oral contraceptives

Procedure
- Restrict food and fluids, except water, for 8 to 12 h before the test.
- Collect 3 to 5 ml of venous blood in a red-top tube. Avoid heat since CRP is thermolabile.

Factors Affecting Laboratory Results

- Pregnancy (third trimester) could elevate the CRP level.
- Oral contraceptives and intrauterine contraceptive devices might elevate the CRP level.

Nursing Implications

- Recognize that an elevated serum CRP level is associated with an active inflammatory process and tissue destruction (necrosis). The CRP and hs CRP may be elevated in cardiovascular and peripheral diseases, rheumatoid arthritis, chronic infections.
- Assess for signs and symptoms of an acute inflammatory process, such as pain and swelling in joints, heat, redness, or increased body temperature.
- Assess for signs and symptoms of cardiovascular and peripheral diseases; also for chest pain associated with coronary artery disease (CAD).
- Compare the serum hs CRP with serum cholesterol and serum lipoprotein tests. An elevated serum hs CRP and serum cholesterol profile may indicate a high risk of coronary artery disease (CAD).
- Compare the results of the serum CRP level. If the titer is decreasing, the client is responding to treatment and/or the acute phase is declining. The CRP titer may be compared to the ESR. The serum CRP level will elevate and return to normal faster than the ESR.
- Notify the health care provider of a recurrence (exacerbation) of an acute inflammation. The HCP may wish to order a serum CRP test or a serum hs CRP level.

CREATININE (SERUM AND URINE)

Reference Values

Adult: Serum: 0.5–1.5 mg/dl; 45–132.5 μmol/l (SI units). Females may have slightly lower values due to less muscle mass

   Urine: 1–2 g/24 h

Child: Newborn: 0.8–1.4 mg/dl; infant: 0.7–1.7 mg/dl; 2–6 years: 0.3–0.6 mg/dl, 27–54 μmol/l (SI units); older child: 0.4–1.2 mg/dl, 36–106 μmol/l (SI units; values increase slightly with age due to muscle mass)
Elderly: May have decreased values due to decreased muscle mass and decreased creatinine production

Description.   Creatinine, a by-product of muscle catabolism, is derived from the breakdown of muscle creatine and creatine phosphate. The amount of creatinine produced is proportional to muscle mass. The kidneys excrete creatinine. When 50% or more nephrons are destroyed, serum creatinine level increases. Serum creatinine is especially useful in evaluation of glomerular function.

Serum creatinine is considered a more sensitive and specific indicator of renal disease than BUN. It rises later and is not influenced by diet or fluid intake. Normal BUN/creatinine ratio is 10:1. Values significantly higher than this suggest to be prerenal.

Purpose
- To diagnose renal dysfunction

Clinical Problems
Increased level: Acute and chronic renal failure (nephritis, chronic glomerulonephritis), shock (prolonged), cancers, lupus erythematosus, diabetic nephropathy, CHF, AMI, diet (e.g., beef [high], poultry, and fish [minimal effect])
Drugs that may increase creatinine value: Antibiotics (cephalosporins, amphotericin B, aminoglycosides, kanamycin), ascorbic acid, L-dopa, methyldopa (Aldomet), lithium carbonate

Procedure
- No food or fluid restriction is required. Suggest avoiding red meats the night before the test, since these meats could increase the level.
- Collect 3 to 5 ml of venous blood in a red-top tube.
- List any drugs the client is taking that could elevate the serum level on the laboratory slip.

Nursing Implications

- Relate the elevated creatinine levels to clinical problems. Serum creatinine may be low in clients with small muscle mass, amputees, and clients with muscle disease. Older clients may have decreased muscle mass and a decreased rate of creatinine formation.
- Check the amount of urine output in 24 h. Less than 600 ml/24 h and an elevated serum creatinine can indicate renal insufficiency.
- Compare the BUN and creatinine levels. If both are increased, the problem is most likely kidney disease.
- Limit beef and poultry if the serum creatinine level is very high.

CREATININE CLEARANCE (URINE)

Reference Values
Urine Creatinine Clearance
Adult: 85–135 ml/min. Females may have somewhat lower values
Child: Similar to adult
Elderly: Slightly decreased values than adult due to decreased glomerular filtration rate (GFR) caused by reduced renal plasma flow
Urine creatinine: 1–2 g/24 h

Description.   Creatinine clearance is considered a reliable test for estimating glomerular filtration rate (GFR). With renal dysfunction, creatinine clearance test is decreased.

The creatinine clearance test consists of a 12- or 24-h urine collection and a blood sample. A creatinine clearance less than 40 ml/min is suggestive of moderate to severe renal impairment.

Purposes
- To detect renal dysfunction
- To monitor renal function

Clinical Problems
Decreased level: Mild to severe renal impairment, hyperthyroidism, progressive muscular dystrophy, amyotrophic lateral sclerosis (ALS)

Drugs that may decrease urine creatinine clearance: Phenacetin, steroids, thiazides
Increased level: Hypothyroidism, hypertension (renovascular), exercise, pregnancy
Drugs that may increase urine creatinine clearance: Ascorbic acid, steroids, L-dopa, methyldopa (Aldomet), cefoxitin

Procedure

- Hydrate client well before test.
- Avoid meats, poultry, fish, tea, and coffee for 6 h before the test and during the test, with health care provider's permission.
- List drugs on the laboratory slip that could affect test results.
- **Blood:** Collect 3 to 5 ml of venous blood in a red-top tube the morning of the test or anytime during the test, as specified.
- **Urine:** Have client void and discard the urine before the test begins. Note the time and save all urine for 24 h in a urine container, without preservative. Refrigerate the urine collection or keep in ice. Encourage water intake during the test to have sufficient urine output.
- Toilet paper and feces should not be in the urine.

Nursing Implications
Client Teaching

- Instruct the client not to eat meats, poultry, fish, or drink tea or coffee for 6 h before the test. Check laboratory policy.
- Encourage water intake throughout the test.
- Instruct client not to do strenuous exercise during the test.
- Answer questions.

CREATINE PHOSPHOKINASE (CPK, CK), AND CPK ISOENZYMES (SERUM)

CREATINE KINASE (CK)

Reference Values
Adult: Male: 5–35 mcg/ml, 30–180 international units/l; female: 5–25 mcg/ml, 25–150 international units/l

Child: Newborn: 65–580 international units/l at 30°C. Child: male: 0–70 international units/l at 30°C; female: 0–50 international units/l at 30°C

CPK Isoenzymes
CPK-MM: 94%–100% (muscle)
CPK-MB: 0%–6% (heart)
CPK-BB: 0% (brain)

Description.   Creatine phosphokinase (CPK) is an enzyme found in high concentration in the heart and skeletal muscles and in low concentration in the brain tissue. CPK/CK has two types of isoenzymes: M, associated with muscle; and B, associated with the brain. Electrophoresis separates the isoenzymes into three subdivisions: MM (in skeletal muscle and some in the heart), MB (in the heart), and BB (in brain tissue). When CPK/CK is elevated, a CPK electrophoresis is done to determine which group of isoenzymes is elevated. The isoenzyme CPK-MB could indicate damage to the myocardial cells.

Serum CPK/CK and CPK-MB rise within 4 to 6 h after an acute myocardial infarction, reach a peak in 18 to 24 h (greater than 6 times the normal value), and then return to normal within 3 to 4 days, unless new necrosis or tissue damage occurs.

Purposes
* To suggest myocardial or skeletal muscle disease
* To compare test results with AST and LDH to determine myocardial damage

Clinical Problems
Increased level: Acute myocardial infarction (AMI), skeletal muscle disease, cerebrovascular accident (CVA), and with elevated CPK isoenzymes
CPK-MM isoenzyme: Muscular dystrophy, delirium tremens, crush injury/trauma, surgery and postoperative state, vigorous exercise, IM injections, hypokalemia, hemophilia, hypothyroidism
CPK-MB: AMI, severe angina pectoris, cardiac surgery, cardiac ischemia, myocarditis, hypokalemia, cardiac defibrillation
CPK-BB: CVA, subarachnoid hemorrhage, cancer of the brain, acute brain injury, Reye's syndrome, pulmonary embolism and infarction, seizures

Drugs that may increase CPK value: IM injections, dexamethasone (Decadron), furosemide (Lasix), aspirin (high doses), ampicillin, carbenicillin, clofibrate

Procedure
- No food or fluid restriction is required.
- Collect 5 to 7 ml of venous blood in a red-top tube. Avoid hemolysis. Take blood specimen to the laboratory immediately.
- Note on the laboratory slip the number of times the client has received IM injections in the last 24 to 48 h. Draw blood for a serum CPK/CK level before giving an IM injection.

Nursing Implications
- Avoid IM injections; they may increase serum CPK level.
- Relate elevated serum CPK/CK and isoenzymes to clinical problems. The CPK-MB is useful in making the differential diagnosis of myocardial infarction.
- Indicate whether the client has received an IM injection in the last 24 to 48 h on the laboratory slip, chart, Kardex.
- Assess the client's signs and symptoms of an AMI (e.g., pain; dyspnea; diaphoresis; cold, clammy skin; pallor; and cardiac dysrhythmia).
- Assess anxiety state of client and family. Be supportive.
- Provide measures for alleviating pain.
- Check the serum CPK/CK level at intervals, and notify the physician of serum level changes. High levels of CPK/CK and CPK-MB indicate the extent of myocardial damage.
- Compare serum AST/SGOT and LDH levels with CPK and CPK-MB.

CROSSMATCH (BLOOD)

BLOOD TYPING TESTS, TYPE AND CROSSMATCH
Reference Values
Adult: Compatibility: absence of agglutination (clumping) of cells
Child: Same as adult

Description. The four major blood types (A, B, AB, and O) belong to the ABO blood group system. RBCs have either antigen A, B, or AB, or none (O) on the surface of the cells. Antigens are capable of producing antibodies. The O negative blood person/donor is the universal donor.

ABO blood type and Rh factor are first determined. Then the compatibility of donor and recipient blood is determined by major crossmatch. The major crossmatch is between the donor's RBC and the recipient's serum; check to determine if the recipient has any antibodies to destroy donor's RBC.

Purpose

• To determine blood type

Procedure

• No food or fluid restriction is required.
• Collect 7 to 10 ml of venous blood in a red-top tube.

Nursing Implications

• Observe for signs and symptoms of fluid volume deficit (e.g., tachycardia, tachypnea, pale color, clammy skin, and low blood pressure [late symptoms]). Crystalloid solutions (saline, lactated Ringer's) might be given rapidly to replace fluid volume until a transfusion can be prepared. Usually 15 to 45 min are required to type and crossmatch blood.
• Check the date of the unit of blood. Usually blood should be used within 28 days. Blood that is older than 28 days should not be given to a client having hyperkalemia.
• Monitor the recipient's vital signs before and during transfusions. Signs and symptoms of transfusion reaction can include temperature increase of 1.1°C, chills, dyspnea, and so on.
• Start the blood transfusion at a slow rate for the first 15 min; stay with client and observe for adverse reactions.
• Flush the transfusion tubing with normal saline if other IV solutions are ordered to follow blood.

CRYOGLOBULINS (SERUM)

Reference Values
Adult: Negative
Child: Negative

Description. Cryoglobulins are abnormal immunoglobulins (Ig) that are in the blood and that precipitate at low temperatures and dissolve at warm temperatures. They are present in IgG and IgM groups. When exposed to very cold temperatures, they precipitate in the blood vessels, such as the fingers, and can cause Raynaud's phenomenon with symptoms of pain, coldness of the fingers, cyanosis, and purpura. These abnormal Ig proteins occur in other disease entities such as autoimmune disorders, for example, rheumatoid arthritis, systemic lupus erythematosus (SLE); acute and chronic infections, for example, infectious mononucleosis, streptococcal glomerulonephritis, endocarditis; and lymphoid malignancies, for example, leukemia, lymphoma, multiple myeloma. They also can occur in hepatitis C and Sjögren's syndrome.

Cryoglobulins are classed as Type 1, 2, or 3. Type 2 cryoglobulinemia is the most common, occurring in Raynaud's phenomenon, rheumatoid arthritis, nephrotic syndrome, and sensory-motor neuropathy. Type 1 cryoglobulin is associated with lymphocytic leukemia, lymphoma, and multiple myeloma. The cryoglobulin level could be equal to or greater than 5 mg/ml. Type 3 cryoglobulin is found with streptococcal glomerulonephritis, endocarditis, SLE, chronic infections, infectious mononucleosis, and rheumatoid arthritis.

Purposes
- To assist in diagnosing certain autoimmune disorders, lymphoid malignancies, acute and chronic infections, and Raynaud's phenomenon
- To compare the test results with other laboratory tests

Clinical Problems
Increased level: Raynaud's phenomenon, autoimmune disorders (rheumatoid arthritis, SLE), acute and chronic infections (infectious

mononucleosis, streptococcal glomerulonephritis, endocarditis), certain malignancies (leukemia, lymphomas, multiple myeloma), Sjögren syndrome, hepatitis C, certain renal dysfunctions (nephrotic syndrome, others), and sensory-motor neuropathy.

Procedure

- No food or fluid restriction is required unless indicated. Some institutions' protocols require food and fluid restriction for 4 to 8 h.
- Collect 10 ml of venous blood in a prewarmed syringe/tube to 37°C or 98.6°F in a red-top tube.
- Transport blood specimen immediately in a warm container.
- Blood specimen is refrigerated in the laboratory for 3 to 7 days and checked periodically for precipitation. If precipitation occurs, the blood specimen is rewarmed and if the precipitation is dissolved, cryoglobulin is present.

Factors Affecting Laboratory Results

- Collecting blood in a red-top tube that has not been prewarmed
- Not transporting the blood specimen immediately to the laboratory in a warmed container
- The laboratory not refrigerating the blood specimen

Nursing Implications

- Obtain a history of client's clinical problems.
- Observe for signs and symptoms of SLE (e.g., "butterfly" rash on cheeks and bridge of the nose, arthritis, and urinary insufficiency).
- Observe for signs and symptoms of rheumatoid arthritis (e.g., pain and stiffness in the joints; swollen, red, tender joints; joint deformities, and inability to make a fist and flexion contractures).
- Compare serum cryoglobulins with other laboratory tests.

Client Teaching

- Explain to the client to remain NPO for at least 4 h (some institutions state 8 h) before the test. Check with your health facility.
- Explain the test procedure. The results of the test take several days.

- Inform the client with Raynaud's symptoms to avoid cold temperature and to dress warmly, wearing hat and gloves.
- Answer questions the client may have or refer the questions to appropriate health professionals.

CULTURES (BLOOD, SPUTUM, STOOL, THROAT, WOUND, URINE)

Reference Values
Adult: Negative or no pathogen
Child: Same as adult

Description.   Cultures are taken to isolate the microorganism that is causing the clinical infection. The culture specimen should be taken to the laboratory immediately after collection (no longer than 30 min). It usually takes 24 to 36 h to grow the organisms.

Purpose
- To isolate the microorganism in body tissue or body fluid

Clinical Problems

Specimen	Clinical Condition or Organism
Blood	Bacteremia, septicemia, postoperative shock, fever of unknown origin (FUO)
Sputum	Pulmonary tuberculosis, bacterial pneumonia, chronic bronchitis, bronchiectasis
Stool	*Salmonella* ss, *Shigella* ss, *Escherichia coli, Staphylococcus* ss, *Campylobacter*
Throat	β-hemolytic streptococci, thrush (*Candida* ss), tonsillar infection, *Staphylococcus aureus*
Wound	*S aureus, Pseudomonas aeruginosa, Proteus* ss, *Bacteroides* ss, *Klebsiella* ss, *Serratia* ss
Urine	*E coli, Klebsiella* ss, *Pseudomonas, Serratia* ss, *Shigella* ss, *Candida* ss, *Enterobacter, Proteus*

Procedure

- Hand washing is essential before and after collection of the specimen.
- Send specimen to the laboratory immediately.
- Obtain specimen before antibiotic therapy is started. If the client is receiving antibiotics, the drug(s) should be listed on the laboratory slip.
- Use sterile collection containers or tubes and aseptic technique during collection.
- Check with the laboratory for specific techniques used; there may be variations with procedure.

Blood: Cleanse the client's skin according to the institution's procedure. Usually, the skin is scrubbed first with povidone–iodine (Betadine). Iodine can be irritating to the skin, so it is removed and an application of benzalkonium chloride or alcohol is applied. Cleanse the top(s) of culture bottle(s) with iodine and allow to dry. The bottle(s) should contain a culture medium. Collect 5 to 10 ml of venous blood and place in the sterile bottle. Special vacuum tubes containing a culture medium for blood may be used instead of a culture bottle.

Sputum: Sterile container or cup: obtain sputum for culture early in the morning, before breakfast. Instruct the client to give several deep coughs to raise sputum. Tell the client to avoid spitting saliva secretion into the sterile container. Saliva and postnasal drip secretions can contaminate the sputum specimen. Keep a lid on the sterile container; it should not be completely filled. If a 24-h sputum specimen is needed, then several sterile containers should be used. **Acid-Fast Bacilli (TB culture):** Follow the instructions on the container. Collect 5 to 10 ml of sputum and take the sample immediately to the laboratory or refrigerate the specimen. Three sputum specimens may be requested, one each day for 3 days. Check for proper labeling.

Stool: Collect an approximately 1-inch diameter feces sample. Use a sterile tongue blade, and place the stool specimen in a sterile container with a lid. The suspected disease or organism should be noted on the laboratory slip. The stool specimen should not contain urine. The client should not be given barium or mineral oil, which can inhibit bacterial growth.

Throat: Use a sterile cotton swab or a polyester-tipped swab. The sterile throat culture kit could be used. Swab the inflamed or ulcerated tonsillar or postpharyngeal areas of the throat. Place the applicator in a culturette tube with its culture medium. Do not give antibiotics before taking culture.

Wound: Use a culture kit containing a sterile cotton swab or a polyester-tipped swab and a tube with culture medium. Swab the exudate of the wound, and place the swab in the tube containing a culture medium. Wear sterile gloves when there is an excess amount of purulent drainage.

Urine: Clean-caught (midstream) urine specimen: Clean-caught urine collection is the most common method for collecting a urine specimen for culture. There are noncatheterization kits giving step-by-step instructions. The penis or vulva should be well cleansed. At times, two urine specimens (2 to 10 ml) are requested to verify the organism and in case of possible contamination. Collect a midstream urine specimen early in the morning, or as ordered, in a sterile container. The urine specimen should be taken immediately to the bacteriology laboratory or should be refrigerated. Label the urine specimen with the client's name, date, and exact time of collection. List any antibiotics or sulfonamides the client is taking on the laboratory slip.

Factors Affecting Laboratory Results
- Antibiotics and sulfonamides may cause false-negative results.

Nursing Implications
- Hold antibiotics or sulfonamides until after the specimen has been collected. If these drugs have been given, they should be listed on the laboratory slip.
- Deliver all specimens immediately to the laboratory, or refrigerate the specimen.
- Handle the specimen(s) using strict aseptic technique.
- Keep lids on sterile specimen containers. Sputum cups should not be uncovered by the bedside.

Client Teaching
- Explain the procedure for obtaining the culture specimen. Answer questions. If the client participates in the collection of the specimen (e.g., urine), review the procedure.
- Suggest a culture if a pathogenic organism is suspected. Check the client's temperature.

CYTOMEGALOVIRUS (CMV) ANTIBODY (SERUM)

Reference Values
(Enzyme immunoassay [EIA] for IgG and IgM)
Adult and Child: Negative to less than 0.30: no CMV IgM Ab detected. 0.30–0.59: weak positive for CMV IgM Ab (suggestive of a recent infection in neonates. Significance of this low level in adults is not determined). Greater than 0.60: positive for CMV IgM Ab.

Description.
Cytomegalovirus (CMV) belongs to the herpes virus family; it causes congenital infection in infants. CMV can be found in most body secretions (saliva, cervical secretions, urine, breast milk, and semen). If the pregnant woman is infected with CMV, it crosses the placenta, infecting the fetus. In infants, this virus can cause cerebral tissue malformation and damage. Urine specimens for CMV bodies or throat swabs may be used to detect CMV, but they frequently are not as helpful in detection as the serology test.

Many adults have been exposed to the virus and have developed immunity to CMV. Transmission of the CMV virus to immunocompromised persons such as persons with AIDS is serious. Also, transmission of CMV can be via blood transfusions from CMV-positive donors. Serologic studies (CMV-IgM antibodies and CMV-IgG antibodies) yield results in a shorter period than by culture. Cultures may be used to confirm the findings.

Purpose
- To identify the CMV of possible infected childbearing or pregnant women, infants, or immunocompromised persons

Clinical Problems
Increased: CMV-infected childbearing or pregnant women, infants, persons with AIDS or other immune deficiency, post-transplant organ recipients, following open heart surgery, hepatitis syndromes

Procedure
Serum
- No food or fluid restriction is required.
- Collect 5 to 7 ml of venous blood in a red-top tube. Two blood samples are usually requested; the first blood specimen is drawn during the acute phase, and 10 to 14 days later the second specimen for the convalescent phase.

Culture/Swab
- Obtain a culture of the infected area. Send the specimen immediately to the laboratory. Cultures are usually used to confirm serologic findings.

Factors Affecting Laboratory Results
- A false-positive test result may occur to those with the rheumatoid factor in the serum or those exposed to the EB virus.

Nursing Implications
- Obtain a history from the client of possible herpes-like viral infection.
- Assess the client for chronic respiratory infection or changes in vision. CMV retinitis can occur, which may result in blindness. Antiviral drugs may be used to treat CMV.
- Use aseptic technique when caring for clients infected with CMV.
- Listen to client concerns about the possible effects of this virus on self or infant. Refer questions to appropriate health care provider as necessary.

D-DIMER TEST (BLOOD)

FRAGMENT D-DIMER; FIBRIN DEGRADATION FRAGMENT
Reference Values
Negative for D-Dimer fragments; Positive greater than 250 ng/ml; greater than 250 µg/l (SI units)

Description.   D-Dimer, a fibrin degradation fragment, occurs through fibrinolysis. This test measures the amount of fibrin degradation that occurs. It confirms the presence of fibrin split products (FSPs) and is more specific for diagnosing disseminated intravascular coagulation (DIC) than FSPs. However, both D-Dimer and FSP tests are frequently used to determine DIC in client.

D-Dimer levels are increased when a fibrin clot is broken down by the thrombolytic drug, tissue plasminogen activator (tPA), streptokinase.

Purpose
- To detect the presence of DIC in a client

Clinical Problems
Increased levels: Disseminated intravascular coagulation (DIC); pulmonary embolism; arterial, coronary, and venous thrombosis; possible myocardial infarction; neoplastic disease; surgery up to post second day; late pregnancy; sickle cell crisis

Procedure
- There is no food or fluid restriction.
- Collect 7 ml of venous blood in a blue-top tube. Avoid hemolysis; invert tube gently, do not shake the tube.
- Apply pressure to the venepuncture site especially if the client has a bleeding tendency. Pressure may need to be applied for up to 5 min.
- Blood specimen should be taken to the laboratory within 4 h.

Nursing Implications
- Obtain a history of unexplained bleeding or any condition that is included in the Clinical Problems.
- Note signs of sweating, cold and mottled fingers and toes, petechiae, and bleeding. Report adverse signs and symptoms immediately.
- Check the monitor vital signs.

Client Teaching
- Explain to the client and family the purposes of the test.

DEXAMETHASONE SUPPRESSION TEST (DST) (PLASMA AND URINE)

ADRENOCORTICOTROPIC HORMONE (ACTH) SUPPRESSION TEST

Reference Values

Greater than 50% reduction of plasma cortisol and urine 17-hydroxycorticosteroids (17-OHCS)

Rapid or overnight screening test: Plasma cortisol: 8 AM: less than 10 mcg/dl; 4 PM: less than 5 mcg/dl. Urine 17-OHCS (5-h specimen): less than 4 mg/5 h.

Increased dexamethasone dose: *Low dose:* Plasma cortisol is one half of client's baseline level. Urine 17-OHCS: less than 2.5 mg/24 h/second day. *High dose:* plasma cortisol and urine 17-OHCS are one half of client's baseline level.

Note: High dose is given if results do not change with low dose of dexamethasone

Description.   Dexamethasone (Decadron) is a potent glucocorticoid. The dexamethasone suppression distinguishes between adrenal hyperplasia and adrenal tumor as the cause of adrenal hyperfunction and is used to diagnose and manage depression. When given dexamethasone, there is a reduction (suppression) in ACTH secretion (negative feedback), thus causing a lower plasma and urine cortisol. Low-dose and high-dose dexamethasone are used to distinguish between adrenal hyperplasia and adrenal tumor (nonsuppress at low or high doses). Adrenal hyperplasia will suppress at high doses but not at low doses.

In psychiatry the DST is useful in diagnosing affective diseases, such as endogenous depression (melancholia). In approximately 50% of these clients, suppression of plasma cortisol does not occur.

Purpose

- To distinguish between adrenal hyperplasia and adrenal tumor as the cause of adrenal hyperfunction

Clinical Problems

Plasma cortisol or urine 17-OHCS nonsuppression: Adrenal tumor, ectopic ACTH-producing tumor, bilateral adrenal hyperplasia (except with high steroid doses), affective disorders (endogenous depression), severe stress, anorexia nervosa, trauma, pregnancy, unstable diabetes

Drugs that may cause false negatives: Synthetic steroid therapy, high doses of benzodiazepines

Drugs that may cause false positives: Phenytoin, barbiturates, meprobamate, carbamazepine

Procedure

- Avoid tea, caffeinated coffee, and chocolates. No other food or fluid restriction is required.
- Refrigerate urine for 17-OHCS levels.
- Obtain a baseline plasma cortisol and urine 17-OHCS 24 h before the test.

Rapid or Overnight Screening Test

- Restrict food and fluids after midnight. Check with laboratory policy.
- Give dexamethasone 1 mg or 5 mcg/kg PO at 11 PM.
- Start at 7 AM, a 5-h urine test for 17-OHCS. Draw blood at 8 AM for plasma cortisol. Obtain a urine OHCS at 12 noon.

Increased dexamethasone dose: 2 days of low or high doses of dexamethasone (Decadron)

Low Dose

- Give dexamethasone, 0.5 mg every 6 h for 2 days (total 4 mg).
- Obtain a plasma cortisol level at 8 AM, 4 PM and 11 PM and 24-h urine OHCS after 2-day low-dose test. If no suppression, the high-dose test may be recommended.

High Dose

- Give dexamethasone, 2 mg every 6 h for 2 days (total 16 mg).
- Obtain a plasma cortisol level at 8 AM, 4 PM, and 11 PM and 24-h urine OHCS after 2-day high-dose test.

Factors Affecting Laboratory Results

- Ingestion of excess coffee, tea, and chocolates could increase steroid release.

Nursing Implications

- Administer dexamethasone at specified times on time. Milk or antacids may be required to decrease gastric irritation.
- Provide ample time for the client to ask questions. Refer unknown answers to appropriate health professionals.
- Report anxiety, stress, fever, or infection to the health care provider.
- Assess for side effects of dexamethasone resulting from high doses (e.g., gastric discomfort, weight gain, peripheral edema).
- Monitor electrolytes during low- and high-dose tests. Steroids cause serum potassium loss and serum sodium excess.
- Check blood glucose with Chemstrip bG for hyperglycemia while the client is taking high doses of dexamethasone. This drug is a glucocorticosteroid and can elevate blood glucose levels.
- Be supportive of client and family members during this time-consuming test procedure. Cooperation from client and family members is needed for accurate results.

DIFFERENTIAL WHITE BLOOD CELL (WBC) COUNT (*SEE* WHITE BLOOD CELL DIFFERENTIAL)

DIGOXIN (SERUM)

LANOXIN

Reference Values

Adult: Therapeutic: 0.5–2 ng/ml; 0.5–2 nmol/l (SI units); infant: 1–3 ng/ml; child: same as adult

  Toxic: greater than 2 ng/ml; greater than 2.6 nmol/l (SI units);
Infant: greater than 3.5 ng/ml
Child: Same as adult

Description.   Digoxin, a form of digitalis, is a cardiac glycoside given to increase the force and velocity of myocardial contraction. Serum plateau levels of digoxin occur 6 to 8 h after an oral dose, 2 to 4 h after IV administration, and 10 to 12 h after IM administration.

The half-life of digoxin is 35 to 40 h, with a shorter half-life in neonates and infants.

Purpose
- To monitor digoxin levels

Clinical Problems
Decreased level: Decreased gastrointestinal absorption or gastrointestinal motility
Drugs that may decrease digoxin level: Antacids, Kaopectate, metoclopramide (Reglan), barbiturates, cholestyramine (Questran), spironolactone (Aldactone)
Increased level: Digoxin overdose, renal disease, liver disease
Drugs that may increase digoxin level: Diuretics, amphotericin B, quinidine, reserpine (Serpasil), succinylcholine, sympathomimetics, corticosteroids

Procedure
- No food or fluid restriction is required.
- Collect 1 to 5 ml of venous blood in a red-top tube.
- Obtain a blood sample 6 to 10 h after administration of oral digoxin or prior to next digoxin dose or as ordered.

Factors Affecting Laboratory Results
- Administering digoxin IM might cause the absorption rate to be erratic.

Nursing Implications
- Report nontherapeutic levels to health care provider STAT.
- Obtain a blood sample for serum digoxin during predicted plateau levels for oral, IV, and IM administration or as ordered. Administering digoxin IM might cause the absorption rate to be erratic.

- Take apical pulse for 1 min prior to administering digoxin. If the pulse rate is below 60 per min, do not give the digoxin and notify the health care provider.
- Check serum potassium and magnesium levels. Hypokalemia and hypomagnesemia enhance the action of digoxin and could cause digitalis toxicity.
- Observe for signs and symptoms of digitalis toxicity (e.g., pulse rate less than 60 per min, anorexia, nausea, vomiting, headache, visual disturbance).

Client Teaching

- Instruct the client to take pulse rate before taking digoxin and to call the health care provider if the rate is less than 60 beats per min in adults and less than 70 in children.

DILANTIN (PHENYTOIN) (SERUM)

DIPHENYLHYDANTOIN

Reference Values

Adult: Therapeutic range: as an anticonvulsant: 10–20 mcg/ml, 39.6–79.3 µmol/l (SI units); as antiarrhythmic agent: 10–18 mcg/ml, 39.6–71.4 µmol/l (SI units); in saliva: 1–2 mcg/ml, 4–9 µmol/l

Toxic range: Greater than 20 mcg/ml, greater than 79.3 µmol/l (SI units)

Child: Toxic range: Greater than 15–20 mcg/ml, 56–79 µmol/l (SI units)

Description. Dilantin (phenytoin) is primarily used for inhibiting grand mal seizures. It is not effective in petit mal seizures. Dilantin is also used as an antiarrhythmic drug for decreasing force of myocardial contraction, improving atrioventricular conduction depressed by a digitalis preparation. Half-life in adults is an average of 24 h and in children an average of 15 h. Frequent monitoring is suggested to avoid toxic level.

Purpose

- To monitor phenytoin levels

Clinical Problems

Decreased level: Pregnancy, infectious mononucleosis
Drugs that may decrease Dilantin level: Alcohol, folate, carbamazepine (Tegretol)
Increased level: Dilantin overdose, uremia, liver disease
Drugs that may increase Dilantin level: Aspirin, dicumarol, sulfonamides, phenylbutazone (Butazolidin), thiazide diuretics, tranquilizers, isoniazid (INH), phenobarbital, propoxyphene (Darvon)

Procedure

- No food or fluid restriction is required.
- Collect 5 to 7 ml of venous blood in a red-top tube. Avoid hemolysis.
- List on the laboratory slip drugs client is taking that could affect test results.

Nursing Implications

- Report immediately nontherapeutic and toxic levels to the health care provider.
- Record dose, route, and last time the drug was given on the requisition slip.
- Observe for signs and symptoms of Dilantin toxicity (e.g., nystagmus, slurred speech, ataxia, drowsiness, lethargy, confusion, and rash).

D-XYLOSE ABSORPTION TEST (BLOOD AND URINE)

Reference Values

Adult: 25 g: Blood: 25–75 mg/dl/2 h (= 45 mg/dl/2 h)
Urine greater than 3.5 g/5 h; greater than 5 g/24 h
5 g: Blood: 8–28 mg/dl (= 15.7 mg/dl)
Urine: 1.2–2.4 g/5 h (= 1.8 g)
Child: Blood: 30 mg/dl/1 h

Description. The D-xylose absorption test determines the absorptive capacity of the small intestine. After ingestion of D-xylose, a pentose sugar, serum and urine D-xylose levels are measured. Usually, a low serum D-xylose level, less than 25 mg/dl, and a low urine D-xylose level, less than 3.0 g, are indicative of malabsorption syndrome. A common cause of a decreased D-xylose value is small intestinal bacterial overgrowth.

The test may cause mild diarrhea and abdominal discomfort. Both blood and urine specimens need to be obtained. Poor renal function can result in an elevated blood D-xylose level.

Various clinical problems such as vomiting, hypomotility, dehydration, alcoholism, rheumatoid arthritis, severe congestive heart failure, ascites, and poor renal function could cause low urine D-xylose levels that are not secondary to intestinal malabsorption. To verify a positive test result, endoscopic examination and biopsy frequently are necessary.

Purpose
- To aid in the diagnosis of gastrointestinal disturbance/disorder

Clinical Problems
Decreased level: Celiac disease, small-bowel ischemia, small-bowel bacterial overgrowth, Whipple's disease, Zollinger–Ellison syndrome, multiple jejunal diverticula, radiation enteritis, massive intestinal resection, diabetic neuropathy, diarrhea, lymphoma

Procedure
- Restrict foods for 8 h for adults and for 4 h for children prior to the test. Foods that contain pentose, such as fruits, jams, jellies, and pastries, should be withheld for 24 h prior to the test.
- Client ingests 25 g of D-xylose dissolved in 8 ounces (240 ml) of water. An additional 8 ounces of water should follow the mixture of D-xylose and water. Child's dose is based on weight: 0.5 g/kg but not more than 25 g. (Five g of D-xylose may be given instead of 25 g.)
- Collect 10 ml of venous blood in a gray-top tube. Blood specimens are drawn at 30, 60, and 120 min or at 2 h only after D-xylose ingestion.
- Discard urine specimen before test. Keep all urine refrigerated; at the end of 5 h, send the urine collection to the laboratory.
- Note client's age on the laboratory slip. Older adults with mild renal impairment can have a decreased 5-h test result.

- Note on the laboratory slip if the client is taking aspirin, NSAIDs (nonsteroidal anti-inflammatory drugs), or atropine. These drugs can decrease intestinal absorption.

Nursing Implications

- Explain the blood and urine test procedures to the client.
- Be supportive to the client and family members. Client compliance during the procedure is essential for accurate test results.
- Report to the health care provider if the client is having severe diarrhea, vomiting, and dehydration. These clinical problems could cause a decreased urine D-xylose level.

Client Teaching

- Closely monitor that the test procedure is correctly followed by the client during the 5 h.
- Instruct the client that food is restricted but fluids are not. Instruct the client not to eat foods containing pentose (see Procedure).
- Instruct the client to save all urine during the 5-h urine test. Refrigerate the urine collection.
- Instruct the client to withhold aspirin, all other NSAIDs, atropine and/or atropine products, with health care provider's approval, for 24 h before the test.

ENCEPHALITIS VIRUS ANTIBODY (SERUM)

Reference Values

Titer: Less than 1:10. Definite confirmation of the virus: a fourfold rise in titer level between the acute and convalescent blood specimens

Description.   Encephalitis is inflammation of the brain tissue, which is frequently due to an arbovirus transmitted by a mosquito after the mosquito has been in contact with an animal host. There are several groups of arbovirus causing encephalitis. The animal host varies according to location.
Eastern equine encephalitis virus: It is mainly found in the eastern United States from New Hampshire to Texas. Transmission is by the

mosquito from animal hosts: birds, ducks, fowl, and horses. Symptoms include fever, frontal headaches, drowsiness, nausea and vomiting, abnormal reflexes, rigidity, and bulging of the fontanel in infants. The mortality rate of 65% to 75% is one of the highest for viral encephalitis.

California encephalitis virus: Incidence is highest in children in the north central states of the United States. It is transmitted by infected mosquitoes and ticks. Symptoms include fever, severe headaches, stiff neck, and sore throat.

St. Louis encephalitis virus: This virus occurs most frequently in the southern, central, and western United States. It is a group B arbovirus and is transmitted by an infected mosquito. The animal host is the bird. The symptoms of headache, stiff neck, and abnormal reflexes may be mild or severe.

Venezuelan equine encephalitis virus: Incidence of this virus is most common in South America, Central America, Mexico, Texas, and Florida. It is a group A arbovirus and is transmitted by an infected mosquito. The animal hosts are the rodent and horse. Symptoms can be mild, such as flu-like symptoms, or severe, such as disorientation, paralysis, seizures, and coma.

Western equine encephalitis virus: Occurrence is primarily west of the Mississippi, particularly California, in the summer months and early fall. The virus is transmitted by infected mosquitoes infected by animal hosts: birds, squirrels, snakes, and horses. Symptoms include sore throat, stiff neck, lethargy, stupor, and coma in severe cases.

Purposes

- To detect the presence of an elevated encephalitis virus antibody titer that indicates an inflammation of the brain tissue caused by an arboviral infection
- To screen for an arbovirus

Clinical Problems

Increased titer: Viral encephalitis (identified strain), meningoencephalitis

Procedure

- No food or fluid restriction is required.
- Collect 3 to 5 ml of venous blood in a red-top tube. Two blood specimens should be taken at least 2 to 3 weeks apart: the first during the

acute phase of the viral infection, and the second during the convalescent phase.
• CSF may be tested for identifying the virus.

Nursing Implications
• Obtain a history of client's contact with mosquitoes. Ascertain when
the client first became ill.
• Assess for symptoms associated with encephalitis, such as fever,
frontal headaches, sore throat, stiff neck, lethargy.
• Listen to the client's concern. Answer the client's questions or refer
the questions to other health care providers.

ENTEROVIRUS GROUP (SERUM)

Reference Values
Norm: Negative
Positive: Fourfold rise in titer between the acute and convalescent period

Description.   The enterovirus group includes many types of viruses that
are found in the alimentary tract. Examples of those serotype viruses
include coxsackie A and B, echovirus, and poliomyelitis virus. Testing for
the enterovirus group is usually indicated when there is an epidemic outbreak of one of these viruses. Other methods for enteroviral testing include
specimens from oropharynx, stool, and CSF.

Purpose
• To identify the presence of an enterovirus associated with an epidemic
outbreak such as coxsackie A and B

Clinical Problem
Positive titer: Enteroviral infections

Procedure
• No food or fluid restriction is required.

- Collect 3 to 5 ml of venous blood in a red-top tube. Usually two blood specimens are required: the first at the acute phase, and the second during the convalescent phase (2 to 3 weeks between the two phases).

Nursing Implications

- Obtain a history of an alimentary tract infection. Symptoms may vary, so the client's description of the symptoms should be recorded.
- Assess the client's vital signs. Report abnormal findings.

ERYTHROCYTE SEDIMENTATION RATE (ESR) (BLOOD)

SEDIMENTATION (SED) RATE

Reference Values

Adult: Westergren method: less than 50 years old: male: 0–15 mm/h, female: 0–20 mm/h; greater than 50 years old: male: 0–20 mm/h, female: 0–30 mm/h. Wintrobe method: male: 0–9 mm/h; female: 0–15 mm/h
Child: Newborn: 0–2 mm/h; 4–14 years old: 0–20 mm/h

Description.   The ESR test measures the rate at which RBCs settle out of unclotted blood in millimeters per hour (mm/h). The ESR test is nonspecific.

The C-reactive protein (CRP) test is considered more useful than the ESR test because CRP increases more rapidly during an acute inflammatory process and returns to normal faster than ESR.

Purpose

- To compare with other laboratory tests for diagnosing inflammatory conditions (see Clinical Problems)

Clinical Problems

Decreased level: Polycythemia vera, CHF, sickle cell anemias, infectious mononucleosis, factor V deficiency, degenerative arthritis, angina pectoris
Drugs that may decrease ESR value: Ethambutol (Myambutol), quinine, aspirin, cortisone preparations

Increased level: Rheumatoid arthritis; rheumatic fever; acute myocardial infarction (AMI); cancer of the stomach, colon, breast, liver, and kidney; Hodgkin's disease; multiple myeloma; lymphosarcoma; bacterial infections; gout; acute pelvic inflammatory disease; systemic lupus erythematosus (SLE); erythroblastosis fetalis; pregnancy (second and third trimesters); surgery; burns

Drugs that may increase ESR value: Dextran, methyldopa (Aldomet), penicillamine (Cuprimine), theophylline, oral contraceptives, procainamide (Pronestyl), vitamin A

Procedure

- Hold medications that can cause false-positive results for 24 h before the test with health care provider's permission.
- No food or fluid restriction is required.
- Collect 5 to 7 ml of venous blood in a lavender-top tube and keep the specimen in a vertical position.

Nursing Implications

- Answer the client's questions about the significance of an increased ESR level. An answer could be that other laboratory tests are usually performed in conjunction with the ESR test for adequate diagnosis of a clinical problem.
- Compare ESR with CRP tests results.

ESTETROL (E$_4$) (PLASMA AND AMNIOTIC FLUID)

Reference Values
Pregnancy

Plasma	
Weeks of Gestation	*pg/ml*
20–26	40–210
30	Greater than 350
36	Greater than 900
40	Greater than 1050

Amniotic Fluid	
Weeks of Gestation	*ng/ml*
32+	0.8
40+	13.0

Description. Estetrol (E$_4$) is an effective indicator of fetal distress during the third trimester of pregnancy. E$_4$ increases during gestation. One test alone should not determine fetal distress; several tests, such as estriol (E$_3$) and human placental lactogen, are usually performed to verify the possible diagnosis.

Purpose
- To detect the occurrence of fetal distress

Clinical Problems
Decreased level: Fetal distress, intrauterine fetal death, anencephalic fetus, fetal malformations

Procedure
- No food or fluid restriction is required.
- Collect 5 to 7 ml of venous blood in a red-top tube.

Nursing Implications
- Obtain a history of client's signs and symptoms related to the pregnancy.
- Monitor fetal heart rate.
- Compare serum E$_4$ with serum E$_3$ and human placental lactogen. Report laboratory values to the health care provider.
- Listen to the client's and family's concerns. Refer unknown answers to client's and family's questions to the appropriate health professionals.

ESTRADIOL (E$_2$) (SERUM)

Reference Values
Adult: Female: Follicular phase: 20–150 pg/ml
   Midcycle phase: 100–500 pg/ml
   Luteal phase: 60–260 pg/ml

Menopause: less than 30 pg/ml
Male: 15–50 pg/ml
Child (6 months to 10 years old):   3–10 pg/ml

Description.   Estradiol (E$_2$) is a more potent estrogen than estrone (E$_1$) and estriol (E$_3$). This serum test is ordered for determining the presence of gonadal dysfunction. It is useful for evaluating menstrual and fertility problems in the female. Estradiol is produced mostly by the ovaries and also by the adrenal cortex and the testes. The serum estradiol levels are likely to be increased in males who have testicular or adrenal tumors and in females with estrogen-secreting ovarian tumors. Because serum estradiol level of prepubertal children may not be accurate, the serum test may need to be repeated.

Purposes
- To determine the presence of gonadal dysfunction
- To evaluate menstrual and fertility problems in the female

Clinical Problems
Decreased level: Primary and secondary hypogonadism, amenorrhea due to anorexia nervosa, ovarian insufficiency, pituitary insufficiency
Drugs that may decrease estradiol value: Oral contraceptives, megestrol
Increased level: Estrogen-producing tumors, gynecomastia (male), testicular tumor, liver failure, renal failure
Drugs that may increase estradiol value: Diazepam, clomiphene

Procedure
- No food or fluid restriction is required.
- Record the phase of the menstrual cycle on the laboratory slip.
- Collect 5 to 7 ml of venous blood in a red-top tube.

Nursing Implications
- Obtain a history of signs and symptoms related to the clinical problem.
- Allow the female or male to express her/his feelings regarding symptoms and test findings. Refer client's questions to health professionals when appropriate.

ESTRIOL (E$_3$) (SERUM AND URINE)

Reference Values
Pregnancy

Serum			*Urine*	
Weeks of Gestation	*ng/dl*		*Weeks of Gestation*	*mg/24 h*
25–28	25–165		25–28	6–28
29–32	30–230		29–32	6–32
33–36	45–370		33–36	10–45
37–38	75–420		37–40	15–60
39–40	95–450			

Description.   E$_3$ is a major estrogenic compound produced largely by the placenta. It increases in maternal serum and urine after 2 months of pregnancy and continues at high levels until term. If toxemia, hypertension, or diabetes is present after 30 weeks' gestation, E$_3$ levels are monitored. A decline in serum or urine E$_3$ levels suggests fetal distress caused by placental malfunction.

Serum estriol is replacing urine estriol because specimen collection is easier and there is no 24-h waiting period. The advantage of the 24-h urine estriol is avoidance of estriol value variations that usually occur within a day.

Purposes
- To monitor estriol levels
- To determine fetal distress after 30 weeks' gestation
- To compare test results with estetrol test results regarding fetal distress

Clinical Problems
Decreased level: Fetal distress, diabetic pregnancy, pregnancy with hypertension, impending toxemia
Increased level: Urinary tract infection, glycosuria
Drugs that may increase estriol value: Antibiotics (ampicillin, neomycin), hydrochlorothiazide (HydroDIURIL), cortisone preparations

Procedure

- No food or fluid restriction is required.

Serum

- Collect 5 to 7 ml of venous blood in a red-top tube.

Urine

- Collect urine for 24 h in a large container with preservative.
- Label with the client's name, the date, and the exact times of collection (e.g., 3/26/09, 8 AM to 3/27/09, 8:03 AM).
- Two 24-h urine specimens (taken a day apart) are usually ordered for more valid results.

Nursing Implications

- Monitor the fetal heart rate, the client's blood pressure, and sugar in the urine. Hypertension and diabetes could cause placental dysfunction, leading to fetal distress.
- Report glycosuria and urinary tract infection during pregnancy; both could cause a false result.
- Be supportive of client and family.

ESTROGEN (SERUM AND URINE—24 H)

Reference Values

Adult: Serum: female: early menstrual cycle: 60–200 pg/ml; midmenstrual cycle: 120–440 pg/ml; late menstrual cycle: 150–350 pg/ml; postmenopausal: less than 30 pg/ml. Male: 40–115 pg/ml

Child: 1–6 years old: 3–10 pg/ml; 8–12 years old: less than 30 pg/ml

Adult: Urine: female: preovulation: 5–25 mcg/24 h; follicular phase: 24–100 g/24 h; luteal phase: 22–80 mcg/24 h; postmenopausal: 0–10 mcg/24 h. Male: 4–25 mcg/24 h

Child: Less than 12 years old: 1 mcg/24 h; postpuberty: same as adult

Description.   There are over 30 estrogens identified in the body but only three measurable types of estrogens: estrone (E_1), estradiol (E_2), and estriol (E_3). Total serum estrogen reflects E_1, mostly E_2, and some E_3. For fetal well-being during pregnancy, serum E_3 is used.

The 24-h urine estrogen test is useful for diagnosing ovarian dysfunction. Client's age and the phase of the menstrual cycle should be known.

Purpose
- To diagnose ovarian dysfunction and other health problems (see Clinical Problems)

Clinical Problems
Decreased level: Ovarian failure or dysfunction, infantilism, primary hypogonadism, Turner's syndrome, intrauterine death in pregnancy, menopausal and postmenopausal symptoms, pituitary insufficiency, anorexia nervosa, psychogenic stress
Drugs that may decrease estrogen value: Some phenothiazines, vitamins
Increased level: Ovarian tumor, adrenocortical tumor or hyperplasia, some testicular tumors, pregnancy (gradual increase from the first trimester on)
Drugs that may increase estrogen value: Tetracycline

Procedure
- No food or fluid restriction is required.
- Note on laboratory slip the phase of client's menstrual cycle.

Serum
- Collect 5 to 7 ml of venous blood in a red-top tube.
- Indicate on the laboratory slip the phase of the menstrual cycle.

Urine
- Collect a 24-h urine sample in a refrigerated container. The urine container should contain a preservative.
- Label with the client's name, the date, and the exact time of collection (e.g., 5/2/09, 7:02 AM to 5/3/09, 7:01 AM). No toilet paper or feces should be in the urine collection.

Nursing Implications
- Indicate on the laboratory slip if the client is taking steroids, oral contraceptives, or estrogens.
- Obtain a history of menstrual problems and the present menstrual cycle.

Client Teaching
- Encourage ventilation of feelings through provision of a private, calm environment.
- Teach the client to keep accurate records on the time of menstruation, how long each menstrual period lasts, and the amount of menstrual flow.

Urine
- Collect specimen in container with preservative.
- Follow strictly the date and times for the urine collection.

ESTRONE (E₁) (SERUM AND URINE)

Reference Values

Serum	Urine
Adult	
Female:	Female:
Follicular phase: 30–100 pg/ml	Follicular phase: 4–7 mcg/24 h
Ovulatory phase: Greater than 150 pg/ml	Ovulatory phase: 11–30 mcg/24 h
Luteal phase: 90–160 pg/ml	Luteal phase: 10–22 mcg/24 h
Postmenopausal: 20–40 pg/ml	Postmenopausal: 1–7 mcg/24 h
Male: 10–50 pg/ml	
Child (1–10 years old): Less than 10 pg/ml	

Description.   Estrone (E_1) is a potent estrogen; however, estrone and estriol (E_3) are not as potent as estradiol (E_2). E_1 is a metabolite of E_2. During the third trimester of pregnancy, the E_1 levels can increase up to tenfold the level for a nonpregnant female. E_1 is the major estrogen occurring after menopause. The serum estrone test is frequently ordered with other estrogen tests.

Purposes
- To determine ovarian failure
- To check occurrence of menopause
- To compare test results with other laboratory estrogen tests

Clinical Problems
Decreased level: Ovarian failure or dysfunction, intrauterine death in pregnancy, menopausal and postmenopausal symptoms

Procedure
Serum
- No food or fluid restriction is required.
- Note on the laboratory slip the phase of the client's menstrual cycle.
- Collect 7 ml of venous blood in a red-top tube.

Urine
- Collect a 24-h urine sample in a collection container that contains a boric acid preservative.
- Label the urine with the client's name, date, and exact time of collection.

Nursing Implications
- Obtain a history of signs and symptoms related to the clinical problem.
- Report laboratory value of E_1 and other estrogen factors to the health care provider. Compare serum total estrogen and serum E_1 results.
- Be supportive to the client and family. Refer client's and family's questions to health professionals when appropriate.

FACTOR ASSAY (PLASMA)

COAGULATION FACTORS, BLOOD CLOTTING FACTORS

Reference Values
Adult and Child
Factor I (fibrinogen):   200–400 mg/dl, minimal for clotting: 75–100 mg/dl

Factor II (prothrombin): Minimal hemostatic level: 10%–15% concentration

Factor III (thromboplastin): Variety of substances

Factor IV (calcium): 4.5–5.5 mEq/l or 9–11 mg/dl

Factor V (proaccelerin): 50%–150% activity; minimal hemostatic level: 5%–10% concentration

Factor VI: Not used

Factor VII (proconvertin stable factor): 65%–135% activity; minimal hemostatic level concentration

Factor VIII (antihemophilic factor [AHF], VIII-A): 55%–145% activity; minimal hemostatic level: 30%–35% concentration

Factor IX (Christmas factor, IX-B): 60%–140% activity; minimal hemostatic level: 30% concentration

Factor X (Stuart factor): 45%–150% activity; minimal hemostatic level: 7%–10% concentration

Factor XI (plasma thromboplastin antecedent [PTA] XI-C): 65%–135% activity; 20%–30% minimal hemostatic level: 20%–30% minimal hemostatic level: 20%–30% concentration

Factor XII (Hageman factor): Minimal hemostatic level: 0% concentration

Factor XIII (fibrin stabilizing factor [FSF]): Minimal hemostatic level: 1% concentration

Description.   Factor assays (coagulation factors) are ordered for identification of defects in the blood coagulation mechanism due to a lack of one or more of the 12 plasma factors. A deficiency in one or more factors usually causes bleeding disorders.

Purpose
- To identify the blood factor that is causing the bleeding or blood disorder

Clinical Problems
The associated clinical problems and the causes of these problems are outlined in the following table.

COAGULATION FACTOR DEFICIENCIES

Factor	Clinical Problems (Decreased Levels)	Rationale
I	Hypofibrinogenemia Severe liver disease Disseminated intravascular coagulation (DIC) Leukemia	Deficiency of fibrinogen and fibrinolysis
II	Hypoprothrombinemia Severe liver disease Vitamin K deficiency Drugs: salicylates (excessive), anticoagulants, antibiotics (excessive), hepatotoxic drugs	Impaired liver function, vitamin K deficit
III	Thrombocytopenia	Low platelet count
IV	Hypocalcemia Malabsorption syndrome Malnutrition Hyperphosphatemia	Low calcium intake in diet
V	Parahemophilia Severe liver disease DIC	Congenital problem, impaired liver function
VI	Not used	
VII	Hepatitis Hepatic carcinoma Hemorrhagic disease of newborn Vitamin K deficiency Drugs: antibiotics (excessive), anticoagulants	Impaired liver function, certain drugs affecting the clotting time, vitamin K deficit
VIII	Hemophilia A (classic) Von Willebrand's disease DIC Multiple myeloma Lupus erythematosus	Congenital disorder (sex linked) occurring mostly in males; circulating factor VIII inhibitors

(continued)

Factor	Clinical Problems (Decreased Levels)	Rationale
IX	Hemophilia B (Christmas disease) Hepatic disease Vitamin K deficiency	Congenital disorder (sex linked) occurring mostly in males; circulating factor IX inhibitors
X	Severe liver disease Hemorrhage disease of newborn DIC Vitamin K deficiency	Impaired liver function; vitamin K deficit
XI	Hemophilia C Congenital heart disease Intestinal malabsorption of vitamin K Liver disease Drugs: anticoagulants	Congenital deficiency in both males and females; circulating factor XI inhibitors
XII	Liver disease	
XIII	Agammaglobulinemia Myeloma Lead poisoning Poor wound healing	Circulating factor XIII inhibitors; mild bleeding tendency

Procedure

- No food or fluid restriction is required.
- Collect 5 to 7 ml of venous blood in a blue-top tube. Apply pressure to the venipuncture. Deliver blood specimen to laboratory immediately.

Nursing Implications

- Obtain a familial history of bleeding disorders and a history of the client's bleeding tendency.
- Observe the venipuncture site for oozing of blood.
- Observe and report signs of bleeding (e.g., purpura; petechiae; or frank, continuous bleeding).

FASTING BLOOD SUGAR (FBS) (*SEE GLUCOSE-FASTING BLOOD SUGAR*)

FEBRILE AGGLUTININS (SERUM)

Reference Values
Adult (febrile, titers): *Brucella:* less than 1:20, less than 1:20–1:80 (individuals working with animals); tularemia: less than 1:40; Widal (*Salmonella*): less than 1:40 (nonvaccinated; Weil-Felix (*Proteus*): less than 1:40
Child: Same as adult

Description. Febrile agglutination tests (febrile group) identify infectious diseases causing fever of unknown origin. Isolating the invading organism (pathogen) is not always possible, especially if the client has been on antimicrobial therapy, so indirect methods are used to detect antibodies in the serum. Detection of these antibodies is determined by the titer of the serum in highest dilution that will cause agglutination (clumping) in the presence of a specific antigen. The test should be done during the acute phase of the disease (maybe several times) and then done about 2 weeks later. A single agglutination titer is of minimal value. These tests can be used to confirm pathogens already isolated or to identify the pathogen present late in the disease (after several weeks).

Diseases commonly associated with febrile agglutination tests are brucellosis (undulant fever), salmonellosis, typhoid fever, paratyphoid fever, tularemia, and certain rickettsial infections (typhus fever).

Purpose
- To detect elevated titer caused by febrile agglutinins denoting a specific pathogen

Clinical Problems

Test	Pathogen(s) Antigen(s)	Increased Levels
Brucella	Brucella abortus (cattle) B suis (hogs) B melitensis (goats)	Brucellosis titer greater than 1:100
Pasteurella (tularemia)	Pasteurella tularensis	Tularemia (rabbit fever) titer. greater than 1:80
Widal	Salmonella O (somatic)	Salmonellosis
	Salmonella H (flagellar)	Typhoid fever
	O and H portions of the organism act as antigens to stimulate antibody production	Paratyphoid fever titer: O antigen—greater than 1:80 suspicious, greater than 1:160 definite; H antigen—greater than 1:40 suspicious, greater than 1:80 definite
	Salmonella VI (capsular)	Nonvaccinated or vaccinated over 1 year before
Weil-Felix	Proteus X	Rickettsial diseases
	Proteus OX19	Epidemic typhus
		Tick-borne typhus (Rocky Mountain spotted fever)
	Proteus OX2	Boutonneuse tick fever
		Queensland tick fever
		Siberian tick fever
	Proteus OXK	Scrub typhus titer—greater than 1:30 significant, greater than 1:60 definite

Procedure

- No food or fluid restriction is required.
- Collect 5 ml of venous blood in a red-top tube. Avoid hemolysis.
- Draw blood before starting antimicrobial therapy, if possible. If the client is receiving drugs for an elevated temperature, write the names of the drugs on the laboratory slip.
- The blood sample should be refrigerated if it is not tested immediately or frozen if it is to be kept 24 h or longer.

Factors Affecting Laboratory Results

- Vaccination could increase the titer level.
- Antimicrobial therapy could decrease the titer level.

Nursing Implications

- Obtain a history of the client's occupation, geographic location prior to the fever, and recent vaccinations. Exposure to animals and ticks could be suggestive of the causative organism.
- Record on the laboratory slip and in the client's chart whether the client has been vaccinated against the pathogen within the last year. Vaccinations can increase the antibody titer.
- Be aware that leukemia, advanced carcinoma, some congenital deficiencies, and general debilitation could cause false-negative results.
- Monitor the temperature every 4 h when elevated.
- Remind the health care provider of the need to repeat the tests when the fever persists and/or titer levels are suspicious. Titer levels could rise fourfold in 1 to 2 weeks.
- Check to determine whether the blood sample has been taken before you give antibiotics or other drugs to combat fever for a suspected organism. Antibiotic therapy could depress the titer level.

Client Teaching

- Instruct the client to keep a record of temperatures and to notify the health care provider of changes in body temperature.

FECAL FAT (STOOL)

Reference Values
Quantitative
Adult: 2 to 7 g/24 h; 7–25 mmol/day (SI units)
Child: Less than 1 year old: less than 1.0 g/24 h

Qualitative
Adult: Neutral fat: less than 50 globules/high-power field (HPF)
Fatty acids: less than 100 globules/high-power field (HPF)

Description.   Fecal fat test is conducted to confirm the diagnosis of steatorrhea (malabsorption of fat). Clients having steatorrhea have a higher fat content in the stools. The cause of steatorrhea may be due to an impairment of intestinal absorption of fat, deficiency of pancreatic digestive enzymes, or a decrease in bile production. Causes of fat absorption impairment could be Crohn's disease, celiac disease, Whipple's disease, or sprue. Causes of maldigestion could be pancreatic duct obstruction or bile duct obstruction that may be due to gallstones or a tumor. The pancreatic enzymes such as amylase, lipase, and trypsin are not able to mix with the food to promote fat digestion. Without digestion, the fats cannot be absorbed.

Collection of stool specimen is usually for 24 h; however, a 2- or 3-day stool collection may be ordered. Also a random specimen may be ordered for a qualitative test.

Purposes
- To determine the presence of high fat content in the stool
- To determine the cause of the high fat content in the stool
- To confirm the diagnosis of steatorrhea

Clinical Problems
Increased levels because of malabsorption: Celiac disease, sprue, Whipple's disease, cystic fibrosis, Crohn's disease, radiation enteritis
Increased levels because of maldigestion: Pancreatic obstruction, bile duct obstruction, gallstones, cancer, surgical removal of a section of the intestine
Drugs that may increase steatorrhea: Colchicine, neomycin, kanamycin, lincomycin, methotrexate

Procedure
- There is no fluid restriction unless indicated by the laboratory.
- The client may be requested to eat a high-fat diet (100 g of fat per day) for 3 days before the test. Procedure may be different; consult with the laboratory.
- Collect a random or 24–72-h stool specimen and send the specimen immediately to the laboratory. Use a tongue blade to move stool to specimen container.
- Watery stools (diarrhea) can be used for fecal fat analysis.
- Stool collected at home or at the medical facility should be refrigerated before sending to the laboratory. Once it is removed from the refrigerator, it should be sent immediately.
- Record client's name, date, and duration of collection time on the specimen container and/or laboratory slip.

Factors Affecting Laboratory Results
- Drugs: Ingestion of mineral oil, psyllium-based (fiber) laxatives such as Metamucil, rectal suppositories, cascara
- Ingestion of low-fat caloric food
- Ingestion of a high-fiber diet
- A recent barium GI study

Nursing Implications
- Obtain a history of GI problems. Record the type of diet (food) the client is eating.
- Obtain a list of client's medication. Note those drugs that can affect the test results.
- Ask the client if she/he has had any previous diagnostic testing that requires barium intake.
- Review the procedure with the client. An ingestion of 50–100 g of fat for 3 days prior to the test may have been prescribed. Check with the laboratory.

Client Teaching
- Inform the client of how to collect the stool. The stool should be refrigerated unless it is to be taken immediately to the laboratory.
- Instruct the client not to urinate in the stool container. Toilet paper should not be put in the stool container.
- Instruct the client not to take an enema or laxative during stool collection because it can alter the test results.
- Inform the client whether the test is for a random stool collection or a 1- to 3-day collection period.
- Be supportive of the client. Answer questions or refer them to other health professionals.

FERRITIN (SERUM)

Reference Values
Adult: Female: less than 40 y: 10–120 ng/ml, 10–120 mcg/l (SI units); greater than 40 y: 10–235 ng/ml, 10–235 mcg/l (SI units); Postmenopausal: 10–310 ng/ml, 10–310 mcg/l (SI units)

Male: 15–445 ng/ml, 15–445 mcg/l

Child: Newborn: 20–200 ng/ml, 20–200 mcg/l (SI units); 1 month: 200–550 ng/ml, 200–550 mcg/l (SI units); Infant: 40–200 ng/ml, 40–200 mcg/l (SI units); 1–16 years: 8–140 ng/ml, 8–140 mcg/l (SI units)

Description. Ferritin, an iron-storage protein, is produced in the liver, spleen, and bone marrow. The ferritin levels are related to the amount of iron stored in the body tissues. It will release iron from tissue reserve as needed and will store excess iron to prevent damage from iron overload.

Serum ferritin level is useful in evaluating the total body storage of iron. It can detect early iron deficiency anemia and anemias due to chronic disease that resemble iron deficiency. Serum ferritin is not affected by hemolysis and drugs.

Purposes
- To evaluate the amount of iron stored in the body
- To detect early iron deficiency anemia

Clinical Problems
Decreased level: Iron deficiency anemia, inflamed bowel disease, gastrointestinal surgery, pregnancy
Increased level: Anemias (hemolytic, pernicious, thalassemia, megaloblastic), metastatic carcinomas, leukemias, lymphomas, hepatic diseases (cirrhosis, hepatitis, cancer of the liver), iron overload (hemochromatosis), acute and chronic infection and inflammation, chronic renal disease, hyperthyroidism, polycythemia, rheumatoid arthritis
Drugs that may increase serum ferritin level: Oral or injectable iron drugs

Procedure
- Collect 2 to 5 ml of venous blood in a red-top tube.
- Food and fluids are not restricted.
- Note on the laboratory slip if the client is taking iron preparations.

Nursing Implications
- Compare serum ferritin level with serum iron and transferrin percent saturation. Serum ferritin levels tend to be more reliable in determining

iron deficiencies than serum iron levels. Serum ferritin levels decrease before iron stores are depleted.

- Assess if the client is taking iron preparations. They can influence test results.

Client Teaching
- Explain to the client the purpose of the test.
- Explain to the client the importance of intake of various groups of nutritional foods.

FETAL HEMOGLOBIN (Hb F) (BLOOD)

HEMOGLOBIN F

Reference Values
From total hemoglobin:
Adult: 0%–2%
Child: Newborn: 60%–90%; 1–5 months: less than 70%; 6–9 months: less than 5%; greater than 1 year: less than 2%

Description. For newborns, an elevated Hb F is normally found in the red blood cells (RBCs). By the time the infant is 6 months old, the Hb F should be less than 5% and the remaining hemoglobin should be comprised of Hb A_1 and Hb A_2. If the Hb F remains elevated after 6 months, hemoglobinopathy should be considered such as minor or major thalassemias.

Purpose
- To diagnose various hemoglobinopathies, such as minor or major thalassemia

Clinical Problems
Increased levels: Thalassemias (minor or major), sickle cell anemia, acquired aplastic anemia (from drugs, toxins, etc.), hyperthyroidism, acute or chronic leukemia especially juvenile myeloid leukemia, multiple myeloma, hemoglobin H disease, hereditary presence of Hb F

Procedure

- There is no food or fluid restriction.
- Collect 7 to 10 ml of venous blood in a lavender- or green-top tube. Fill the tube. Invert the tube gently. Avoid hemolysis (do NOT shake tube).
- Collect capillary blood from a young child in a microcollection tube.

Factors Affecting Laboratory Results

- Hemolysis of the blood sample.
- Blood specimen that is older than 3 h may cause a false-positive result.

Nursing Implications
Client Teaching

- Explain the test procedure to the client or parent. Blood specimen can be taken from a finger or earlobe.
- Listen to client's concerns. Refer questions to which the answers are unknown to other health care professionals.

FIBRIN DEGRADATION FRAGMENT *(SEE D-DIMER TEST)*

FIBRIN (FIBRINOGEN) DEGRADATION PRODUCTS (FDP) (SERUM)

FIBRIN OR FIBRINOGEN SPLIT PRODUCTS (FSP)

Reference Values
Adult: 2–10 mcg/ml
Child: Not usually done

Description.   The FDP test is usually done in an emergency when the client is hemorrhaging as the result of severe injury, trauma, or shock.

Thrombin, which initially accelerates coagulation, promotes the conversion of plasminogen into plasmin, which in turn breaks fibrinogen and fibrin into FDP. The fibrin degradation (split) products act as anticoagulants, causing continuous bleeding from many sites. A clinical condition resulting from this fibrinolytic (clot-dissolving) activity is disseminated intravascular coagulation (DIC).

Purpose
- To aid in the diagnosis of DIC

Clinical Problems
Increased level: DIC caused by severe injury, trauma, or shock; massive tissue damage; surgical complications; septicemia; obstetric complications (abruptio placentae, preeclampsia, intrauterine death, postcesarean birth); acute myocardial infarction (AMI); pulmonary embolism; acute necrosis of the liver; acute renal failure; burns; acute leukemia
Drugs that may increase FDP value: Streptokinase, urokinase

Procedure
- No food or fluid restriction is required.
- Collect 5 to 7 ml of venous blood in a blue-top tube. Avoid hemolysis.
- Draw blood before administering heparin.

Nursing Implications
- Monitor vital signs and report shock-like symptoms (e.g., tachycardia; hypotension; pallor; and cold, clammy skin).
- Observe and report bleeding sites (e.g., chest, nasogastric tube, incisional or injured areas, and others).
- Report progressive discoloration of the skin (e.g., petechiae, ecchymoses).
- Check urine output hourly. Report decreased urine output, less than 25 ml/h, and blood-colored urine.
- Provide comfort and support to the client and family.

FIBRINOGEN (PLASMA)

FACTOR I

Reference Values
Adult: 200–400 mg/dl
Child: Newborn: 150–300 mg/dl; child: same as adult

Description.   Fibrinogen, a plasma protein synthesized by the liver, is split by thrombin to produce fibrin strands necessary for clot formation. A deficiency of fibrinogen results in bleeding. Low fibrinogen levels are life-threatening in *disseminated intravascular coagulation (DIC)* caused by severe trauma or obstetric complications. Markedly prolonged prothrombin time (PT) and partial thromboplastin time (PTT) and a low platelet count suggest a fibrinogen deficiency and signs of DIC. Fibrin degradation products (FDPs) are usually ordered to confirm DIC.

Purposes
- To check for a deficiency of fibrinogen as a cause of bleeding
- To compare test results with FDPs in diagnosing DIC

Clinical Problems
Decreased level: Severe liver disease, hypofibrinogenemia, DIC, leukemia, obstetric complications
Increased level: Acute infections, collagen diseases, inflammatory diseases, hepatitis
Drugs that may increase fibrinogen value: Oral contraceptives

Procedure
- No food or fluid restriction is required.
- Collect 5 to 7 ml of venous blood in a blue-top tube. Avoid hemolysis. Take blood specimen to laboratory within 1 h.

Factors Affecting Laboratory Results
- Postoperative surgery and third trimester of pregnancy could cause a false-positive fibrinogen elevation.

Nursing Implications

- Report if client had blood transfusion within 4 weeks.
- Monitor for signs and symptoms of DIC (e.g., petechiae and ecchymoses, hemorrhage, tachycardia, hypotension).
- Check laboratory results of PT, INR, PTT, and platelet count.
- Notify health care provider if active bleeding occurs.

FOLIC ACID (FOLATE) (SERUM)

Reference Values

Adult: 3–16 ng/ml (bioassay), greater than 2.5 ng/ml (radioimmunoassay [RIA] serum), greater than 200–700 ng/ml (RBC)
Child: Same as adult

Description. Folic acid, one of the B vitamins, is needed for normal RBC and WBC function. Usually, the serum folic acid or folate test is performed to detect folic acid anemia, which is a megaloblastic anemia (abnormally large RBCs). Other causes of serum folic acid deficit are pregnancy, chronic alcoholism, and old age.

Purposes

- To check for folic acid deficiency during early pregnancy
- To detect folic acid anemia

Clinical Problems

Decreased level: Folic acid anemia, vitamin B_6 deficiency anemia, malnutrition, malabsorption syndrome, pregnancy, malignancies, liver disease, celiac sprue disease
Drugs that may decrease folic acid value: Anticonvulsants, folic acid antagonists (methotrexate), oral contraceptives
Increased level: Pernicious anemia

Procedure

- No food or fluid restriction is required. Avoid alcohol.

- Collect 7 to 10 ml of venous blood in a red-top tube. Avoid hemolysis. Send to the laboratory immediately.
- Collect 7 ml of venous blood in a lavender-top tube for RBC folic acid determination. Send it to the laboratory immediately.

Nursing Implications

- Collaborate with the dietitian and client on formulating a diet high in folic acid (e.g., liver, lean meats, milk, eggs, leafy vegetables, bananas, oranges, beans, and whole-wheat bread).
- Observe for signs and symptoms of folic acid deficiency (e.g., fatigue, pallor, nausea, anorexia, dyspnea, palpitations, and tachycardia).

Client Teaching

- Encourage the client to eat foods rich in folic acid, such as liver, lean meats, milk, eggs, leafy vegetables, bananas, oranges, beans, and whole-wheat bread.

FOLLICLE-STIMULATING HORMONE (FSH) (SERUM AND URINE)

Reference Values

Adult: *Serum:* female: follicular phase: 4–30 mU/ml; midcycle: 10–90 mU/ml; luteal phase: 4–30 mU/ml; menopause: 40–170 mU/ml; male: 4–25 mU/ml.

Urine: female: follicular phase: 4–25 international units/24 h; midcycle: 8–60 international units/24 h; luteal phase: 4–20 international units/24 h; menopause: 50–150 international units/24 h; male: 4–18 international units/24 h

Child (prepubertal): *Serum:* 5–12 mU/ml; *urine:* less than 10 international units/ml

Description.   FSH, a gonadotrophic hormone from the pituitary gland, stimulates the growth and maturation of the ovarian follicle to produce estrogen in females and to promote spermatogenesis in males. Infertility disorders can be determined by a serum and urine FSH test. Increased and decreased FSH levels can indicate gonad failure due to pituitary dysfunction.

Purposes
- To check for FSH-producing pituitary tumor
- To compare serum and urine FSH levels for determining the cause of infertility

Clinical Problems
Decreased level: Neoplasms of the ovaries, testes, adrenals; polycystic ovarian disease; hypopituitarism; anorexia nervosa
Drugs that may decrease FSH value: Estrogens, oral contraceptives, testosterone
Increased level: Gonadal failure, such as menopause, precocious puberty, FSH-producing pituitary tumor, Turner's syndrome, Klinefelter's syndrome, orchiectomy, hysterectomy, primary testicular failure

Procedure
- No food or fluid restriction is required.
- State phase of menstrual cycle or if menopausal on the laboratory slip.
- Note on the laboratory slip if the client is taking oral contraceptives or any type of hormones.

Serum
- Rest 30 min to 1 h before blood is drawn.
- Collect 5 to 7 ml of venous blood in a red-top tube. Avoid hemolysis.

Urine
- Collect a 24-h urine specimen in a large container with a preservative. The pH of the 24-h urine specimen should be maintained between 5 and 6.5 (glacial acetic acid or boric acid may be added).
- Label container with the client's name, the dates, and the exact times of urine collection (e.g., 5/10/09, 8 AM to 5/11/09, 8:01 AM).
- Avoid getting feces and toilet paper in the urine.

Nursing Implications
Client Teaching

- Instruct the client to rest prior to a serum test, since exercise can increase FSH release.
- Answer client questions concerning the test. Be supportive of client and family.

FTA-ABS (FLUORESCENT TREPONEMAL ANTIBODY ABSORPTION) (SERUM)

Reference Values
Adult: Nonreactive (negative)
Child: Nonreactive (negative)

Description. The FTA-ABS test is the treponemal antibody test, which uses the treponemal organism to produce and detect these antibodies. This test is most sensitive, specific, and reliable for diagnosing syphilis. It is more sensitive than the Venereal Disease Research Laboratory (VDRL) or rapid plasma reagin (RPR) tests. Test results can remain positive after treatment or forever, and it does not indicate the stage and activity of the disease.

Purpose
- To aid in the diagnosis of syphilis

Clinical Problems
Reactive: Primary and secondary syphilis; false positives (rare): lupus erythematosus, pregnancy, acute genital herpes

Procedure
- No food or fluid restriction is required.
- Collect 3 to 5 ml of venous blood in a red-top tube. Avoid hemolysis.
- A borderline FTA-ABS should be repeated.

Nursing Implications
- Keep information confidential except for what is required by law.
- Encourage medical care for sexual partner(s) if test is positive.
- Check the results of other serology tests for syphilis. A positive VDRL could be false positive because of acute or chronic illness.
- Recognize that a positive FTA-ABS result can occur after treatment (penicillin, erythromycin) for months or several years.
- Assess for signs and symptoms of syphilis. The primary stage begins with a small papule filled with liquid, which ruptures, enlarges, and becomes a chancre. With secondary syphilis, a generalized rash (macular and papular) develops (found on the arms, palms, face, and soles of the feet).

FUNGAL ORGANISMS; FUNGAL ANTIBODY TEST; FUNGAL DISEASE; MYCOTIC INFECTIONS (SMEAR, SERUM, CULTURE—SPUTUM, BRONCHIAL, LESION)

Reference Values
Adult: Negative, serum: less than 1:8
Child: Same as adult

Description.   There are more than 45,000 species of fungi, but about 45 species of fungi (0.01%) are considered pathogenic to humans. Fungal infections are more common today and can be classified as (1) superficial and cutaneous mycoses (tinea pedis, athlete's foot; tinea capitis, ringworm of the scalp), (2) subcutaneous mycoses, and (3) systemic mycoses (histoplasmosis, blastomycosis).

The persons most susceptible to fungal infections are those with debilitating or chronic diseases (e.g., diabetes) or those who are receiving drug therapy (e.g., steroids, prolonged antibiotics, antineoplastic agents, and oral contraceptives).

Purpose
- To assist in the diagnosis of selected fungal organisms

Clinical Problems
Positive response: Actinomycosis, histoplasmosis, blastomycosis, coccidioidomycosis, cryptococcosis meningitis, candidiasis (moniliasis, thrush), aspergillosis

Procedure
Serum
- No food or fluid restriction is required. Suggest NPO for 12 h. Check with your laboratory.
- Collect 7 ml of venous blood in a red-top tube.
- Obtain serum antibody test 2 to 4 weeks after exposure to organism.

Culture
- Follow directions from the special laboratory on collection of the specimen.

Organism	Disease Entity	Tests
Actinomyces israelii	Actinomycosis	Smear and culture of lesion
		Biopsy
Histoplasma capsulatum	Histoplasmosis	Sputum
		Histoplasmin skin test
		Serum test: complement fixation or latex agglutination
Blastomyces dermatitidis	Blastomycosis	Culture
		Smear, wet-mount examination of the material from the lesion
		Biopsy, histologic examination
		Skin test
		Serum test: complement fixation
Coccidioides immitis	Coccidioidomycosis	Culture
		Sputum smears
		Skin test
		Serum test: complement fixation (sensitive), latex agglutination (very sensitive)
Cryptococcus neoformans	Cryptococcosis meningitis	Culture of CSF
		Serum test: latex agglutination (sensitive)

(continued)

Organism	Disease Entity	Tests
Candida albicans	Candidiasis (moniliasis thrush)	Smear and culture of the skin, mucous membrane, and vagina
Aspergillus fumigatus	Aspergillosis	Sputum culture
		Skin test
		Serum IgE level and complement fixation

Nursing Implications
- Associate mycotic infections with high-risk clients having chronic illnesses or debilitating diseases.
- Obtain a history from the client as to where he or she has been living and his or her occupation.
- Monitor the client's temperature.
- Report clinical signs and symptoms of respiratory problems (e.g., cough, sputum, dyspnea, and chest pain).
- Check the color of the sputum. Certain fungi can be identified by the color of their secretions.
- Assess the neurologic status when cryptococcosis is suspected. Report headaches and changes in sensorium, pupil size and reaction, and motor function.

Client Teaching
- Inform the client to wear a mask when exposed to chicken feces. *H capsulatum* spores in the feces can be inhaled.

GAMMA-GLUTAMYL TRANSFERASE (GGT) (SERUM)

GAMMA-GLUTAMYL TRANSPEPTIDASE (GGTP OR GTP)

Reference Values
Adult: Male: 4–23 international units/l, 9–69 units/l at 37°C (SI units); female: 3–13 international units/l, 4–33 units/l at 37°C (SI units)
Values may differ among institutions.

Child: Newborn: 5× higher than adult; premature:10× higher than adult; child: similar to adult
Elderly: Slightly higher than adult

Description.   The enzyme GGT is found primarily in the liver and kidney. GGT is sensitive for detecting a wide variety of hepatic diseases. The serum level will rise early and will remain elevated as long as cellular damage persists.

High levels of GGT occur after 12 to 24 h and heavy alcohol intake. Levels may remain increased for several days to weeks after alcohol intake stops.

Purposes
- To detect the presence of a hepatic disorder
- To monitor the liver enzyme GGT during the liver disorder and treatment
- To compare with other liver enzymes for identifying liver dysfunction

Clinical Problems
Increased level: Cirrhosis of the liver, acute and subacute necrosis of the liver, alcoholism, acute and chronic hepatitis, cancer (liver, pancreas, prostate, breast, kidney, lung, and brain), infectious mononucleosis, renal disease, acute myocardial infarction (AMI) [fourth day], acute pancreatitis, CHF
Drugs that can increase GGT value: Aminoglycosides, phenytoin (Dilantin), phenobarbital, warfarin (Coumadin)

Procedure
- No food or fluid restriction is required.
- Collect 3 to 5 ml of venous blood in a red-top tube. Avoid hemolysis.

Nursing Implications
- Compare serum GGT with serum alkaline phosphatase (ALP), leucine aminopeptidase (LAP), and alanine aminotransferase (ALT or SGPT). The GGT test tends to be more sensitive for detecting liver dysfunction than the others.

- Observe for signs and symptoms of liver damage (e.g., restlessness, jaundice, twitching, flapping tremors, spider angiomas, bleeding tendencies, purpura, ascites).

Client Teaching

- Teach the client to maintain a well-balanced diet with adequate protein and carbohydrate.

GASTRIN (SERUM OR PLASMA)

Reference Values

Adult: Fasting: less than 100 pg/ml; nonfasting: 50–200 pg/mL
Child: not usually performed

Description. Gastrin is a hormone secreted by the G cells of the pyloric mucosa which stimulates the secretion of gastric juices, namely hydrochloric acid (HCl). A very small amount of gastrin is secreted by the islets of Langerhans in the pancreas. Gastrin values follow a circadian rhythm, with the highest values occurring during the day, especially during meals. Hypersecretion of HCl inhibits gastrin secretion.

This test is usually ordered to diagnose pernicious anemia and gastric ulcer (mildly increased serum levels), and Zollinger–Ellison syndrome (high serum levels). Zollinger–Ellison syndrome may be due to pancreatic gastrinoma.

Gastrin stimulation tests aid in differentiating between Zollinger–Ellison syndrome and hypergastrinemia due to other causes. Either calcium infusion or secretion is administered intravenously. A marked increase in serum gastrin values occurs with Zollinger–Ellison syndrome and not with other probable causes of hypergastrinemia.

Purposes

- To aid in the diagnosis of pernicious anemia
- To aid in the diagnosis of gastric ulcer
- To differentiate between Zollinger–Ellison syndrome and hypergastrinemia from other causes

Clinical Problems
Decreased level: Vagotomy, hypothyroidism
Drug that may decrease serum gastrin value: Atropine sulfate
Increased level: Pernicious anemia, Zollinger–Ellison syndrome, malignant neoplasm of the stomach, peptic ulcer, chronic atrophic gastritis, cirrhosis of the liver, acute and chronic renal failure
Drugs that may increase serum gastrin value: Calcium products, insulin, catecholamines, caffeine

Procedure
- Food and fluids (except water) are restricted for 12 h before the test.
- Collect 5 to 7 ml of venous blood in a red- or lavender-top tube.

Factors Affecting Laboratory Results
- IV infusion of calcium elevates the serum gastrin level.

Nursing Implications
- For the gastrin stimulation test, infuse calcium gluconate intravenously over a period of 3 to 4 h. Blood sample is taken before the test and then drawn every 30 min to 1 h during the infusion. For the secretin test, infuse secretin intravenously over 1 h. Obtain a blood sample before the test and then every 15 to 30 min for 1 h as prescribed by the health care provider.
- Check the serum gastrin value. In Zollinger–Ellison syndrome, the serum level may reach 2,800 to 300,000 pg/ml.

Client Teaching
- Instruct the client that food and beverages are restricted (with the exception of water) for 12 h before the test. A fasting blood sample is usually ordered.

GLUCAGON (PLASMA)

Reference Values
Adult: 50–200 pg/ml, 50–200 ng/l (SI units)
Newborn: 0–1,750 pg/ml, 0–1,750 ng/l (SI units)

Description.   Glucagon is secreted by the alpha cells of the pancreas. It functions as a counterregulatory hormone to insulin in regulating glucose metabolism. In response to hypoglycemia, glucagon increases blood glucose level by converting glycogen to glucose.

Very high glucagon levels (500–1,000 pg/ml) occur in glucagonoma, pancreatic alpha cell tumor.

Purposes
- To detect an increase or deficit in the serum glucagon
- To screen for glucagonoma

Clinical Problems
Decreased level: Glucose tolerance test during first hour, idiopathic glucagon deficiency, loss of pancreatic tissue

Increased level: Glucagonoma, acute pancreatitis, severe diabetic ketoacidosis, trauma, infections, pheochromocytoma

Drugs that may increase glucagon level: Glucocorticoids, insulin, sympathomimetic amines

Procedure
- Collect 5 to 7 ml of venous blood in a lavender-top tube. Avoid hemolysis. Chill the tube with ice and take to the laboratory immediately.
- Food and fluids are restricted for 10 to 12 h prior to the test.
- Have client relax for 30 min prior to the test.
- Withhold drugs such as insulin, cortisone, growth hormones, and epinephrine, with health care provider's permission, until the test is completed.

Factors Affecting Laboratory Results
- Infections, trauma, steroids, insulin, excessive exercise, uncontrolled diabetes mellitus, acute pancreatitis, and/or undue stress may elevate glucagon level.

Nursing Implications
- Compare serum glucose and insulin levels. Glucose and insulin influence plasma glucagon levels.

- Record on the laboratory slip and report if client has taken large doses of steroids in the last 24 h.
- Observe for signs and symptoms of hyperglycemia.

Client Teaching

- Instruct the client to relax in chair or lie down for at least 30 min prior to the test. Stress and activity could cause false-positive test results.

GLUCOSE—FASTING BLOOD SUGAR (FBS) (BLOOD)

Reference Values

Adult: *Serum and plasma:* 70–110 mg/dl; 3.9–6.1 mmol/l (SI units)
Whole blood: 60–100 mg/dl; 3.3–5.5 mmol/l (SI units)
Panic values: Less than 40 mg/dl; less than 2.2 mmol/l (SI units)
greater than 700 mg/dl; greater than 38.5 mmol/l (SI units)

Gestational diabetes: Greater than 140 mg/dl; greater than 7.9 mmol/l (SI units)

Elderly: *Serum:* 70–120 mg/dl; 3.9–6.7 mmol/l (SI units)

Newborn: 30–80 mg/dl; 1.7–4.4 mmol/l (SI units)

Child: 60–100 mg/dl; 3.3–5.5 mmol/l (SI units)

Description.   Glucose is formed from dietary carbohydrates and is stored as glycogen in the liver and skeletal muscles. Insulin and glucagon, two hormones from the pancreas, affect the blood glucose level. Insulin is needed for cellular membrane permeability to glucose and food transportation of glucose into the cells. Without insulin, glucose cannot enter the cells. Glucagon stimulates glycogenolysis (conversion of stored glycogen to glucose) in the liver.

A decreased blood sugar level (hypoglycemia) results from inadequate food intake or too much insulin. When elevated blood sugar (hyperglycemia) occurs, there is not enough insulin; this condition is known as diabetes mellitus. A fasting blood sugar level greater than 125 mg/dl usually indicates diabetes, and to confirm the diagnosis when the blood sugar is borderline or slightly elevated, a feasting (postprandial) blood sugar and/or a glucose tolerance test may be ordered.

Today, there are various home glucose monitoring devices available to monitor blood sugar such as Accu-check bG, Glucometer, MediSense Optium, and others. These glucose monitoring devices can be used for fasting blood sugar and can be used throughout the day to check blood sugars.

Purposes
- To confirm a diagnosis of prediabetic state or diabetic mellitus
- To monitor blood glucose levels for diabetic clients taking an antidiabetic agent (insulin or oral hypoglycemic drug)

Clinical Problems
Decreased level: Hypoglycemic reaction (insulin excess); cancer (stomach, liver, lung), adrenal gland hypofunction, malnutrition, alcoholism, cirrhosis of the liver, strenuous exercise, erythroblastosis fetalis (hemolytic disease), hyperinsulinism.

Drugs that may decrease glucose value: Insulin excess, acetaminophen, alcohol, propranolol, and hypoglycemic agents.

Increased level: Diabetes mellitus, diabetes acidosis, adrenal gland hyperfunction (Cushing's syndrome), acute myocardial infarction, stress, crushed injury, burns, infections, renal failure, hypothermia, exercise, acute pancreatitis, cancer of the pancreas, heart failure, acromegaly, postgastrectomy (dumping) syndrome, extensive surgery.

Drug that may increase glucose value. ACTH; cortisone preparations; diuretics (hydrochlorothiazide [HydroDIURIL], furosemide [Lasix], ethacrynic acid [Edecrin]), anesthesia drugs, levodopa. estrogen, lithium, epinephrines, phenytoin, high doses of salicylates.

Procedure
- NPO except water for 10–12 h before the test.
- Withhold insulin and oral hypoglycemic agents.
- Collect 3 to 5 ml of venous blood in a gray- or red-top tube. Blood is drawn between 7 AM and 9 AM.
- Give insulin as ordered and after the blood sample is taken.

Factors Affecting Laboratory Results

- Drugs—cortisone, thiazide, and the "loop" diuretics can cause an increase in blood sugar.
- Trauma—stress can cause an increase in blood sugar.
- The Clinitest for determining urine glucose (glycosuria) may be falsely positive if the client is taking excessive amounts of aspirin, vitamin C, and certain antibiotics (cephalosporin), because the test is not specific for glucose but for all reducing substances.
- High doses of vitamin C could cause false-negative results when using urine glucose testing tapes (e.g., Tes-Tape).

Nursing Implications

- Hold morning insulin and drugs until the blood specimen is taken.
- Record on the laboratory slip if the client has been taking daily cortisone preparations, thiazides, or loop diuretics.

Decreased Level

- Recognize clinical problems associated with a low blood sugar level. Excessive doses of insulin, skipped meals, and inadequate food intake are the common causes of hypoglycemia.
- Observe for signs and symptoms of hypoglycemia (nervousness, weakness, confusion, cold and clammy skin, diaphoresis, and increased pulse rate).

Client Teaching

- Instruct the client to carry lumps of sugar or candy at all times. Most diabetic persons have warnings when hypoglycemia occurs.
- Teach the client to adhere to the American Dietetic Association (ADA) diet, as prescribed. Explain the Exchange Lists for meal planning.
- Encourage the client to contact the American Diabetic Association for literature and information concerning their meeting dates.
- Explain to the client that strenuous exercise can lower the blood sugar. Carbohydrate or protein intake should be increased before exercise or immediately after exercise; the health care provider should be contacted for food instruction.

- Encourage the client to take insulin 0.5 to 1 h before breakfast and to eat meals on time.
- Teach clients with a hypoglycemic problem (blood sugar less than 50 mg/dl) to eat food high in protein and fat and low in carbohydrate. Too much sugar stimulates insulin secretion.

Increased Level

- Recognize clinical problems associated with high blood sugar levels. Diabetes mellitus, Cushing's syndrome, and stressful situations (trauma, burns, extensive surgery) are the common causes of hyperglycemia.
- Consider drugs (such as cortisone, thiazides, and "loop" diuretics) as the cause of a slightly elevated blood sugar level. If blood sugar becomes too high, notify the health care provider—drug dosages may need to be decreased or insulin may need to be ordered or increased.
- Observe for signs and symptoms of hyperglycemia (excessive thirst [polydipsia], excessive urination [polyuria], excessive hunger [polyphagia], and weight loss). If the blood sugar is greater than 500 mg/dl, Kussmaul's breathing (rapid, deep, vigorous breathing) caused by acidosis may be observed.

Client Teaching

- Instruct the client to test his or her blood before meals. Demonstrate how to use Chemstrip bG techniques or others.
- Explain to the client that infections can increase the blood sugar level and that medical advice should be sought.

GLUCOSE-6-PHOSPHATE DEHYDROGENASE (G6PD) (BLOOD)

Reference Values

Adult: Screen test: negative; quantitative test: 8–18 international units/g Hb, 125–281 units/dl packed RBC, 251–511 units/10^6 cells, 1,211–2,111 milli-international units/ml packed RBC (varies with methods used)
Child: Similar to adult

Description.   G6PD is an enzyme present in the RBCs. A G6PD deficit is a sex-linked genetic defect carried by the female (X) chromosome, which will, in conjunction with infection, disease, and drugs, make a person susceptible to developing hemolytic anemia. A screen test is usually done before the quantitative test.

Purpose
- To screen for hemolytic anemia

Clinical Problems
Decreased level: Hemolytic anemia, infections (bacterial and viral), septicemia, diabetes acidosis

Drugs that may decrease G6PD value: Aspirin, ascorbic acid, acetanilid, nitrofurantoin (Furadantin), phenacetin, primaquine, thiazide diuretics, probenecid (Benemid), quinidine, sulfonamides, vitamin K, tolbutamide (Orinase)

Procedure
- No food or fluid restriction is required.
- Screening test for G6PD is methemoglobin reduction (Brewer's test) or ascorbate and fluorescent spot test and others.
- Collect a small amount of capillary blood in a heparinized microhematocrit tube, or collect 5 ml of venous blood in a lavender- or green-top tube. Avoid hemolysis.

Nursing Implications
- Obtain a familial history of RBC enzyme deficiency.
- Observe for signs of hemolysis, such as jaundice of the sclera and skin.
- Check for decreased urinary output (expected to be at least 25 ml/h or 600 ml/day). Prolonged hemolysis can be toxic to the kidney cells.
- Record oxidative drugs (see drug list). Hemolysis usually occurs 3 days after taking an oxidative drug. Hemolytic symptoms will disappear 2 to 3 days after the drug has been stopped.

Client Teaching
- Instruct the susceptible person to read labels on over-the-counter (OTC) medicines and not to take drugs that contain phenacetin and

aspirin. Most of these drugs, if taken continuously, can cause hemolytic anemia.

GLUCOSE—POSTPRANDIAL (FEASTING BLOOD SUGAR) (BLOOD)

TWO-HOUR POSTPRANDIAL BLOOD SUGAR (PPBS)

Reference Values
Adult: *Serum and plasma:* less than 140 mg/dl/2 h; less than 7.8 mmol/l (SI units)

Whole blood: less than 120 mg/dl/2 h; less than 6.7 mmol/l (SI units)

Elderly: *Serum:* less than 160 mg/dl; less than 8.9 mmol/l (SI units)

Whole blood: less than 140 mg/dl; less than 7.8 mmol/l (SI units)

Child: *Serum:* less than 140 mg/dl; less than 6.7 mmol/l (SI units)

Description.   A 2-h PPBS or feasting sugar test is usually done to determine the patient's response to a high-carbohydrate intake 2 h after a meal (breakfast or lunch). This test is a screening test for diabetes, normally ordered if the fasting blood sugar was high normal or slightly elevated. A serum glucose greater than 140 mg/dl or a blood glucose greater than 120 mg/dl is abnormal, and further tests may be needed.

A glucose tolerance test may be prescribed for a client who has a feasting blood sugar (PPBS) between 140 and 200 mg/dl to confirm diabetes mellitus. If the feasting blood sugar is greater than 200 mg/dl, a glucose tolerance test is not suggested and diabetes mellitus is confirmed.

Purpose
See Glucose—Fasting Blood Sugar

Clinical Problems
Decreased level: See Glucose—Fasting Blood Sugar
Increased level: See Glucose—Fasting Blood Sugar

Procedure
- Food is restricted for 2 h after breakfast or lunch before the test, but water is not.
- A high-carbohydrate meal might be requested at breakfast or lunch.
- Collect 3 to 5 ml of venous blood in a gray- or red-top tube 2 h after the client finishes eating breakfast or lunch. If the nurse does not draw the blood, the laboratory needs to be notified when the client finished breakfast or lunch.

Factors Affecting Laboratory Results
- Smoking may increase the serum glucose level.
- See Glucose—Fasting Blood Sugar.

Nursing Implications
- Determine the breakfast foods that the client likes and dislikes and notify the dietary department.

Client Teaching
- If the client is not hospitalized, instruct the person to be at the laboratory 0.5 to 2 h after breakfast or lunch.

Increased Level
- See Glucose—Fasting Blood Sugar.

GLUCOSE SELF-MONITORING (SELF-TESTING) DEVICES (BLOOD AND URINE)

GLUCOSE FINGER-STICK, GLUCOSE CAPILLARY TEST

Reference Values
Adult: *Blood:* 60–110 mg/dl, 3.3–6.1 µmol/l (SI units)
Child: *Blood:* 50–85 mg/dl, 2.7–4.7 µmol/l (SI units)
Urine: Negative

Description. To control blood glucose levels, glucose monitoring devices are available for checking blood glucose levels. The glucose monitoring devices can be used in institutions such as hospitals, and the clients with type 1 diabetes mellitus and the clients with type 2 diabetes mellitus can use it in their homes for managing diabetes mellitus. The test takes about 2 min, test results are reliable, and the cost is approximately 1/20th of a laboratory test.

The use of reagent strips for urine testing (e.g., Clinistix, Diastix, Tes-Tape, and Clinitest tablets) is less desirable for glucose accuracy than the self-monitoring metered devices. Clients who are unable to perform a finger-stick and use the meter machine should use the urine testing method to evaluate blood glucose levels.

Purpose

- To check the blood glucose level

Clinical Problems

Decreased level: Insulin overdose
Increased level: Diabetes mellitus, hyperalimentation, excessive stress
Drugs that may increase glucose value: Steroids, thiazide diuretics

Procedure

- NPO prior to the test unless otherwise instructed.

Blood

Finger-stick capillary method

- Check procedure on the specific glucose monitoring device.
- Cleanse the finger site with alcohol; wipe dry.
- Puncture the lateral side of the finger. Wipe off first drop of blood. Do not "milk" the finger.
- Let a large drop of blood drop onto the reagent strip. The blood should cover the pad of the strip.
- Place the reagent strip into the meter for reading. Follow directions on the meter.
- Apply pressure to the site until bleeding has stopped.

Heelstick: Use the same method for obtaining a finger-stick; however, hold the heel in a dependent position to allow the blood drop to accumulate.

The use of a capillary tube to obtain the blood specimen may be necessary for blood glucose testing.

Urine

Clinitest: Dip the reagent strip into the urine specimen, remove the strip, wait 10 seconds, read by comparing strip to the color blocks.

Diastix: Dip the reagent strip in the urine specimen, remove the strip, wait 30 seconds, read by comparing strip to the color chart.

Tes-Tape: Tear off 1½ inches of reagent tape, dip into the urine specimen, remove tape, wait 60 seconds, read tape by comparing the dark part of tape to color chart.

Factors Affecting Laboratory Results

Blood

- A blood drop that is insufficient for the test.
- Milking the finger can cause false-low results.

Urine

- Stale urine interferes with test results.
- Drugs that may cause a false-negative result include levodopa, aspirin, ascorbic acid, tetracycline, and methyldopa.

Nursing Implications

- Obtain a history regarding the client's glucose testing method including the past glucose testing results.

Client Teaching

- Discuss the procedure (blood and/or urine) with the client. Have the client demonstrate the procedure.
- Discuss the course of action the client should take if the test result is abnormal.
- Instruct the client to take insulin or the oral hypoglycemic agent at the prescribed time.
- Tell the client to report immediately signs and symptoms of hypoglycemia or hyperglycemia.
- Instruct the client to keep accurate records of the glucose tests.
- Encourage the client to keep all medical appointments.

GLUCOSE TOLERANCE TEST—ORAL (OGTT) (SERUM) AND IV (IV-GTT)

Reference Values
Adult:

ORAL GTT

Time	Serum (mg/dl)	mmol/l	Blood (mg/dl)	mmol/l
Fasting	70–110	3.9–6.1	60–100	3.3–5.5
0.5 h	Less than 160	Less than 8.9	Less than 150	Less than 8.3
1 h	Less than 170	Less than 9.4	Less than 160	Less than 8.9
2 h	Less than 125	Less than 6.9	Less than 115	Less than 6.9
3 h	Fasting levels		Fasting levels	

IV GLUCOSE TOLERANCE TEST

Time	Serum (mg/dl)	mmol/l
Fasting	70–110	3.9–6.1
5 min	Less than 250	Less than 13.8
0.5 h	Less than 155	Less than 8.5
1 h	Less than 125	Less than 6.9

Child: Infant: lower blood sugar level than adult; less than 6 years: similar to adult

Description.   A GTT is done to diagnose diabetes mellitus in persons having high normal or slightly elevated blood sugar values. The test may be indicated when there is a familial history of diabetes, in women having babies weighing 10 pounds or more, in persons having extensive surgery or injury, and in obese persons. The test should not be performed if the fasting blood sugar (FBS) is over 200 mg/dl. The peak glucose level for the OGTT is 0.5 to 1 h after the ingestion of 100 g of glucose, and the blood sugar should return to normal range in 3 h. OGTT can be a 3- to 6-h test.

An IV GTT may be done if the person cannot eat or tolerate the oral glucose. The blood glucose returns to the normal range in 2 h after IV GTT.

Purpose
* To confirm the diagnosis of diabetes mellitus

Clinical Problems
Decreased level: Hyperinsulinism, adrenal gland insufficiency, malabsorption, protein malnutrition
Increased level: Diabetes mellitus, latent diabetes, adrenal gland hyper function (Cushing's syndrome), stress, infections, extensive surgery or injury, acute myocardial infarction (AMI), cancer of the pancreas, insulin resistance condition
Drugs that may increase OGTT values: Steroids, oral contraceptives, estrogens, thiazide diuretics, salicylates

Procedure
* Restrict food and fluids except for water for 12 h before the test.
* NPO except for water during test. No coffee, tea, or smoking are allowed during test.
* Collect 5 ml of venous blood in a red- or gray-top tube for the FBS. Collect a fasting urine specimen.
* Record on laboratory slip if client has been taking cortisone preparations, thiazide diuretics, or oral contraceptives daily.
* Give 100 g of glucose solution. Some health care providers will give glucose according to body weight (1.75 g/kg), as in pediatrics.
* Obtain blood and urine specimens 0.5, 1, 2, 3 h or longer after glucose intake.

Nursing Implications
* Check previous FBS results before the test. A known diabetic normally does not have this test performed.
* Notify the laboratory of exact time the client drank the glucose solution.
* Minimize activities during the test.
* Identify factors affecting glucose results (e.g., emotional stress, infection, vomiting, fever, exercise, inactivity, age, drugs, and body weight). These should be reported to the health care provider.

Client Teaching
- Explain to the client that he or she may perspire or feel weak and giddy during the 2- to 3-h test. This is frequently transitory; however, the nurse should be notified, and these symptoms should be recorded. They could be signs of hyperinsulinism.
- Explain the procedure for the test.

GLYCOSYLATED HEMOGLOBIN (*SEE* HEMOGLOBIN A$_1$C [BLOOD])

GROWTH HORMONE (GH), HUMAN GROWTH HORMONE (hGH) (SERUM)

SOMATOTROPHIC HORMONE (STH)

Reference Values
Adult: Male: less than 5 ng/ml; female: less than 10 ng/ml (norms vary with method)
Child: Less than 10 ng/ml

Description.   Human growth hormone (hGH) is secreted from the anterior pituitary gland and regulates the growth of bone and tissue. Growth hormone levels are elevated by exercise, deep sleep, protein food, and fasting. Highest levels occur during sleep. GH levels are decreased with obesity and in corticosteroid therapy.

A low serum hGH level may be a cause of dwarfism. Elevated hGH levels can cause gigantism in children and acromegaly in adults. From a single blood sample to determine the serum growth hormone level, a positive diagnosis cannot be made; therefore, growth hormone stimulation or suppression test might be suggested. A glucose loading GH suppression test should suppress hGH secretion. Failure to suppress hGH levels confirms gigantism (children) or acromegaly (adult).

Purposes
- To determine the presence of human growth hormone deficit or excess
- To aid in the diagnosis of dwarfism, gigantism, or acromegaly

Clinical Problems

Decreased level: Dwarfism in children, hypopituitarism

Drugs that may decrease hGH value: Cortisone preparations, glucose, phenothiazines

Increased level: Gigantism (children), acromegaly (adult), major surgery, stress, exercise, uncontrolled diabetes mellitus, premature and newborn infants

Drugs that may increase hGH value: Estrogens, insulin, amphetamines, glucagon, levodopa, beta blockers, methyldopa (Aldomet), oral contraceptives

Procedure

- Restrict food and fluids except for water for 8 to 10 h.
- Have the client rest for 30 min to 1 h before taking a blood sample.
- Collect 3 to 7 ml of venous blood in a red-top tube, preferably in the early morning. Avoid hemolysis. Deliver the blood specimen immediately to the laboratory because hGH has a short half-life.

Factors Affecting Laboratory Results

- Stress, exercise, food (protein), and deep sleep could cause an elevated hGH level.

Nursing Implications

- Obtain a history of the client's activities and behavior that could affect the test results, such as stress, exercise, and food intake.

Client Teaching

- Instruct the client not to eat 8 to 10 h before the test. Encourage the client to rest and not to exercise prior to the test.
- Encourage the client to express his/her feeling as it relates to the test and health problem. Be supportive to client and family.

HAPTOGLOBIN (HP) (SERUM)

Reference Values

Adult: 60–270 mg/dl, 0.6–2.7 g/l (SI units)

Child: Newborn: 0–10 mg/dl (absent in 90%); infant: 0–30 mg/dl, then gradual increase

Description.   Haptoglobins are α_2 globulins in the plasma, and these globulin molecules combine with free (released) hemoglobin during hemolysis (RBC destruction). A haptoglobin–hemoglobin complex occurs, and the iron in the hemoglobin is able to be conserved. A decreased level of serum haptoglobin indicates hemolysis. After a hemolytic transfusion reaction, the serum haptoglobin level begins to fall within a few hours. It may take several days before the haptoglobin level returns to normal. A hemolytic process may be masked in persons taking steroids.

Purposes
- To identify the occurrence of hemolysis
- To assist in the diagnosis of selected health problems (see Clinical Problems)

Clinical Problems
Decreased level: Hemolysis, anemias (pernicious, vitamin B_6 deficiency, hemolytic, sickle cell), severe liver disease (hepatic failure, chronic hepatitis), thrombotic thrombocytopenic purpura, disseminated intravascular coagulation (DIC), malaria
Increased level: Inflammation, acute infections, malignancies (lung, large intestine, stomach, breast, liver), Hodgkin's disease, ulcerative colitis, chronic pyelonephritis (active stage), rheumatic fever, acute myocardial infarction
Drugs that may increase haptoglobin value: Steroids (cortisone), estrogens, oral contraceptives, dextran

Procedure
- No food or fluid restriction is required.
- Collect 5 to 7 ml of venous blood in a red-top tube. Avoid hemolysis.

Nursing Implications
- Assess the client's vital signs. Report abnormal vital signs, especially if the client is having breathing problems related to a reduced oxygen-carrying capacity.

- Assess the client's urinary output. Excess amounts of free hemoglobin may cause renal damage.
- Check the serum haptoglobin level. The haptoglobin level may be masked by steroid therapy and inflammation. If hemolysis is suspected, the serum level may be normal instead of low due to steroids or inflammation. Notify the health care provider of the findings.

HELICOBACTER PYLORI (SERUM, CULTURE, BREATH ANALYSIS)

Reference Values
Negative findings
Positive: Elevated titer level using ELISA testing, presence of *H pylori*, urea breath test

Description.   The Gram-negative bacillus *Helicobacter pylori* is found in the gastric mucous layer of the epithelium in about 50% of the population by age 55. The majority of persons with the infection remain asymptomatic. *H pylori* was first identified in 1983 as a cause of peptic ulcer disease. It is recognized as a primary cause of chronic gastritis, and it may progress over years to gastric cancer or gastric lymphoma. *H pylori* is associated with 70% to 85% of clients with gastric ulcers and with 90% to 95% of clients with duodenal ulcers.

Eradication of *H pylori* for asymptomatic clients usually is not suggested or prescribed but is definitely indicated for perforated, bleeding, or refractory ulcers. Treatment to eradicate the infection includes using either a dual, triple, or quadruple drug therapy program using a variety of drug combinations. Dual drug therapy (omeprazole and amoxicillin) for 14 days has fewer side effects but is not as effective in eradicating *H pylori* as the use of triple or quadruple therapy. Quadruple therapy has a 7-day treatment course which eliminates some of the side effects. After the drug therapy program, a 6-week standard acid suppression drug (histamine-2 blocker) usually is recommended.

Purposes
- To detect the cause of the gastrointestinal disorder
- To determine the presence of *H pylori*

Clinical Problems
Increased titer or positive culture: Presence of *H pylori* causing acute or chronic gastritis, peptic ulcer disease, gastric carcinoma, gastric lymphoma

Procedure
Serum (Enzyme-Linked Immunosorbent Assay [ELISA] Serology Test)
- No food or fluid restriction is required.
- Collect 7 ml of venous blood in a red-top tube.
- Use of a variety of commercial diagnostic kits.

Culture or Biopsy (Endoscopy)
- Obtain a culture or biopsy using endoscopy for detection of urease produced by *H pylori*.

Urea Breath Test
- Use the urea breath test to diagnose urease, which is given off by *H pylori*. It has a sensitivity of 92% to 94%.

Nursing Implications
- Obtain a familial history of gastrointestinal disorders, such as gastritis or peptic ulcer disease.
- Record symptoms client has related to gastritis or peptic ulcer disease, such as pain, abdominal cramping, gastroesophageal reflux disease (GERD), dyspepsia (heartburn), anorexia, nausea, vomiting, GI bleeding, and tarry stools.

Client Teaching
- Encourage the client to avoid smoking (if client smokes) because smoking reduces bicarbonate content in the GI tract, allows reflux of the duodenum into the stomach, and slows the healing process.
- Listen to client's concerns. Answer client's questions or refer unknown answers to other health care providers.

HEMATOCRIT (Hct) (BLOOD)

Reference Values
Adult: Male: 40%–54%, 0.40–0.54 (SI units); female: 36%–46%, 0.36–0.46 (SI units); *panic value:* less than 15% and greater than 60%
Child: Newborn: 44%–65%; child: 1–3 years: 29%–40%; 4–10 years: 31%–43%

Description. The hematocrit (Hct) is the volume of packed RBCs in 100 ml of blood, expressed as a percentage. It is the proportion of RBCs to plasma. The test is prescribed to measure the concentration of RBCs, also called erythrocytes, in the blood. To obtain an accurate hematocrit, the client should NOT be dehydrated.

Purposes
* To check the volume of red blood cells in the blood
* To monitor the volume of RBCs to plasma during a debilitating illness

Clinical Problems
Decreased level: Acute blood loss, anemias, leukemias, Hodgkin's disease, lymphosarcoma, multiple myeloma, chronic renal failure, cirrhosis of the liver, malnutrition, vitamin B and C deficiencies, pregnancy, systemic lupus erythematosus (SLE), rheumatoid arthritis, peptic ulcer, bone marrow failure
Drugs that may decrease Hct value: Penicillin, chloramphenicol
Increased level: Dehydration/hypovolemia, severe diarrhea, polycythemia vera, diabetic acidosis, pulmonary emphysema (later stage), transient cerebral ischemia (TIA), eclampsia, trauma, surgery, burns

Procedure
* No food or fluid restriction is required.

Venous Blood
* Collect 3 to 5 ml of venous blood in a lavender-top tube. Mix well. Tourniquet should be on for less than 2 min.
* Do not take blood specimen from the same arm as IV.

Capillary Blood

- Collect capillary blood using the microhematocrit method. Blood is obtained from a finger-prick, using a heparinized capillary tube.

Factors Affecting Laboratory Results

- If blood is collected from an extremity that has an IV line, the hematocrit will most likely be low. Avoid using such an extremity.
- If blood is taken to check the hematocrit immediately after moderate to severe blood loss and transfusions, the hematocrit could be normal.
- Age of the client should be known; newborns normally have higher hematocrits because of hemoconcentration.

Nursing Implications
Decreased Level

- Assess for signs and symptoms of anemia (e.g., fatigue, paleness, and tachycardia).
- Assess changes in vital signs for shock (e.g., tachycardia, tachypnea, and normal or decreased blood pressure).
- Recommend a repeat hematocrit several days after moderate/severe bleeding or transfusions. A hematocrit taken immediately after blood loss and after transfusions may appear normal.

Increased Level

- Assess for signs and symptoms of dehydration/hypovolemia (e.g., a history of vomiting, diarrhea, marked thirst, lack of skin turgor, and shock-like symptoms).
- Assess changes in urinary output; urine output of less than 25 ml/h or 600 ml daily could be due to dehydration.

HEMOGLOBIN (Hb OR Hgb) (BLOOD)

Reference Values
Adult: Male: 13.5–18 g/dl; 8.4–11.2 mmol/l (SI units); Female: 12–15 g/dl; 7.45–9.31 mmol/l (SI units)

Child: *Newborn:* 14–24 g/dl. *Infant:* 10–17 g/dl. *Child:* 11–16 g/dl

Description. Hemoglobin, a protein substance in red blood cells, is composed of iron, which is an oxygen carrier. A hemoglobin test aids in assessing the presence of anemia. Hemoglobin (erythrocyte) indices are needed to determine the type of hemoglobin disorder (see Hemoglobin Electrophoresis). Hematocrit is approximately three times the hemoglobin value if the hemoglobin is within normal level.

Abnormally high hemoglobin levels may be due to hemoconcentration resulting from dehydration. Low hemoglobin values are related to clinical problems, such as anemia.

Purposes
- To monitor the hemoglobin value in red blood cells
- To assist in diagnosing anemia
- To suggest the presence of body fluid deficit due to an elevated hemoglobin level

Clinical Problems
Decreased level: Anemias, cancers, kidney diseases, excess IV fluids, Hodgkin's disease
Drugs that may decrease hemoglobin value: Antibiotics, aspirin, antineoplastic drugs, doxapram (Dopram), indomethacin (Indocin), sulfonamides, primaquine, rifampin, trimethadione (Tridione)
Increased level: Dehydration/hemoconcentration; polycythemia; high altitudes; chronic obstructive lung disease (COLD), such as emphysema and asthma; CHF; severe burns
Drugs that may increase hemoglobin value: Methyldopa (Aldomet), gentamicin

Procedure
- No food or fluid restriction is required.
- The tourniquet should be on less than a minute.
- Do not take the blood sample from the extremity receiving IV fluids.

Venous Blood
- Collect 3 to 5 ml of venous blood in a lavender-top tube. Avoid hemolysis. Pediatric tube can also be used.

Capillary Blood
- Puncture the cleansed earlobe, finger, or heel with a sterile lancet. Do not squeeze the puncture site tightly, for serous fluid and blood would thus be obtained. Wipe away the first drop of blood. Collect drops of blood in micropipettes with small rubber tops or microhematocrit tubes. Expel blood into the tubes with diluents.

Factors Affecting Laboratory Results
- Taking blood from an arm or hand receiving IV fluids could dilute blood sample.
- Leaving the tourniquet on for more than a minute will cause hemostasis, which will result in a falsely elevated hemoglobin.
- Living in high altitudes will increase hemoglobin levels.
- Decreased fluid intake or fluid loss will increase hemoglobin levels due to hemoconcentration, and excessive fluid intake will decrease hemoglobin levels due to hemodilution.

Nursing Implications
Decreased Level
- Recognize clinical problems and drugs that could cause a decreased hemoglobin level (e.g., anemia with Hgb less than 10.5 g/dl).
- Observe the client for signs and symptoms of anemia (e.g., dizziness, tachycardia, weakness, dyspnea at rest). Symptoms vary with decreased hemoglobin level.
- Check the hematocrit if the hemoglobin level is low.

Increased Level
- Observe for signs and symptoms of dehydration (e.g., marked thirst, poor skin turgor, dry mucous membranes, and shock-like symptoms [tachycardia, tachypnea, and, later, a decreased blood pressure]).
- Instruct the client to maintain an adequate fluid intake.

HEMOGLOBIN A₁c (Hgb A₁c OR Hb A₁c) (BLOOD)

GLYCOSYLATED HEMOGLOBIN (Hgb A₁a, Hgb A₁b, Hgb A₁c), GLYCOHEMOGLOBIN

Reference Values

Total glycosylated hemoglobin: 5.5%–9% of total Hgb (Hb)

Adult: Hgb (Hb) A₁c: Nondiabetic: 2%–5%. Diabetic control: 2.5%–6%; high average: 6.1%–7.5%. Diabetic uncontrolled: greater than 8.0%

Child: Hgb (Hb) A₁c: Nondiabetic: 1.5%–4%

Description.   Hemoglobin A (Hgb or Hb A) composes 91% to 95% of total hemoglobin. A glucose molecule is attached to Hb A₁, which is a portion of hemoglobin A. This process of attachment is called *glycosylation* or *glycosylated hemoglobin* (or *hemoglobin A₁*). There is a bond between glucose and hemoglobin. Formation of Hb A₁ occurs slowly over 120 days, the life span of red blood cells (RBCs). Hb A₁ is composed of three hemoglobin molecules—Hb A₁a, Hb A₁b, and Hb A₁c—of which 70% Hb A₁c is 70% glycosylated (absorbs glucose). The amount of glycosylated hemoglobin depends on the amount of blood glucose available. When the blood glucose level is elevated over a prolonged period of time, the red blood cells (RBCs) become saturated with glucose; glycohemoglobin results.

A glycosylated hemoglobin represents an average blood glucose level during a 1- to 3-month period. This test is used mainly as a measurement of the effectiveness of diabetic therapy. Fasting blood sugar reflects the blood glucose level at a one-time fasting state, whereas the Hgb or Hb A₁c is a better indicator of diabetes mellitus control. However, a false decreased Hb A₁c level can be caused by a decrease in red blood cells.

An elevated Hb A₁c greater than 8% indicates uncontrolled diabetes mellitus, and the client is at a high risk of developing long-term complications, such as nephropathy, retinopathy, neuropathy, and/or cardiopathy. Total glycohemoglobin may be a better indicator of diabetes control for clients with anemias or blood loss.

Purposes

- To monitor and evaluate diabetes mellitus control
- To provide information regarding the presence of diabetes mellitus

Clinical Problems

Decreased level: Anemias (pernicious, hemolytic, sickle cell), thalassemia, long-term blood loss, chronic renal failure

Increased level: Uncontrolled diabetes mellitus, hyperglycemia, recently diagnosed diabetes mellitus, alcohol ingestion, pregnancy, hemodialysis

Drugs that may increase Hb A1c value: Prolonged cortisone intake, ACTH

Procedure

- Schedule client 6 to 12 weeks from the last Hb A$_1$c test.
- Food restriction prior to the test is not required but is suggested.
- Collect 5 ml of venous blood in a lavender- or green-top tube. Avoid hemolysis; send specimen immediately to the laboratory.

Factors Affecting Laboratory Results

- Anemias may cause a low-value result.
- Hemolysis of the blood specimen can cause an inaccurate test result.
- Heparin therapy may cause a false test result.

Nursing Implications

- Monitor blood and/or urine glucose levels. Compare monthly fasting blood sugar with glycosylated hemoglobin (Hb A$_1$c) test result.
- Determine client's compliance to diabetic treatment regimen.
- Check the dose of daily insulin or oral hypoglycemic agent.
- Recognize clinical problems that can cause a false glycosylated hemoglobin result (see Clinical Problems).
- Observe for signs and symptoms of hyperglycemia.
- Report any complications client has due to diabetes mellitus.

Client Teaching

- Inform the client that fasting prior to the test may or may not be prescribed. The laboratory person should be told if the client has not fasted prior to the test.

- Explain the purpose of the test.
- Instruct the client to comply with the diabetic treatment regimen, such as prescribed insulin, diet, and glucose monitoring.

HEMOGLOBIN ELECTROPHORESIS (BLOOD)

HGB OR HB ELECTROPHORESIS

Reference Values
Adult: **Hb A$_1$:** 95%–98% total Hb; **A$_2$:** 1.5%–4%; **F:** less than 2%; **C:** 0%; **D:** 0%, **S:** 0%
Child: Newborn: **Hb F:** 50%–80% total Hb; 6 months: **Hb F:** 8%; Child: **Hb F:** 1%–2% after 6 months

Description.   Hemoglobin electrophoresis is useful for identifying more than 150 types of normal and abnormal hemoglobin. Many abnormal hemoglobin types do not produce harmful diseases; the common hemoglobinopathies are identified through electrophoresis.
Hemoglobin S: Hb S is the most common hemoglobin variant. If both genes have Hb S, sickle cell anemia will occur; but if only one gene has Hb S, then the person simply carries the sickle trait. Approximately 1% of the black population in the United States has sickle cell anemia, and 8% to 10% carry the sickle cell trait.

Purpose
- To detect abnormal hemoglobin type in the red blood cells (e.g., sickle cell anemia, which is characterized by the S-shaped hemoglobin)

Clinical Problems

Hemoglobin Type	Increased Level
Hemoglobin F	Thalassemia (after 6 months)
Hemoglobin C	Hemolytic anemia
Hemoglobin S	Sickle cell anemia

Procedure

- No food or fluid restriction is required.
- Collect 3 to 5 ml of venous blood in a lavender-top tube. Send immediately to the laboratory. Abnormal hemoglobin is unstable.

Nursing Implications

- Observe for signs and symptoms of sickle cell anemia. Early symptoms are fatigue and weakness. Chronic symptoms are fatigue, dyspnea on exertion, swollen joints, bones that ache, and chest pains.

Client Teaching

- Encourage genetic counseling.
- Instruct the client to take rest periods, to minimize strenuous activity, and to avoid high altitudes and extreme cold.
- Encourage client to avoid infections.
- Suggest a medical alert bracelet or card.

HEPATITIS PROFILE (HEPATITIS A, B, C, D, E)

Five major types of hepatitis virus can be identified through laboratory testing: hepatitis A virus (HAV), hepatitis B virus (HBV), hepatitis C virus (HCV), hepatitis D virus (HDV), and hepatitis E virus (HEV). These hepatitis viruses can be detected by testing serum antigens, antibodies, DNA, RNA, and/or the immunoglobulins IgG and IgM. The following table differentiates between the hepatitis viruses according to method of transmission, incubation time, jaundice, acute and chronic phases of the disease, carrier status, immunity, and mortality rate.

Hepatitis A virus (HAV).   Hepatitis A virus is transmitted primarily by oral–fecal contact. Jaundice is an early sign of HAV, which can occur a few days after the viral infection and may last up to 12 weeks. The antibodies to hepatitis A, anti-HAV-IgM and anti-HAV-IgG, are used to confirm the phase of the hepatitis A infection. Anti-HAV-IgM denotes an acute phase of the infection, while anti-HAV-IgG indicates recovery, past infection, or immunity. Approximately 45% to 50% of clients having HAV may have a positive anti-HAV-IgG for life.

Hepatitis B virus (HBV).

The hepatitis B virus was once called serum hepatitis. There are numerous laboratory tests for diagnosing the acute or chronic phase of HBV. These include hepatitis B surface antigen (HBsAg), antibody to HBsAg (anti-HBs), hepatitis Be antigen (HBeAg), antibody to HBeAg (anti-HBe), and antibody to core antigen (anti-HBc-total).

HbsAg: The earliest indicator for diagnosing hepatitis B viral infection is the hepatitis B surface antigen. This serum marker can be present as early as 2 weeks after being infected, and it persists during the acute phase of the infection. If it persists after 6 months, the client could have chronic hepatitis and be a carrier. The hepatitis B vaccine will not cause a positive HBsAg. Clients who have a positive HBsAg should NEVER donate blood.

Antibody to hepatitis B surface antigen (anti-HBs): With HBV, the acute phase of viral hepatitis B usually lasts for 12 weeks; therefore, HBsAg is absent and anti-HBs (antibodies to HBsAg) develop. This serum marker indicates recovery and immunity to the hepatitis B virus. An anti-HBs-IgM would determine if the client is still infectious. An anti-HBs titer of greater than 10 mIU/ml and without HBsAg presence, confirms that the client has recovered from HBV.

Hepatitis B e antigen (HBeAg): This serum marker occurs only with HBsAg. It usually appears 1 week after HBsAg and disappears before anti-HBs. If HBeAg is still present after 10 weeks, the client could be developing a chronic carrier state.

Antibody to HBeAg (anti-HBe): The presence of anti-HBe indicates the recovery phase.

Antibody to core antigen (anti-HBc): The anti-HBc may occur with a positive HBsAg approximately 4 to 10 weeks after acute HBV. An elevated anti-HBc-IgM titer indicates the acute infection process. Anti-HBc can detect clients who have been infected with HBV. This serum marker may persist for years, and clients with a positive anti-HBc should not give blood.

Hepatitis C virus (HCV).

HCV is formerly non-A, non-B hepatitis. It is transmitted parenterally. It occurs more frequently with post-transfusion hepatitis, but also should be considered with drug addicts, needle sticks, hemodialysis, and hemophilias. Approximately half of the acute cases of HCV become chronic carriers.

Antibody to hepatitis C virus (anti-HCV):   HCV is confirmed by the anti-HCV test. Anti-HCV does not indicate immunity as it can with anti-HBs and anti-HBe.

Hepatitis D virus (HDV).   Hepatitis D (delta) virus is transmitted parenterally. HDV can be present only with HBV. It is coated by the HBsAg and depends upon the HBV for replication. HDV is severe and usually occurs 7 to 14 days after an acute, severe HBV infection. It has a low occurrence rate except for IV drug abusers and clients receiving multiple transfusions. Its presence is in the acute phase of HBV or as a chronic carrier of HBV. Of all the types of hepatitis, it has the greatest incidence of fulminant hepatitis and death.

COMPARISON OF THE TYPES OF VIRAL HEPATITIS

Factors Associated with Hepatitis	*Types of Hepatitis*				
	HAV	*HBV*	*HCV*	*HDV*	*HEV*
Method of transmission	Enteral (oral-fecal) Water and food	Parenteral Intravenous Sexual Perinatal	Parenteral Sexual (possible) Perinatal	Parenteral Sexual (possible) Perinatal	Enteral (oral–fecal) Water and food
Incubation time	Abrupt onset; 2–12 weeks	Insidious onset; 6–24 weeks	Insidious onset; 2–26 weeks	Abrupt onset; 3–15 weeks	Abrupt onset; 2–8 weeks
Jaundice	Adult: 70%–80% Child: 10%	20%–40%	10%–25%	Varies	25%–60%
Hepatocellular carcinoma	None	Possible	Possible	Possible	None

(continued)

Types of Hepatitis

Factors Associated with Hepatitis	HAV	HBV	HCV	HDV	HEV
Acute disease: serum markers	Anti-HAV-IgM	HBsAg, HBeAg, Anti-HBe-IgM	Anti-HCV	HDAg	Anti-HEV
Chronic disease: serum markers	None	HBsAg	Anti-HCV (50% of cases)	Anti-HD	None
Infective state: serum markers	None (HAV-RNA)	HBsAg. HBeAg, HBV-DNA	Anti-HCV HCV-RNA	Anti-HD HDV-RNA	None (HEV-RNA)
Fulminant hepatitis	Very low	Very low	Very low	High	Low
Chronic carrier	None	HbsAg (low incidence in adult; high incidence in children)	High incidence	Anti-HDV, HDAg low incidence (10%–15%)	None
Immunity: serum markers	Anti-HAV total, Anti-HAV-IgG	Anti-HBs, Anti-HBc total	None	None	Anti-HEV
Mortality rate	Less than 2%	Less than 2%	Less than 2%	Less than 30%	Less than 2%

Hepatitis D antigen (HDAg):   Detection of HDAg and HDV-RNA indicates the acute phase of HBV and HDV infection. When HBsAg diminishes, so does HDAg. Anti-HDV appears later and may suggest chronic hepatitis D.

Hepatitis E virus (HEV).   HEV is transmitted by oral–fecal contact and not parenterally. The transmission can occur due to unsafe water as well as traveling in Mexico, Russia, India, or Africa. HEV is rare in the United States. Antibodies to hepatitis E (anti-HEV) detect hepatitis E infection.

HEPATITIS A VIRUS (HAV) ANTIBODY (HAV ab, ANTI-HAV) (SERUM)

Reference Values
None detected

Description.
Hepatitis A virus (HAV), previously called *infectious hepatitis,* usually is transmitted by oral–fecal contact. The incubation period for HAV is 2 to 6 weeks, unlike the 7 to 25 weeks for hepatitis B virus. HAV is not associated with chronic liver disease.

Antibodies to hepatitis A virus (IgM and IgG) indicate present or past infection and possible immunity. Anti-HAV IgM (Hav ab IgM) appears early after exposure and is detectable for 4 to 12 weeks. Anti-HAV IgG appears postinfection (greater than 4 weeks) and usually remains present for life. Approximately 50% of the population in the United States have a positive anti-HAV IgG.

Purpose
- To determine the presence or past infection of HAV

Clinical Problems
Positive: Hepatitis A virus (HAV)

Procedure
- No food or fluid restriction is required.
- Collect 3 to 5 ml of venous blood in a red-top tube.

Nursing Implications
- Obtain a history from the client of a possible contact with a person having HAV. Record if the client has eaten shellfish that may have been taken from contaminated water.

Client Teaching

- Explain to the client that HAV is normally transmitted by oral–fecal contact. Inform the client to wash hands after toileting.
- Alert the client that HAV can spread in institutions such as day-care centers, prisons, state mental institutions.

Positive Test

- Rest and nutritional dietary intake are indicated for several weeks according to the severity of the HAV. Fatigue is common. Rest periods are necessary as long as jaundice is present.
- Instruct the client that effective personal hygiene is very important.

HEPATITIS B SURFACE ANTIGEN (HBsAg) (SERUM)

HEPATITIS-ASSOCIATED ANTIGEN (HAA), AUSTRALIAN ANTIGEN TEST

Reference Values
Adult: Negative
Child: Negative

Description. The HBsAg test is done to determine the presence of hepatitis B virus in the blood in either an active or a carrier state. It is routinely performed on donor's blood to identify the hepatitis B antigen. Approximately 5% of persons with diseases other than hepatitis B (serum hepatitis), such as leukemia, Hodgkin's disease, and hemophilia, will have a positive HBsAg test.

In hepatitis B, the antigen in the serum can be detected 2 to 24 weeks (average 4 to 8 weeks) after exposure to the virus. The positive HBsAg may be present 2 to 6 weeks after onset of the clinical disease.

HBsAg test does not diagnose hepatitis A virus. Two tests for hepatitis A are anti-HAV-IgM (indicates an acute infection) and anti-HAV-IgG (indicates a past exposure).

Purposes

- To screen for the presence of hepatitis B in the client's blood
- To detect the presence of hepatitis B in donor's blood

Clinical Problems

Increased level (positive):   Hepatitis B, chronic hepatitis B; less common: hemophilia, leukemia

Procedure

- No food or fluid restriction is required.
- Collect 5 to 7 ml of venous blood in a red-top tube.

Nursing Implications

- Obtain a history of any previous hepatitis infection and report it to the physician.
- Handle blood specimen with strict aseptic technique.
- Follow the institution's isolation procedure in discarding disposable equipment.
- Observe for signs and symptoms of hepatitis (e.g., lethargy, anorexia, nausea and vomiting, fever, dark-colored urine, and jaundice).

Client Teaching

- Instruct the client to get plenty of rest, a nutritional diet, and fluids.

HERPES SIMPLEX VIRUS (HSV) ANTIBODY TEST (SERUM)

Reference Values

Negative: Less than 1:10

Positive: Early primary herpes simplex infection: 1:10 to 1:100. Late primary herpes simplex infection: 1:100 to 1:500. Latent herpes simplex infection: greater than 1:500. Fourfold titer increase between the acute and convalescent period.

Description.   Herpes simplex, a member of the herpesvirus group, is an infectious virus that produces antibody titers. The two types of herpes simplex are herpes simplex virus 1 (HSV-1) and herpes simplex virus 2

(HSV-2). HSV-1 infects the mouth, mostly the mucous membrane around the lip (cold sores), eyes, or upper respiratory tract. HSV-1 commonly occurs to the young as stomatitis (mouth ulcers) prior to the age of 20. HSV-2 is frequently referred to as genital herpes infecting the genitourinary tract. HSV-2 is transmitted primarily through sexual contact and can infect the newborn during vaginal delivery. Neonatal herpes may be mild, resulting in eye infection or skin rash, or it may result in a fatal systemic infection. Congenital herpes is not as common but may be acquired during early pregnancy, resulting in central nervous system disorders causing brain damage. Severe HSV infection can occur in immunosuppressed clients and neonates.

In addition to the serology blood test, a culture may be obtained for HSV-2 using the HERPCHEK test. The scrapings from suspected HSV genital vesicular lesions are obtained.

Antibodies for HSV-1 and HSV-2 begin to rise in 7 days and reach peak titers in 4 to 6 weeks after infection. HSV-IgM usually denotes acute infection, whereas HSV-IgG can indicate the convalescent phase. Those infected may have an increased titer level for 6 months after infection or it may persist throughout their life. Genital herpes (HSV-2) tends to be more severe and needs appropriate medical care, such as an antiviral drug.

Purposes
- To detect the presence of HSV
- To diagnose the convalescent phase of HSV

Clinical Problems
Positive titer: HSV-1, HSV-2, HSV-1 encephalitis, cervicitis, congenital herpes

Procedure
Serum
- No food or fluid restriction is required.
- Collect 3 to 5 ml of venous blood in a red-top tube. Avoid hemolysis. Deliver the blood sample to the laboratory within 1 h. Gloves should be worn when obtaining a blood specimen.

- Indicate on the laboratory slip to test for HSV-1 or HSV-2, or both.
- CSF may be obtained to determine the presence of HSV if HSV-1 encephalitis is suspected.

Culture
- Swab the infected area of the throat, skin, genital area, or eye.
- Obtain respiratory or body secretions through lavage or washing.
- Deliver the specimen immediately to the microbiology lab.

Nursing Implications
- Obtain a history from the client of a possible herpes infection of the mouth (HSV-1) or the genital area (HSV-2). Ascertain when the symptoms first occurred.
- Use gloves when inspecting the area as herpes simplex can be infectious.
- Avoid giving antiviral drugs until the specimen has been obtained.

Client Teaching
- Listen to the client's concerns. If the herpes simplex is HSV-2, the client should be encouraged to have her or his sexual partner tested for HSV-2.
- Encourage the pregnant client to speak with the appropriate health care provider. This helps in alleviating the client's fears and making the client well informed. The health care provider will most likely culture the genital area near the time of birthing.

HETEROPHILE ANTIBODY (SERUM), AND MONO-SPOT

Reference Values
Adult: Normal: less than 1:28 titer; abnormal: greater than 1:56 titer
Child: Same as adult
Elderly: Normal: slightly higher titer than adult

Description.   This is a test primarily for infectious mononucleosis (IM). IM is thought to be caused by the EB virus (EBV).

Heterophiles are a group of antibodies that react to sheep and horse RBCs and, if positive (titer), an agglutination occurs. Titers of 1:56 to 1:224 are highly suspicious of infectious mononucleosis; those of 1:224 or greater are positive for infectious mononucleosis. Elevated heterophile titers occur during the first 2 weeks, peak in 3 weeks, and remain elevated for 6 weeks.

Mono-Spot: There are several commercially prepared tests: Mono-Spot by Ortho Diagnostics; Monoscreen by Glaxo Smith Kline and Monotest by Wapole. Mono-Spot test is usually done first and, if positive, then the titer test.

Purposes
- To check for elevated heterophile titer
- To aid in the diagnosis of infectious mononucleosis

Clinical Problems
Increased level: Infectious mononucleosis, serum sickness, viral infections

Procedure
Heterophile antibody (HA) test: There are several HA tests: Paul–Bunnell test, Davidsohn differential test
- No food or fluid restriction is required.
- Collect 3 to 5 ml of venous blood in a red-top tube.

Mono-Spot test: Follow directions listed on the kit.

Nursing Implications
- Obtain a history of the client's contact with any person or persons recently diagnosed as having infectious mononucleosis.
- Observe for signs and symptoms of infectious mononucleosis (e.g., fever, sore throat, fatigue, swollen glands).
- Determine when the symptoms first occurred. A repeat heterophile or Mono-Spot test may be needed if the first was done too early.

Client Teaching
- Encourage the client to rest, drink fluids, and have a nutritional diet.

HEXOSAMINIDASE (TOTAL, A, AND A AND B) (SERUM AND AMNIOTIC FLUID)

Reference Values
Adult: Total: 5–20 units/l. Hexosaminidase A: 55%–80%

Description.   Hexosaminidase is a group of enzymes (isoenzymes A and B) responsible for the metabolism of gangliosides. It is found in brain tissue. Lack of the hexosaminidase A causes Tay-Sachs disease because of the accumulation of gangliosides in the brain. The total hexosaminidase may be normal or decreased. This test is used to confirm Tay-Sachs disease or to identify Tay-Sachs carriers.

Tay-Sachs disease is an autosomal-recessive disorder resulting in progressive destruction of central nervous system (CNS) cells. It is characterized by mental retardation, muscular weakness, and blindness. It affects primarily the Ashkenazic Jewish population. Death usually occurs before the age of 5 years.

Sandhoff's disease, a variant of Tay-Sachs, progresses more rapidly than Tay-Sachs disease. With this disorder, there is a deficiency of hexosaminidase A and B. It is not prevalent in any ethnic group.

Purposes
- To diagnose a deficit of hexosaminidase A (Tay-Sachs disease) or hexosaminidase A and B (Sandhoff's disease)
- To identify carriers of Tay-Sachs disease or Sandhoff's disease

Clinical Problems
Decreased level: Hexosaminidase A: Tay-Sachs disease. Hexosaminidase A and B: Sandhoff's disease

Procedure
- No food or fluid restriction is required.
- Collect 5 to 7 ml of venous blood in a red-top tube. Avoid hemolysis.
- Collect cord blood from the newborn.

Nursing Implications
Client Teaching

* Inform the Ashkenazic Jewish couple that the hexosaminidase screening test is to determine if they are Tay-Sachs carriers. Explain to the couple that it is a recessive trait and that both must carry the gene for their offspring to get Tay-Sachs disease.
* Have client communicate with health care providers such as the physician, nurse, and/or genetic counselor when both partners have a hexosaminidase A deficiency.
* Be supportive of the partners and child with Tay-Sachs disease. Answer questions or refer them to other health care providers.

HOMOCYSTEINE (SERUM)

Reference Values
Adult: 4–17 µmol/l (fasting)

Description.   Homocysteine is a byproduct of protein. It is an amino acid found in the blood and is formed when eating such protein as eggs, chicken, beef, or cheddar cheese. A deficiency of certain B vitamins, such as B_6, B_{12}, and folate (folic acid), can lead to an accumulation of homocysteine.

A high level of homocysteine has been linked to cardiovascular disease, stroke, and possibly Alzheimer's disease. Also it may promote blood clotting. Research has suggested that an increase in serum homocysteine can damage the inner lining of blood vessels and promote a thickening and loss of flexibility in the blood vessel. Persons who have undergone an angioplasty and have a high level of serum homocysteine generally have restenosis or repeated blockage of the coronary artery. Those who have a low serum homocysteine level usually have a lower rate of reblockage. It has been suggested that a person having an angioplasty take B vitamins following the procedure to decrease the homocysteine level and thus hopefully lower the incidence of restenosis.

Purposes
- To detect the risk of cardiovascular disease including myocardial infarction, stroke
- To detect a possible increased risk of Alzheimer's disease

Clinical Problems
Increased level: Coronary artery disease (CAD), heart attack (MI), thrombosis, stroke, possible Alzheimer's disease, folic acid deficiency
Decreased level: Certain vitamin B drugs, folate

Procedure
- Food and fluids are restricted until after the test.
- Collect 3 to 5 ml of venous blood in a red-top tube.

Factors Affecting Laboratory Results
- Penicillamine reduces the serum homocysteine levels.

Nursing Implications
- Obtain a dietary history of the client. Note if the client takes vitamins, especially B complex vitamins and folic acid.
- Report if the client is having symptoms of cardiovascular disease (e.g., pain).

Client Teaching
- Instruct the client with a high level of serum homocysteine to take vitamins B_6, B_{12}, and folate with the health care provider's consent. These vitamins help to lower the serum homocysteine level.
- Explain to the client that certain foods, such as cheddar cheese, eggs, and beef, can increase the serum homocysteine level when consumed in large quantities.
- Encourage the client to repeat the serum homocysteine test when the test is elevated and measures are taken to lower the serum level.

HUMAN CHORIONIC GONADOTROPIN (HCG) (SERUM AND URINE)

PREGNANCY TEST

Reference Values

Values may be expressed as international units/ml or ng/ml. Check with your laboratory.

Adult: Serum: nonpregnant female: less than 0.01 international units/ml

Pregnant (Weeks)	Values	
1	0.01–0.04	international units/ml
2	0.03–0.10	international units/ml
4	0.10–1.0	international units/ml
5–12	10–100	international units/ml
13–25	10–30	international units/ml
26–40	5–15	international units/ml

Urine: Nonpregnant female: negative
Pregnant: 1–12 weeks: 6,000–500,000 international units/24 h
Many over-the-counter (OTC) pregnancy kits available.
Usually tested 3 days after missed menstrual period.

Description.   HCG is a hormone produced by the placenta. In pregnancy, HCG appears in the blood and urine 14 to 26 days after conception, and the HCG concentration peaks in approximately 8 to 12 weeks. After the first trimester of pregnancy, HCG production declines. HCG is not found in nonpregnant females, in death of the fetus, or after 3 to 4 days postpartum.

Purposes

- To determine if the client is pregnant
- To detect a threatened abortion or dead fetus

Clinical Problems

Decreased level: Nonpregnant, dead fetus, postpartum (3 to 4 days), incomplete abortion, threatened abortion

Increased level: Pregnancy, hydatidiform mole, chorionepithelioma, choriocarcinoma, erythroblastosis fetalis

Drugs that may increase HCG value: Anticonvulsants, hypnotics, phenothiazines, antiparkinsonism drugs

Procedure
Serum
- Perform the pregnancy test no earlier than 5 days after the first missed menstrual period.
- Collect 3 to 5 ml of venous blood in a red-top tube. Avoid hemolysis.

Urine
- Restrict fluids for 8 to 12 h; no food is restricted.
- Take a morning urine specimen (60 ml) with specific gravity greater than 1.010 to the laboratory immediately. A 24-h urine collection may be requested.
- Instruct client to follow directions when using commercial kit.
- Avoid blood in the urine, as false positives could occur.

Factors Affecting Laboratory Results
- Diluted urine (specific gravity less than 1.010) could cause a false-negative test result.
- Protein and blood in the urine could cause false-positive test results.

Nursing Implications
Client Teaching
- Ask the client when she had her last period. The test should be done 5 or more days after the missed period to avoid a false negative. Blood in the urine can cause false-positive result.
- Listen to client's concerns.

HUMAN IMMUNODEFICIENCY VIRUS TYPE 1 (HIV-1) OR HIV* (SERUM)

Note: The retrovirus designated human immunodeficiency virus type 2 (HIV-2) exhibits a pattern of transmission, and causes clinical disease

---

*This test contributed by Jane Purnell Taylor, RN, MSN, updated by Joyce Kee.

features, similar to those of HIV-1. Prevalent in Africa, with equal numbers of infected men and women, HIV-2 is generally spread through heterosexual contact as a classical sexually transmitted disease, often concurrent with other genital lesions. HIV-2 cases in the United States are currently more limited. The long-term concern is that the African pattern may, in the future, be duplicated in North America.

Reference Values
Antibody Screening
HIV-1/2 antibody screen (ELISA, EIA)
Adult: Seronegative for antibodies to HIV-1/2; nonreactive
Child: Seronegative for antibodies to HIV-1/2; nonreactive
HIV-1 Western blot (confirmatory test that directly detects HIV viral gene proteins)
HIV-2 Western blot (confirmatory test that directly detects HIV viral gene proteins)
Adult: Negative
Child: Negative

Antigen Screening
HIV-1 p24 Antigen
Adult: Negative for p24 antigen of HIV; nonreactive
Child: Negative for p24 antigen of HIV; nonreactive
(*Note:* There is no HIV-2 p24 antigen test; confirmatory test for the HIV-1 p24 antigen is a neutralization.)
Viral load tests: Sensitive assay that measures levels of HIV's ribonucleic acid (RNA) in plasma (to predict disease course). Uses polymerase chain reaction (PCR) to amplify HIV RNA. Used as a marker for basing treatment decisions and evaluating effectiveness of anti-HIV drug therapy (rechecked 4–8 weeks after changes in drug therapy as monitoring technique). Expressed as the number of copies of HIV RNA in a 1-ml sample of plasma
Low numbers: Represents suppressed replication
High numbers: Represents increased replication and disease progression

Description.   The retrovirus HIV-1, identified as the cause of acquired immunodeficiency syndrome (AIDS), was first recognized in 1981. However, it is now believed that HIV has existed in human populations for at least 70 years, based on genetic work comparing genetic composition of many current HIV strains and extrapolation back to a common origin. In 26 years since HIV was first identified (June 1981), the HIV has killed more than 25 million people worldwide and has infected 40 million others. In 2005, the number of HIV-positive persons in the United States was 100,000. The infection is expressed along a progressive continuum extending from clinically asymptomatic (although seropositive for HIV-1 antibodies) to expression of a severely damaged (suppressed) immune system [due to T-helper lymphocyte (T4 lymphocyte) destruction] manifested by clinical signs and symptoms, altered laboratory values, and increased susceptibility to AIDS-defining opportunistic infections (including *pneumocystis carinii pneumonia;* chronic cryptosporidiosis; toxoplasmosis; cryptococcosis; disseminated histoplasmosis; mycobacterial infection; disseminated cytomegaloviral infection; chronic mucocutaneous or disseminated herpes simplex viral infection; and esophageal, bronchial, or pulmonary candidiasis that rarely cause disease in an immune-competent person) and rarer forms of cancer (including Kaposi's sarcoma and lymphomas [Non-Hodgkin lymphoma and primary brain lymphoma]).

The incubation time between HIV infection and the development of HIV-1 related disease is highly individualized. Research shows that HIV multiplies rapidly with high viral levels in peripheral blood during the first few weeks of infection. HIV viral antigen may become detectable within approximately 2 to 3 weeks after infection. The outcome is a decrease in CD4+ T lymphocyte count, increased viral load, and the stimulation of the body's immune response; as antibodies to HIV and new CD4+ T lymphocyte cells are produced, the amount of viral load decreases. During the period of initial infection, it is estimated that about half of infected individuals remain asymptomatic, whereas others may experience an influenza-type illness (low-grade fever, muscle aches, sweating, rash, sore throat, headache, fatigue, swollen lymph nodes). These flu-like symptoms may last up to 12 weeks; medical care is seldom sought during this period and possible HIV infection is seldom considered as well. The client recovers, but during this 2 to 12 week period, antibodies against HIV are formed as part of the immune response. The Centers for Disease Control and Prevention counsel that the average length of time for production of antibodies to HIV is 25 days (some earlier and some later) but that most individuals will seroconvert by 3 months, allowing for antibody detection using the ELISA, EIA antibody tests, and Western blot confirmatory test. Depending on individual variables, many clients next enter into a symptomless stage of infection that may last 8 to 11 years on average, during which HIV infection may be unknowingly transmitted. Thus, knowledge of one's HIV status and prevention of transmission is critically important. Addition of the HIV-1 p24 antigen test may identify HIV infection in an individual within 2 weeks (approximately a week earlier than the anti-HIV-1/2 test), thus narrowing the vulnerable period when the virus may be passed to others while antibody-based screening tests cannot detect it. Care is called for, however, because a negative test may mean that there is not yet detectable viral levels.

In 1993, the CDC revised the system by which HIV infection and the definition of AIDS is classified to include the CD4+ T lymphocyte count as a marker for the degree of immunosuppression related to HIV. This new definition adds to the previous operational definition of AIDS that included 23 clinical conditions. Now, the definition includes those individuals with pulmonary tuberculosis, recurrent pneumonia (within a 12-month period), and invasive cervical cancer in addition to laboratory confirmation of HIV infection with a less than 200 CD4+ T lymphocyte/μL or a CD4+ T lymphocyte percentage of total lymphocytes less than 14%. It is expected that the new working definition will promote earlier diagnosis of those at risk and that treatment modalities will be instituted.

Close monitoring and treatment regimens using approved antiretroviral drugs in an individualized "cocktail" combination, known as highly active antiretroviral therapy (HAART), are employed with the goal of reducing viral load and preserving immune function. Included are *protease inhibitors* affecting viral reproduction by interfering with the needed enzyme protease (e.g., ritonavir) in combination. Also included are nucleoside/nucleotide (e.g., zidovudine) and non-nucleoside *reverse transcriptase inhibitors* (affecting enzyme reverse transcriptase needed for HIV to make copies of itself). Tenofovir and emtricitabine are the hope for preventing high-risk persons from becoming infected. The "1-pill HIV cocktail" was approved by the FDA in July 2006. It contains three drugs combined in a once-a-day pill called Atripla, and it is especially effective in treating HIV-1, which is the most common type of HIV. The drug costs over $1,000 for a 30-day supply. The difficulty with drug treatment is that the virus can mutate and can become immune to the drug. Hopefully with the use of multiple drugs in one or more pills, the virus will not become immune as it can be to one specific drug.

Today in the United States, many of the HIV-1 cases are becoming more manageable. Major hurdles to be overcome include development of viral strains resistant to treatment; overwhelmingly expensive drug therapies involving a complex treatment regimen (important to both individuals and the developing countries most afflicted by the AIDS epidemic); product availability; and the ability of the virus to remain hidden (nondetectable) throughout the body (in the brain, testes, lymph nodes) outside the bloodstream. There is still no magic-bullet vaccine available; the first AIDS vaccine to reach human trials was pronounced a failure in early 2003. The infection remains preventable, possibly chronically manageable, but not curable at the present time.

It is estimated by the Center for Disease Control and Prevention that one million Americans are HIV positive; however, many—perhaps 25%— of these individuals (having moderate to high risk factors) are unaware that they are infected, potentially jeopardizing their own health and exposing others. About 40,000 new infections occur each year. AIDS has become the fifth leading cause of death for those aged 25 to 44. A decline is due largely to advances made in treatment therapies. Caution is needed, however, as the hoped-for continued rate of decline (in both new AIDS cases and AIDS-related deaths) is reportedly slowing. These findings raise concern that the benefits of the combination drug therapies referred to as highly active antiretroviral therapy (HAART) in controlling viral progression may have peaked and begun to level off.

As of June 2001, decreases in the number of children diagnosed with AIDS continue as a result of intensive perinatal transmission prevention in the United States; previously up to 91% of pediatric AIDS cases were perinatally acquired. Heterosexual women, minorities (Black Americans, Hispanics), and young adults remain among the most rapidly escalating groups of affected individuals. Overall, of the total number of people with HIV, increases continue to be observed in the heterosexual community, but, as a risk group, men who have sex with men (MSM) show the greatest number of new infections (42%) followed by heterosexuals (33%) and injection drug use (25%). Evidence suggests also that male-to-female transmission of HIV is more likely based on anatomical and social factors including lack of use of barrier-type birth control methods or barrier-method failure. In addition, the baby of an untreated HIV-positive pregnant woman has a 21% to 25% chance of being infected before or during birth, or afterward, if breastfed. Child-to-child transmission of HIV-1 infection in school and day-care settings is rare, as CDC guidelines in regard to injected children remain effective. Risk of HIV infection in the health care setting is small. A national campaign to motivate health care settings to select newer and safer products (particularly protected or needleless equipment) in addition to use of standard precautions is ongoing.

Worldwide, the World Health Organization (WHO) estimates that approximately 95% of new cases occur in individuals who live in the developing world, including Southeast Asia and sub-Saharan Africa, with United Nations estimates of the total number currently infected at 30 million. By the end of 2010, the number of orphaned African children under age 15 who will have lost one or both parents to AIDS is expected to be over 20 million. The pandemic will be stopped only through a reexamination of culture (including gender and sexual customs) and implementation of major prevention strategies, including strategies to promote clean medical care procedures.

Although HIV-1 has been isolated from blood, semen, saliva, vaginal secretions, breast milk, tears, cerebrospinal fluid, amniotic fluid, and urine, actual transmission occurs via infected lymphocytes carried by blood, semen, vaginal secretions, and breast milk. Those *at risk* for acquiring HIV infection include noninfected persons who have unprotected direct sexual contact (vaginal, oral, or rectal) with an infected person of either sex; those who share sex toys; multiple partners; men who have sex with men (MSM); persons with hemophilia or related clotting disorders who have received clotting factor concentrates; other recipients of infected blood or blood products (particularly prior to 1985); persons who have had, or have been treated for, syphilis or gonorrhea during the past 12 months; persons who have had a positive screening test for syphilis in the past 12 months without a negative confirmatory test; persons who have been in jail within the past 12 months; those who share infected needles with others as a component of illicit IV drug use; persons who subsequently have sexual contact with someone included in one or more of these groups; and fetuses or neonates exposed to an infected mother during the perinatal period (possibly secondary to maternal IV drug use or maternal heterosexual contact with an IV drug user).

Screening of blood products by blood banks in the United States was instituted in 1985 using the enzyme-linked immunosorbent assay (ELISA).

Blood banks are required to test donors for antibodies to HIV-1 and -2. Blood banks have also implemented six additional infectious disease tests to ensure safety of the blood reaching hospitals nationally. In March 1996, the FDA-approved HIV-1 p24 antigen test was added to help identify infection earlier (because a person can be infected and have a negative antibody test). To help eliminate the period of risky silent infections in donated blood the FDA has approved the use of the nucleic acid test (NAT), which detects viral genes (genetic RNA) rather than antibodies or antigens. Further work continues to be done using polymerase chain reaction (PCR) technology. Screening of donors and public education has also been enhanced to assure the public concerning blood safety. All blood that tests positive is destroyed. Donors notified of confirmed-positive test results are included on a permanent deferral list and asked not to donate in the future. Nationally, the safety record is positive; the risk of contracting HIV via blood transfusion in this era is estimated at 1 in 500,000 to 800,000 transfusions.

Purposes
- To screen for the presence of HIV infection
- To monitor HIV during drug therapy

Clinical Problems
Seropositive test: Blood shows evidence of infection; blood test detects antibodies to HIV-1/2; or viral antigen is detected (p24 antigen of HIV). Recall that a positive test indicative of HIV infection does not diagnose AIDS (which is defined as a clinical diagnosis with defining characteristics). HIV infection is expressed on a continuum from seropositive asymptomatic infection to disease expression. *Note:* Diagnosing HIV infection in children born to HIV-infected mothers is complicated by maternal antibodies that transplacentally affect the fetus, giving a positive HIV antibody result at birth (although only 16% to 25% in North America and Europe are truly infected); the antibody usually becomes undetectable by 9 months of age (occasionally as long as 18 months). Thus, standard antibody tests are not reliable, and polymerase chain reaction (PCR) and virus culture are the most specific and sensitive means for detection of infection in children whose mothers are infected. These additional tests can identify 90% of actually infected babies within the first 2 months of birth.

Procedure

- A signed consent form for the HIV-1/2 antibody screen is usually required and should include appropriate pre- and post-counseling.
- No food or fluid restriction is required.
- Collect 5 to 10 ml of venous blood in a red-top tube.

Two tests are most commonly employed for HIV-1/2 antibody screening (not for the virus itself). These include ELISA and EIA (enzyme immunoassay). ELISA testing is reliable, specific, and highly sensitive. When a positive HIV-1 test result occurs, the test is generally repeated twice on the same sample; if two out of three of these tests are positive, an HIV-1 Western blot is done as well as an HIV-2 antibody screen. If the HIV-2 antibody screen is positive, an HIV-2 Western blot is performed. A second quickly performed confirmatory test commonly used is the immunofluorescence assay (IFA), but it is slightly less reliable than the Western blot. Collectively, when the ELISA plus Western blot show a persistently positive outcome, the specificity and sensitivity rates are both 99%, and the accuracy rate is 99%. False-positive Western blot results in low-risk populations are possible but less likely than with ELISA. False positives may be retested using an alternate laboratory; false-negative results are usually noted when testing is done prior to seroconversion.

If the client tests positive (reactive) when screening is for the HIV-1 p24 antigen, the test is repeated twice more on the same sample. A separate confirmatory test (called a neutralization) may be performed. If a client tests positive for the antigen but doesn't neutralize, both an antibody and an antigen test may be redone in approximately 4 weeks; at 8 weeks, just an antibody test may be done. It must be recalled that the HIV-1 p24 antigen generally disappears from the blood during the asymptomatic phase and is undetectable.

Additional Information Related to Antibody Testing Available

Some individuals who are willing to be tested may exhibit reluctance on the basis of having to have blood samples taken. These persons may elect to have a test done using either urine or oral fluid samples. The *urine test* is not as sensitive or specific as is blood testing, but the process is similar using the EIA with confirmatory Western blot. Testing is ordered and the result is sent to the client's physician. The *oral-fluid test (Ora Sure c)* is

FDA approved and involves collecting a sample of oral secretions between the gums and cheeks with a collection device followed by analysis using the EIA and confirmatory Western blot as indicated. The test is available at numerous HIV testing sites (locations available via CDC hotline).

In addition, on November 7, 2002, the FDA announced the approval of a new *rapid test* for HIV antibody known as *Ora Quick Rapid HIV-1 Antibody.* The test uses a simple fingerstick giving results in 20 min or less once the sample is mixed in a vial with a developing solution. If HIV-1 antibodies are present, colored red/purple lines appear and the test is indicated as reactive, necessitating confirmation with an additional test of a different type. The data indicate that the rapid test is equally accurate (99.6%) when compared with the EIA. Blood donors are *not* screened using this test. The test was designed to fill a gap in the numbers of people who get tested by other means but do not follow up and obtain results due to the additional time involved. The new test provides an opportunity for immediate client counseling related to risk behavior. Recently, the number of sites where the new rapid test will be available has increased and includes physicians' offices and counseling centers for HIV. The rapid testing is expected to become very helpful in addressing perinatal transmission issues at the level of labor and delivery (if not detected during pregnancy), allowing laboring women to be started on antiretroviral agents and knowledge-based plans for delivery made to protect the fetus.

In addition to the present rapid test, two additional rapid tests are also available: (1) Reveal HIV-1 Antibody Test and (2) Single Use Diagnostic System for HIV-1.

Last, there is only one home-based test kit (Home Access Test), which requires a blood sample be sent to a laboratory with counseling made available and results returned via an ID number provided via phone. There are no FDA-approved home tests that provide for self-testing and results interpretation based on concerns about accuracy and psychological issues.

Nursing Implications

- Ascertain the purpose of being tested for each person screened and assess the risk potential for HIV using information provided. Include sexual histories for older persons in risk assessments as well as the younger ones.

- Obtain a signed consent form from the client for HIV antibody test and/or antigen screening test. If client is pregnant or intrapartum, document consent and/or nonconsent for testing, using an "opt-out" approach.
- Provide clients being screened for HIV antibody or antigen with comprehensive pretest counseling, protection for confidential information obtained, and consistently accurate and comprehensive posttest education, support, and follow-up. Be mindful that health care organizations must now be in compliance with the Health Insurance Portability and Accountability Act of 1996 (HIPAA), limiting who has access to protected health information and requires privacy-maintaining strategies to be in effect.
- Become knowledgeable about commercially available HIV home blood test kits in order to be able to accurately provide advice for clients who may elect self-testing and experience a variety of positive and negative issues as an outcome.
- Recognize the role of education as a highly effective preventive strategy.
- Develop a full knowledge of HIV infection and AIDS-related diseases in order to adequately address actual and potential client concerns in the role of nurse-educator.
- Be prepared to clearly explain and clarify the meaning of test results for clients who may be experiencing a situational crisis associated with the testing process and/or outcome.
- Monitor laboratory reports for indication of decreasing CD4+ T-lymphocyte cell counts; inform the health care provider.
- Assess for signs and symptoms related to clinical progression toward a depressed immune system, including profound involuntary weight loss, chronic diarrhea, chronic weakness, and intermittent or constant fever.
- Implement standard precautions, which combine the major features of universal (blood and body fluid) precautions (designed to reduce risk of blood-borne pathogen transmission) and body substance isolation (designed to reduce the risk of transmission of pathogens from moist body substances), and apply them to all clients regardless of diagnosis or presumed infection status; these precautions apply to blood, all body fluids, secretions, and excretions (except sweat),

regardless of whether visible blood is present, nonintact skin, and mucous membranes.

- In obstetric settings, gloves should be worn whenever handling placentas; also when handling newborns who have not had initial baths; when changing diapers; obtaining urine or fecal samples; and during suctioning, heelsticks for blood glucose determination, and vitamin K administration. Unique to the obstetrical setting, these aspects are included in standard precautionary care.

- Request and use tight-fitting collection containers for all laboratory specimens involving blood and body fluids, followed by placing containers into plastic cover bags for safe handling and transport.

- Be nonjudgmental with HIV/AIDS clients and their families with regard to how the illness may have been acquired. Be prepared to help offer social support.

- Recognize that infants born to HIV/AIDS-infected mothers will exhibit and maintain a positive HIV antibody response (reflecting maternal antibodies) for up to 18 months. However, only 16% to 25% are truly infected. Those who do become infected become symptomatic more quickly than adults and may have a decreased survival period. Many children (both infected and noninfected) may be orphaned if their mothers die, necessitating interdisciplinary planning for the family.

- Recognize actual and/or at-risk clients for HIV/AIDS. HIV-infected clients should be screened for the presence of coinfection with TB. Anergy testing may be necessary.

- Become knowledgeable concerning institutional policies in compliance with CDC guidelines and the OSHA Blood-borne Pathogen Standard concerning needlestick/penetrating injuries and blood or secretion splash incidents.

- Screen women for the presence of frequent vaginal yeast infections.

- Review client records for adequate immunization status; recognize that HIV-infected clients are also high-risk for coinfection with hepatitis B virus. Screen client records for documentation of hepatitis B vaccine; inform the health care provider of findings; tetanus booster should be current within 10 years; documentation should show receipt of annual flu shot and a single dose of pneumococcal vaccine.

Client Teaching

- Provide clients with an overview about HIV and the testing available for antibodies. Inform clients that June 27 each year is National HIV Testing Day, a national campaign to encourage the untested to "take the test, take control." Testing sites are available via the CDC hotline or Web site. Also stress that most women who are tested do *not* have the virus.

- Explain to the client that if a first HIV test indicates a positive response, a repeat test and confirmatory tests will need to be made prior to reaching any conclusions.

- Explain to the client that a confirmed positive HIV antibody test indicates exposure to HIV that has stimulated an immune system response; the person is infected and able to transmit the infection. Explain that a negative test is not a guarantee that infection has not occurred; variables include the time frame in relation to exposure and when the test is done. For both outcomes, plan strategies with the client to ensure risk reduction related to HIV for both self and others; include relationship and sexual boundary setting as part of the discussion.

- Discuss the meaning of test results for the client's desired or planned life events (e.g., sexual contact, marriage, childbearing, breastfeeding, etc.). Refer the client to other health professionals as necessary. Provide the National AIDS Hotline phone number (1-800-342-AIDS) (1-800-342-2437); if needed, suggest Spanish AIDS Hotline (1-800-342-SIDA); Hearing Impaired AIDS Hotline (TDD Service; 1-800-243-7889). Provide these Internet Web sites: American Social Health Association (www.ashastd.org) and Centers for Disease Control (www.cdc.gov/HIV).

- Explain that there is no definitive cure for HIV/AIDS; however, well-being and survival are effected through early intervention strategies, including early diagnosis and the use of combination drug therapy.

- Teach awareness and prevention to at-risk clients who demonstrate knowledge deficits about HIV/AIDS, particularly in primary care settings.

- Stress elimination of substance abuse, especially involving needles and syringes, and to expose oneself to only low-risk sexual behavior as a preventive strategy; explain that sexual abstinence is 100%

effective. Stress that condom use is also recommended for oral-penile and oral-vaginal contact.

- Suggest that clients facing elective surgery discuss autologous transfusion with their health care providers to allay fears related to blood transfusions. Stress the current safety record related to blood transfusions.
- Explain to members in the community that casual contact with a person with HIV/AIDS does not put them at high risk for contracting HIV/AIDS. However, intimate sexual contact (oral, genital, rectal) with a person with HIV/AIDS puts the individual at high risk.
- Address anxiety and fear reactions about HIV/AIDS within the public sector. Stress that HIV/AIDS is not spread by talking to, shaking hands with, sharing glasses with, embracing, sharing spoons with, or sharing a household with an HIV/AIDS-infected client. Stress that there are no known cases transmitted by general mouth-to-mouth kissing with intact mucous membranes, as saliva is low in lymphocytes; nor spread by insect bites.
- Encourage clients with HIV/AIDS to identify persons with whom they have had sexual contact. At times, clients are more likely to tell the nurse names of partners than they are to tell the health care provider.
- Encourage childbearing-age women and all pregnant clients to voluntarily and routinely be tested for their HIV status to prolong life (if HIV positive), prevent HIV transmission to newborns during pregnancy, assist with childbearing decisions, and allow for early intervention with any subsequent offspring.
- Explain to HIV-positive pregnant clients that the American College of Obstetricians and Gynecologists (ACOG) currently recommends (effective July 1999) that *all* HIV-positive pregnant women should be offered scheduled C-section deliveries at 38 weeks' gestation to decrease the risk of transmission to the newborn; also that HIV risk to the infant can be further reduced to less than 2% with a scheduled C-section.
- Inform infected pregnant women who labor with an anticipated vaginal delivery that internal fetal monitoring will not be used during labor (to maintain fetal skin integrity and prevent exposure to potentially bloody amniotic fluid).

- Explain that breastfeeding is permitted if a client is initially negative and remains so at the time of delivery; breastfeeding is not initiated when the mother is untested for HIV or determined to be positive, because breast milk contains HIV-infected lymphocytes, colostrum has high concentrations, and maternal nipples may become sore and crack, with potential HIV exposure for the neonate.
- Inform families that HIV-infected infants and children will need to receive all routine immunizations *except* oral polio vaccine. Only injectable killed polio vaccine should be given. These babies should also receive flu shots in the fall of the year. Hepatitis B vaccine should also be given.
- Inform women clients to seek gynecologic evaluation if an infection is persistent and/or unresponsive to nonprescription treatment (e.g., Monistat-7 and/or Gyne-Lotrimin). Teach clients to wear cotton underwear and avoid douching. Tell clients to not douche prior to a gynecologic examination because PAP tests and specimen quality may be adversely affected.
- Advise clients not to use the toothbrushes or razors of high-risk or HIV/AIDS-infected individuals because of the possibility of blood contamination; women should be taught to safely dispose of menstrual blood-containing items.
- Inform clients not to share needles and syringes used for tattooing and/or body piercing.
- Clarify for clients the availability of newer rapid HIV tests. These tests are designed to detect antibodies; however, antibodies may not be present up to 3 months after exposure. The rapid test does not mean an individual may be tested immediately following exposure via risky behavior.
- Stress how the medications are to be taken by the clients placed on a complex medication regimen following HIV/AIDS diagnosis. Explain how these medications address and control viral load levels and thus the need for them to adhere to the medication plan.
- Be prepared to individualize and discuss specific personal behavior and adherence to drug regimen with each client. Emphasize the importance of following disease progression and immune status by systematic viral load measurement and CD4+ cell counts.

HUMAN LEUKOCYTE ANTIGENS (HLA) (SERUM)

HLA TYPING, ORGAN-DONOR TISSUE TYPING

Reference Values

Histocompatibility match or nonmatch; no norms

Description.   The human leukocyte antigens (HLA) are on the surface membranes of leukocytes, platelets, and many tissue cells. This antigenic system is very complex as it relates to tissue compatibility for transplantation and immune response. There are five different antigens that belong to the HLA system; A, B, C, D, and DR (D-related). Each of these antigens contains many groups (20 A antigens, 40 B antigens, 8 C antigens, 12 D antigens, and 10 DR antigens) that can be HLA phenotyped to determine histocompatibility.

The four main purposes for HLA testing are: (1) organ transplantation; (2) transfusion; (3) disease association, such as juvenile rheumatoid arthritis, ankylosing spondylitis, myasthenia gravis, Addison's disease, and insulin-dependent diabetes mellitus; and (4) paternity testing may be verified when the putative father has one haplotype (phenotyping) that is identical to the child. This test may be useful in genetic counseling when associated with susceptibility to certain diseases.

Purposes

- To screen for histocompatibility in tissue typing
- To determine paternity of the child

Clinical Problems

Positive histocompatibility: Tissue compatibility for grafts and organ transplants, father of the child

Procedure

- No food or fluid restriction is required.
- Collect 5 to 7 ml of venous blood in a green-top tube. Avoid hemolysis. Blood samples should be analyzed immediately.

Factors Affecting Laboratory Results

• Blood transfusion in the last 3 days could affect test results.

Nursing Implications
Client Teaching

• Encourage the client to express concerns related to the health problem.
• Listen to client's and family's concerns. Refer questions to appropriate health professionals if necessary.

HUMAN PLACENTAL LACTOGEN (hPL) (PLASMA OR SERUM)

CHORIONIC SOMATOMAMMOTROPIN

Reference Values
Nonpregnant female: Less than 0.5 µg/ml
Pregnant female

Weeks of Gestation	Reference Values
5–7	1.0 mcg/ml
8–27	Less than 4.6 mcg/ml
28–31	2.4–6.0 mcg/ml
32–35	3.6–7.7 mcg/ml
36–term	5.0–10.0 mcg/ml

Male: Less than 0.5 mcg/ml

Description.   Human placental lactogen (hPL) is a hormone secreted by the placenta and can be detected in the maternal blood after 5 weeks of gestation. During pregnancy, the hPL increases slowly. This test is useful for evaluating placental function and fetal well-being, especially from the 28th week to term. A decreased hPL level, less than 4.0 mcg/ml, during the third trimester of pregnancy is indicative of fetal distress, retarded fetal growth, threatened abortion, toxemia, or post-fetal maturity. A serum estriol and nonstress test are frequently ordered to verify the hPL test result.

Purposes
- To evaluate placental function
- To determine fetal well-being after 28th week to term

Clinical Problems
Decreased level: Fetal distress, toxemia of pregnancy, threatened abortion, trophoblastic neoplastic disease (hydatidiform mole, choriocarcinoma)
Increased level: Multiple pregnancy, diabetes mellitus, bronchogenic carcinoma, liver tumor, lymphoma

Procedure
- No food or fluid restriction is required.
- Collect 5 to 7 ml of venous blood in a red- or green-top tube. Avoid hemolysis.
- hPL value fluctuates; therefore, the test may need to be repeated.

Nursing Implications
- Record the gestation week on the laboratory slip.
- Correlate the serum/plasma human placental lactogen result with the serum or urine estriol level. The hPL value can fluctuate daily, so the hPL test is usually repeated. Other tests for detecting fetal distress may also be ordered.
- Be supportive of the client and family. Allow the client time to express her concerns. Be a good listener. Direct appropriate questions to other health professionals, such as the physician or midwife.

17-HYDROXYCORTICOSTEROIDS (17-OHCS) (URINE)

PORTER-SILBER CHROMOGENS

Reference Values
Adult: Male: 3–12 mg/24 h; female: 2–10 mg/24 h; average: 2–12 mg/24 h
Child: Infant to 1 year: less than 1 mg/24 h; 2 to 4 years: 1–2 mg/24 h; 5–12 years: 6–8 mg/24 h
Elderly: Lower than adult

Description.   17-OHCS are metabolites of adrenocortical steroid hormones, mostly of cortisol, and are excreted in the urine. Because the excretion of the metabolites is diurnal, varying in rate of excretion, a 24-h urine specimen is necessary for accuracy of test results. This test is useful for assessing adrenocortical hormone function.

Purposes
* To assess adrenocortical hormone function
* To detect disorders caused by deficit or excess of adrenocortical hormone

Clinical Problems
Decreased level: Addison's disease, androgenital syndrome, hypopituitarism, hypothyroidism, liver disease

Drugs that may decrease urine 17-OHCS: Calcium gluconate, dexa methasone (Decadron), phenytoin (Dilantin), promethazine (Phenergan), reserpine (Serpasil)

Increased level: Cushing's syndrome, adrenal cancer, hyperpituitarism, hyperthyroidism, extreme stress, eclampsia

Drugs that may increase urine 17-OHCS: Antibiotics (penicillin and erythromycin), cortisone, acetazolamide (Diamox), ascorbic acid, thiazide diuretics, phenothiazides, digoxin, estrogen, colchicine, hydroxyzine (Atarax), iodides, oral contraceptives, quinidine, spironolactone (Aldactone), paraldehyde

Procedure
* Withhold drugs (with health care provider's approval) for 3 days before the test to prevent false results. Any drugs given should be listed on the laboratory slip.
* No food or fluid is restricted except for coffee and tea. Fluid intake should be encouraged.
* Collect urine in a large container/bottle, and add an acid preservative to prevent bacterial degradation of the steroids. The urine collection should be refrigerated if no preservative is added. No toilet paper or feces should be in the urine.

- Label container with client's name, date, and exact time of collection (e.g., 9/23/09, 7:30 AM to 9/24/09, 7:30 AM).

Nursing Implications
- Encourage the client to increase fluid intake, except coffee, during the 24-h test.
- If levels are decreased, observe for signs and symptoms of hypoadrenalism (e.g., fatigue, weakness, weight loss, bronze coloration of the skin, postural hypotension, cardiac dysrhythmia, craving for salty food, and fasting hypoglycemia).
- If levels are elevated, observe for signs and symptoms of hyperadrenalism (e.g., "moon face," "buffalo hump," fluid retention, hypertension, hyperglycemia, petechiae or ecchymosis, and hirsutism).

5-HYDROXYINDOLEACETIC ACID (5-HIAA) (URINE)

5-OH-INDOLEACETIC ACID

Reference Values
Adult: Qualitative random samples: negative; quantitative 24-h: 2–10 mg/24 h
Child: Usually not done

Description.   5-HIAA, a metabolite of serotonin, is excreted in the urine as the result of carcinoid tumors found in the appendix or in the intestinal wall. Serotonin is a vasoconstricting hormone secreted by the argentaffin cells of the gastrointestinal (GI) tract and is responsible for peristalsis. Carcinoid tumor cells, which secrete excess serotonin, are of low-grade malignancy; removal ensures an 80% to 90% cure. Some noncarcinoid tumors may produce high levels of 5-HIAA.

Purposes
- To confirm carcinoid tumor of the intestine
- To compare with other laboratory tests for confirmation of carcinoid tumor

Clinical Problems

Drugs that may decrease urine 5-HIAA: ACTH, heparin, imipramine (Tofranil), phenothiazines, methyldopa (Aldomet), MAO inhibitors, promethazine (Phenergan)

Increased level: Carcinoid tumors of the appendix and intestine, carcinoid tumor with metastasis (greater than 100 mg/24 h), sciatica pain, skeletal and smooth muscle spasm

Drugs that may increase urine 5-HIAA: Acetophenetidin (Phenacetin), reserpine (Serpasil), methamphetamine (Desoxyn)

Foods that may increase urine 5-HIAA: Banana, pineapple, plums, avocados, eggplant, walnuts

Procedure

- Eliminate the foods and drugs listed above for 3 days before the test. Check with health care provider.

Qualitative Random Urine Sample (Screening)

- Collect a random urine sample and take to the laboratory immediately. The random urine test is usually done first.

Quantitative 24-h Urine Collection

- Collect urine for 24 h in a large container with an acid preservative. Urine collection should have a pH less than 4.0.

Nursing Implications

- Check the 5-HIAA result of the random urine test. A repeat test may be needed if the client has taken drugs that can depress the 5-HIAA. If the urine test is positive, the health care provider may order the 5-HIAA 24-h urine test.

Client Teaching

- Instruct the client not to eat food listed or to take drugs for 3 days before test without health care provider's permission. Foods and drugs taken should be listed on the laboratory slip.

IMMUNOGLOBULINS (Ig) (SERUM)

IgG, IgA, IgM, IgD, IgE

Reference Values

Values may differ in institutions.

	Total Ig (99%: mg/dl)	IgG (80%: mg/dl)	IgA (15%: mg/dl)	IgM (4%: mg/dl)	IgD (0.2%: mg/dl)	IgE (0.0002: U/ml)
Adult	900–2,200	650–1,700	70–400	40–350	0–8	Less than 40 (IgE 0–120 mg/dL)
6–16 years	800–1,700	700–1,650	80–230	45–260		Less than 62
4–6 years	700–1,700	550–1,500	50–175	22–100		Less than 25
1–3 years	400–1,500	300–1,400	20–150	40–230		Less than 10
6 months	225–1,200	200–1,100	10–90	10–80		
3 months	325–750	275–750	5–55	15–70		
Newborn	650–1,450	700–1,480	0–12	5–30		

Description.   Immunoglobulins (Ig) are classes of proteins referred to as antibodies. They are divided into five groups found in gamma globulin (IgG, IgA, IgM, IgD, and IgE) and can be separated by the process of immunoelectrophoresis. As individuals are exposed to antigens, immunoglobulin (antibody) production occurs, and with further exposure to the same antigen, immunity results.

IgG: IgG results from secondary exposure to the foreign antigen and is responsible for antiviral and antibacterial activity. This antibody passes through the placental barrier and provides early immunity for the newborn.

IgA: IgA is found in secretions of the respiratory, GI, and genitourinary (GU) tracts, tears, and saliva. It protects mucous membranes from viruses and some bacteria. IgA does not pass the placental barrier. Those having congenital IgA deficiency are prone to autoimmune disease.

IgM: IgM antibodies are produced 48 to 72 h after an antigen enters the body and are responsible for primary immunity. IgM does not pass the placental barrier. It is produced early in life, after 9 months.

IgD: Unknown
IgE: Increases during allergic reactions and anaphylaxis

Purposes

- To identify the occurrence of total or a specific elevated immunoglobulin
- To associate a specific immunoglobulin elevation with a health problem (see Clinical Problems)

Clinical Problems

Ig	Decreased Level	Increased Level
IgG	Lymphocytic leukemia	Infections (all types)
	Agammaglobulinemia	Severe malnutrition
	Preeclampsia	Chronic granulomatous infection
	Amyloidosis	Hyperimmunization
		Liver disease
		Rheumatic fever
		Sarcoidosis
IgA	Lymphocytic leukemia	Autoimmune disorders
	Agammaglobulinemia	Rheumatic fever
	Malignancies	Chronic infections
		Liver disease
IgM	Lymphocytic leukemia	Lymphosarcomas
	Agammaglobulinemia	Brucellosis
	Amyloidosis	Trypanosomiasis
		Infectious mononucleosis
		Rubella virus in newborns
IgE		Allergic reactions (asthma)
		Skin sensitivity
		Drugs: tetanus toxoid and antitoxin, gamma globulin

Procedure

- No food or fluid restriction is required. Some laboratories request NPO 12 h before the test. Check with your laboratory.
- Collect 5 to 7 ml of venous blood in a red-top tube.

- Record on the laboratory slip if client has received any vaccination or immunization (including toxoid) in the last 6 months; any blood transfusion, gamma globulin, or tetanus antitoxin in the last 6 weeks.

Factors Affecting Laboratory Results
- Immunizations and toxoids received in the last 6 months and blood transfusions received in the last 6 weeks can affect test results.

Nursing Implications
- Obtain vaccination, immunization, transfusion, and gamma globulin history.

Client Teaching
- Instruct the client to avoid infections.

INSULIN (SERUM), INSULIN ANTIBODY TEST

Reference Values
Adult: Serum insulin: 5–25 μU/ml, 10–250 μIU/ml.

Insulin antibody test: less than 4% serum binding of beef or pork

Description.   Insulin, hormone from the beta cells of the pancreas, is essential in transporting glucose to the cells. Increased glucose levels stimulate insulin secretion. Serum insulin and blood glucose levels are compared to determine the glucose disorder. Serum insulin level is valuable in diagnosing insulinoma (islet cell tumor) and islet cell hyperplasia, and in evaluating insulin production in diabetes mellitus (DM). Insulin values are more helpful during an OGTT (oral glucose tolerance test) for diagnosing an early pre-hyperglycemic DM state. A normal fasting insulin level and a delayed rise in GTT curves occur frequently with a mildly diabetic individual. In insulinoma the serum insulin is high, and blood glucose is less than 30 mg/dl.

Insulin antibody test: This test is ordered when a diabetic, taking pork or beef insulin, requires larger and larger insulin dosages. Insulin antibodies develop as the result of impurities in animal insulins. These antibodies are of immunoglobulin types such as IgG (most common), IgM, and IgE. The IgG antibodies neutralize the insulin, thus preventing glucose metabolism. IgM antibodies can cause insulin resistance, and IgE may be responsible for allergic effects.

Purposes
- To assist in the detection of an early pre-hyperglycemic diabetes mellitus state
- To check for the presence of insulin antibody that can affect insulin absorption and dosage

Clinical Problems
Decreased level: Diabetes mellitus (insulin-dependent diabetes mellitus [IDDM] or type 1), hypopituitarism

Drugs that may decrease insulin value: Beta blockers (e.g., propranolol), cimetidine, calcitonin, loop and thiazide diuretics (i.e., furosemide, hydrochlorothiazide), phenytoin, calcium channel blockers, phenobarbital

Increased level: Insulinoma, non–insulin-dependent diabetes mellitus (NIDDM or type 2), liver disease, Cushing's syndrome (hyperactive adrenal cortex), acromegaly, obesity (may double its value)

Drugs that may increase insulin value: Cortisone preparations, oral contraceptives, thyroid hormones, epinephrine, levodopa, terbutaline (Brethine), tolazamide (Priscoline), oral antidiabetic drugs (e.g., tolbutamide [Orinase], acetohexamide [Dymelor])

Procedure
- Restrict food and fluids for 10 to 12 h with the exception of water. Insulin secretion reaches its peak in 30 min to 2 h after meals.
- Withhold medications that may affect test results, such as insulin and cortisone, until after the test.
- Collect 3 to 5 ml of venous blood in a red-top tube. Avoid hemolysis. If the test is to be conducted with OGTT, draw blood specimen for serum insulin before administering glucose.

Nursing Implications
- Obtain a history of clinical symptoms related to a glucose disorder. Report client's complaints.

- Report if the client's insulin dosage has increased over a period of time due to an increase in blood sugar. This may result from insulin antibody formation.

Client Teaching
- Instruct the client to report signs and symptoms of insulin reaction, such as nervousness, sweating, weakness, rapid pulse rate, and/or confusion.

INTERNATIONAL NORMALIZED RATIO (INR) (PLASMA)

Reference Values
Oral anticoagulant therapy: 2.0–3.0 INR
Higher value for mechanical heart value: 3.0–4.5 INR

Description.   The International Normalized Ratio (INR) was devised to monitor more correctly anticoagulant therapy for clients receiving warfarin (Coumadin) therapy. The World Health Organization (WHO) recommends the use of INR for a more consistent reporting of prothrombin time results. The INR is calculated by the use of a nomogram demonstrating the relationship between the INR and the PT ratio. Usually both PT and INR values are reported for monitoring Coumadin therapy.

Refer to Prothrombin Time (PT) for the Purpose, Clinical Problems, Procedure, Factors Affecting Laboratory Results, Nursing Implications, and Client Teaching.

IRON (Fe), TOTAL IRON-BINDING CAPACITY (TIBC), TRANSFERRIN, TRANSFERRIN SATURATION (SERUM)

IRON-BINDING CAPACITY (IBC)
Reference Values

Description.   Iron is absorbed from the duodenum and upper jejunum; the amount absorbed usually covers the amount of iron that has been lost. The average daily iron intake is 10 to 20 mg.

	Serum Iron	TIBC	Serum Transferrin	Transferrin Saturation
Adult	50–150 mcg/dl	250–450 mcg/dl	200–430 mcg/dl	30%–50% (male)
	10–27 mol/l (SI units) Males slightly higher			20%–35% (female)
Elderly Child	60–80 mcg/dl	Less than 50 mcg/dl		
Newborn Infant	100–270 mcg/dl	60–175 mcg/dl 100–400 mcg/dl	125–275 mcg/dl	
6 months– 2 years	40–100 mcg/dl	100–135 mcg/dl		
Greater than 2 years		40–100 mcg/dl		

Iron is coupled with the iron-transporting protein *transferrin.* Transferrin is responsible for transporting iron to the bone marrow for the purpose of hemoglobin synthesis (see Transferrin). The storage compound for iron is ferritin (see Ferritin). Serum iron levels are elevated when there is excessive red blood cell destruction (hemolysis), and levels are decreased in iron deficiency anemia.

Total iron-binding capacity (TIBC) measures the maximum amount of iron that can bind to the protein transferrin. The level of TIBC decreases with age. Usually, serum iron and TIBC are determined together.

Transferrin can be measured as serum and as percentage of saturation (transferrin saturation). The transferrin saturation is the ratio between serum iron and TIBC relating to the availability of transferrin in binding with iron. Transferrin saturation is given in percent.

Serum iron, TIBC, transferrin, and transferrin saturation values are needed to adequately diagnose iron deficiency anemia and other disorders. The table on the next page gives the various tests used for diagnosing health problems related to iron and transferrin imbalances.

Purposes
- To determine a probable cause of iron excess (e.g., hemolysis) or deficit (e.g., iron deficiency anemia)

SERUM IRON, TIBC, TRANSFERRIN, AND TRANSFERRIN SATURATION

Serum Iron	TIBC	Transferrin	Transferrin Saturation	Health Problems
Low	High	High	Low	Iron deficiency anemia
Low	Low	Low	Normal	Chronic Illness: cancer, infection, cirrhosis
High	Normal or low	Low	Very high	Iron therapy overload

- To compare serum iron and TIBC for diagnosing iron deficiency anemia

Clinical Problems
Decreased Level
Serum iron: Iron deficiency anemia; cancer of the stomach, small and/or large intestines, rectum, and breast; rheumatoid arthritis; bleeding peptic ulcer; chronic renal failure; pregnancy; low-birth-weight infants; protein malnutrition; chronic blood loss (GI, uterine)

TIBC: Hemochromatosis (excess iron deposits in organs and tissues), anemias (hemolytic, pernicious, sickle cell), renal failure, cirrhosis of the liver, rheumatoid arthritis, infections, cancer of the GI tract

Transferrin: Anemia of chronic disease, hepatic damage, renal disease, cancer, acute or chronic infection

Transferrin saturation: Chronic iron deficiency anemia, anemia of chronic disease

Drugs that may decrease TIBC value: Cortisone preparations, dextran, testosterone

Increased Level
Serum iron: Hemochromatosis, anemias (hemolytic, pernicious, and folic acid deficiency), liver damage, thalassemia, lead toxicity

TIBC: Iron deficiency anemia, acute chronic blood loss, polycythemia

Drugs that may increase TIBC value: Oral contraceptives, iron preparations

Transferrin: Iron deficiency

Transferrin saturation: Anemias (hemolytic, sideroblastic), hemochromatosis, iron overload

Procedure
- No food or fluid restriction is required.
- Collect 5 to 7 ml of venous blood in a red-top tube. Avoid hemolysis; false elevated readings can occur.

Factors Affecting Laboratory Results
- Oral iron medications and recent blood transfusion.

Nursing Implications
Decreased Level
- Observe for signs and symptoms of iron deficiency anemia (e.g., pallor, fatigue, headache, tachycardia, dyspnea on exertion).

Client Teaching
- Encourage the client to eat foods rich in iron (e.g., liver, shellfish, lean meat, egg yolk, dried fruits, whole grain, wines, and cereals). Milk has little or no iron.
- Recommend rest and avoidance of strenuous activity.
- Instruct how to take iron supplements. Iron should be given following meals or snacks because it irritates the gastric mucosa. Orange juice (ascorbic acid) promotes iron absorption.
- Explain that iron supplements can cause constipation and that stools will have a tarry appearance.

Increased Level
- Observe for signs and symptoms of hemochromatosis (e.g., bronze pigmentation of the skin, cardiac dysrhythmias, and heart failure).

17-KETOSTEROIDS (17-KS) (URINE)

Reference Values
Adult: Male: 5–25 mg/24 h; female: 5–15 mg/24 h

Child: Infant: less than 1 mg/24 h; 1–3 years: less than 2 mg/24 h; 3–6 years: less than 3 mg/24 h; 7–10 years: 3–4 mg/24 h; 10–12 years: 1–6 mg/24 h. Adolescent: male: 3–15 mg/24 h; female: 3–12 mg/24 h
Elderly: 4–8 mg/24 h

Description.   17-KS are metabolites of male hormones that are secreted from the testes and adrenal cortex. In men, approximately one third of the hormone metabolites come from the testes and two thirds from the adrenal cortex. In women, nearly all of the excreted hormones (androgens) are derived from the adrenal cortex. Since most of the 17-KS are from the adrenal cortex, this test is useful for diagnosing adrenal cortex dysfunction.

Purpose
* To assist in the diagnosis of adrenal cortex dysfunction

Clinical Problems
Decreased level: Adrenal cortical hypofunction (Addison's disease), hypogonadism, hypopituitarism, myxedema, nephrosis, severe debilitating diseases
Drugs that may decrease urine 17-KS: Thiazide diuretics, estrogen, oral contraceptives, reserpine, chlordiazepoxide (Librium), probenecid (Benemid), promazine, meprobamate (Miltown), quinidine, prolonged use of salicylates
Increased level: Adrenal cortical hyperfunction (adrenocortical hyperplasia, Cushing's syndrome, adrenocortical carcinoma); testicular neoplasm; ovarian neoplasm; hyperpituitarism; severe stress or infection, or both
Drugs that may increase urine 17-KS: ACTH, antibiotics, phenothiazines, dexamethasone (Decadron), spironolactone (Aldactone)

Procedure
* No food or fluid restriction is required.
* If possible, drugs that interfere with test results should not be given for 48 h before the test with health care provider's approval.
* Collect a 24-h urine specimen in a large container and keep refrigerated. An acid preservative is usually added to keep the urine at a pH

less than 4.5, thus preventing steroid decomposition by bacterial growth.

- List on the laboratory slip the client's sex and age.
- Postpone test if female has her menstrual period. Blood in urine can cause false-positive results.

Nursing Implications
- Encourage the client to increase fluid intake.

Decreased Level
- Observe for signs and symptoms of adrenal gland insufficiency (e.g., weakness, weight loss, polyuria, hypotension, tachycardia).
- Record fluid intake and output. Report if client's urine output is greater than 2,000 ml/24 h. Diluted urine can cause a false-negative test result.
- Monitor weight loss. In Addison's disease, sodium is not retained. Weight loss and dehydration usually occur.

Client Teaching
- Suggest medical alert bracelet or card.

Increased Level
- Observe for signs and symptoms of adrenal gland hyperfunction (e.g., "moon face," cervical–dorsal fat pad ["buffalo hump"], weight gain, bleeding tendency, hyperglycemia).
- Check serum potassium and blood glucose levels. Hypokalemia and hyperglycemia frequently occur; potassium supplements and insulin or a low-carbohydrate diet may be indicated.

LACTIC ACID (BLOOD)

Reference Values
Adult: Arterial blood: 0.5–2.0 mEq/l, 11.3 mg/dl, 0.5–2.0 mmol/l (SI units)

Venous blood: 0.5–1.5 mEq/l, 8.1–15.3 mg/dl, 0.5–1.5 mmol/l (SI units)

Panic range: greater than 5 mEq/l, greater than 45 mg/dl, greater than 5 mmol/l (SI units)

Description.   Increased secretion of lactic acid occurs following strenuous exercise, and acute or prolonged hypoxemia (tissue hypoxia). A major
cause of metabolic acidosis is excess circulating lactic acid.

Shock and severe dehydration cause cell catabolism (cell breakdown) and an accumulation of acid metabolites, such as lactic acid. When
the anion gap is greater than 18 mEq/l, pH less than 7.25, and the $PaCO_2$
remains within normal range (35–45 mm Hg), blood lactic acid level
should be checked to determine if lactic acidosis is present.

Purpose

- To detect the presence of acidosis related to shock, trauma, or severe
  illness (also see Anion Gap)

Clinical Problems

Decreased level: High lactic dehydrogenases (LDH) value
Increased level: Shock, severe dehydration, severe trauma, keto acidosis, severe infections, neoplastic conditions, hepatic failure, renal disease,
chronic alcoholism, severe salicylate toxicity

Procedure

- Collect 5 to 7 ml of blood in a green- or gray-top tube.
- Instruct the client to avoid hand clenching, which can lead to a
  buildup of lactic acid caused by a release of lactic acid from muscle
  of the clenched hand.
- Avoid using a tourniquet if possible; it could increase the blood lactic
  acid level.
- Deliver the blood specimen on ice to the laboratory immediately.

Factors Affecting Laboratory Results

- Use of tourniquet could elevate lactic acid value.

Nursing Implications

- Obtain a history of the clinical problem as described by the client,
  family, or referral report.
- Compare laboratory values that may indicate acidotic state, such as
  low pH, low bicarbonate, normal $PaCO_2$, or low serum CO_2.

- Observe for signs and symptoms of acidosis, such as dyspnea or Kussmaul's breathing, increased pulse rate.
- Be supportive of client and family. If shock is present, anxiety and fear are common.

LACTIC DEHYDROGENASE (LDH OR LD); LDH ISOENZYMES (SERUM)

Reference Values
Adult: Total LDH: 100–190 international units/l, 70–250 international units/l, 70–200 international units/l (differs among institutions)

LDH isoenzymes: LDH_1: 14%–26%; LDH_2: 27%–37%; LDH_3: 13%–26%; LDH_4: 8%–16%; LDH_5: 6%–16%. Differences of 2% to 4% are usually normal.
Child: Newborn: 300–1,500 international units/l; child: 50–150 international units/l

Description.   LDH is an intracellular enzyme present in nearly all metabolizing cells, with the highest concentrations in the heart, skeletal muscle, RBCs, liver, kidney, lung, and brain. Two subunits, H (heart) and M (muscle), are combined in different formations to make five isoenzymes.

- LDH_1: cardiac fraction; H, H, H, H; in heart, RBCs, kidneys, brain (some)
- LDH_2: cardiac fraction; H, H, H, M; in heart, RBCs, kidneys, brain (some)
- LDH_3: pulmonary fraction; H, H, M, M; in lungs and other tissues: spleen, pancreas, adrenal, thyroid, lymphatics
- LDH_4: hepatic fraction; H, M, M, M; liver, skeletal muscle, kidneys and brain (some)
- LDH_5: hepatic fraction; M, M, M, M; liver, skeletal muscle, kidneys (some)

Serum LDH and LDH_1 are used for diagnosing acute myocardial infarction (AMI). A high serum LDH (total) occurs 12 to 24 h after an

AMI, reaches its peak in 2 to 5 days, and remains elevated for 6 to 12 days. It is a useful test for diagnosing a delayed reported myocardial infarction. A flipped LDH_1/ LDH_2 ratio, with LDH_1 higher indicates a myocardial infarction.

Purposes
- To aid in the diagnosis of myocardial or skeletal muscle damage
- To compare test results with other cardiac enzyme tests (e.g., CPK, AST)
- To check LDH isoenzyme results to determine organ involvement

Clinical Problems
Increased level: AMI, acute pulmonary embolus and infarction, cerebral vascular accident (CVA), acute hepatitis, cancers, anemias, acute leukemias, shock, skeletal muscular diseases, heat stroke
Drugs that may increase LDH value: Narcotics

Procedure
- No food or fluid restriction is required.
- Collect 5 to 7 ml of venous blood in a red-top tube. Avoid hemolysis.
- List narcotics or IM injections given in the last 8 h on the laboratory slip.

Nursing Implications
- Obtain a history of the client's discomfort. A complaint of severe indigestion for several days could be indicative of a myocardial infarction.
- Assess for signs and symptoms of an AMI (e.g., pale or gray color; sharp, stabbing pain or heavy pressure pain; shortness of breath [SOB], diaphoresis, nausea and vomiting; and indigestion).

Client Teaching
- Instruct the client to notify the nurse of any recurrence of chest discomfort.

LACTOSE AND LACTOSE TOLERANCE TEST (SERUM OR PLASMA, URINE)

Reference Values
Serum/Plasma: Less than 0.5 mg/dl, less than 14.5 μmol/l (SI units)
Urine: 12–40 mg/dl
Lactose test: Tolerance: fasting serum glucose plus 20–50 mg/dl
Intolerance: fasting serum glucose plus less than 20 mg/dl

Description.   Lactose is a disaccharide sugar. Milk is rich in lactose; one glass of milk may contain 12 g of lactose. For lactose to be absorbed, lactase (an intestinal enzyme) converts lactose to glucose and galactose. With a deficiency of the lactase enzyme, diarrhea, flatus, and abdominal cramping commonly occur due to excess lactose in the intestine.

When lactose intolerance is suspected, a lactose tolerance test is usually conducted. A large amount of lactose is ingested, and serum glucose levels are drawn at specified times. If the serum glucose level is more than 20 mg/dl, greater than the fasting glucose level, lactose is tolerated and is being converted into glucose; if the increase in the serum glucose level is less than 20 mg/dl of the fasting glucose, lactose intolerance is occurring. Milk products should be avoided to decrease lactose intolerance.

Purposes
- To compare serum and urine lactose results for determining lactose deficit
- To diagnose lactose intolerance

Clinical Problems
Decreased glucose level: Excess lactose in intestine, lactose intolerance
Increased glucose level: Normal lactose tolerance

Procedure
Lactose Tolerance Test
- Restrict food and fluids for 8 to 12 h before the test.
- Administer 50 to 100 g of lactose in 200+ ml of water. The amount of lactose is determined by the laboratory. Fifty grams of lactose is equivalent to a quart of milk.

- Collect four venous blood specimens, 5 ml each, in gray-top tubes. The first blood specimen should be collected before the test. After oral administration of lactose solution, collect the next three blood samples 0.5, 1, and 2 h after lactose ingestion.
- Conduct test adjacent to bathroom in the event that diarrhea due to lactose intolerance occurs.

Nursing Implications

- Explain to the client the test procedure. Instruct the client to remain NPO for 8 to 12 h (as determined by the institution's protocol) before the test. Tell the client that he or she will have four blood specimens collected within 2 to 2.5 h.

Client Teaching

- Instruct the client who has a lactose intolerance to avoid milk products. Suggest lactose-free milk. Calcium supplements may be necessary.
- Instruct the client not to exercise 8 h before the test and not to smoke during the test because smoking can increase the blood glucose level.

LATEX ALLERGY TESTING (SERUM)

LATEX-SPECIFIC IgE

Reference Values
Negative: Less than 0.35 international units/ml by EIA
Positive: Greater than 0.35 international units/ml by EIA

Description. Many persons, including health care professionals, are allergic to latex-containing medical products, such as gloves, catheters, bandages. Allergic reactions can range from mild to severe. Clients, including health personnel, who have a questionable allergy to latex should be tested for latex allergy. For health professionals who are allergic to latex there are nonallergic gloves that can be used.

Since 1987, health care providers have been required to wear gloves as a standard precaution to protect self and others from organisms. It is predicted that 10%–15% of health care providers are allergic to latex.

The Latex Allergy test measures IgE latex sensitivity. There are two types of allergic reactions to latex; type IV is allergic contact dermatitis caused by chemicals in the process of manufacturing latex, and type 1 occurs from the proteins in the natural latex product. Latex actually comes from the rubber tree and is collected from the tree before it hardens and becomes rubber.

Purpose
- To detect sensitivity to the use of latex products by clients or health professionals

Clinical Problems
Increased level: Allergy to latex products, industrial exposure to latex, use of latex catheter (retention latex catheters), multiple surgeries requiring latex products.

Procedure
- No food or fluid restriction is required.
- Collect 5 to 7 ml of venous blood in a red-top tube.

Factors Affecting Laboratory Results
- None known

Nursing Implications
- Obtain a history of allergy to latex products, such as gloves, retention catheters.
- Note if the client has swelling or itching from latex exposure to hands or body.
- Note if there is hand eczema present.
- Record the presence of latex allergy on client's chart.

Client Teaching
- Explain to the client and health professional with allergic reaction to latex to avoid contact with latex products. Inform them that there are nonallergic products available.

- Encourage client to read labels before purchasing products that may contain latex.
- Instruct clients that, when asked if they are allergic to drugs, they should include latex products if they have a latex allergy.

LEAD (BLOOD)

Reference Values

Adult: Normal: 10–20 mcg/dl; acceptable: 20–40 mcg/dl; excessive: 40–80 mcg/dl; toxic: greater than 80 mcg/dl

Child: Normal: 10–20 mcg/dl; acceptable: 20–30 mcg/dl; excessive: 30–50 mcg/dl; toxic: greater than 50 mcg/dl

Description. Excessive lead exposure due to occupational contact is hazardous to adults; however, most industry will accept a 40 mcg/dl blood lead level as a normal value. Lead toxicity can occur in children from eating chipped lead-based paint.

Lead is usually excreted rapidly in the urine, but if excessive lead exposure persists, the lead will accumulate in the bone and soft tissues. Chronic lead poisoning is more common than acute poisoning.

Purpose

- To check for lead toxicity

Clinical Problems

Increased level: Lead gasoline, fumes from heaters, lead-based paint, unglazed pottery, batteries, lead containers used for storage, heat stroke

Procedure

- No food or fluid restriction is required.
- Collect 5 to 7 ml of venous blood in a lavender- or green-top tube.
- Urine may be requested for a 24-h quantitative test; a lead-free container must be used.

Nursing Implications

- Observe for signs and symptoms of lead poisoning (e.g., lead colic [crampy abdominal pain], constipation, occasional bloody diarrhea, behavioral changes [from lethargy to hyperactivity, aggression, impulsiveness], tremors, and confusion).
- Monitor the urinary output, as lead toxicity can decrease kidney function. A urine output less than 25 ml/h should be reported.
- Monitor medical treatment for removing lead from the body (e.g., chelation therapy).
- Provide adequate fluid intake.

Client Teaching

- Instruct those in high-risk groups to have their blood lead levels monitored.
- Instruct client(s) that paint chips from woodwork in house may contain lead and that some children have tendencies to eat paint chips.

LE CELL TEST; LUPUS ERYTHEMATOSUS CELL TEST (BLOOD)

LUPUS TEST, LE PREP, LE PREPARATION, LE SLIDE CELL TEST

Reference Values

Adult: Negative, no LE cells
Child: Negative

Description.   LE cell test, a screening test for systemic lupus erythematosus (SLE), is a nonspecific test. Positive results have been reported in those having rheumatoid arthritis, scleroderma, and drug-induced lupus, such as penicillin, tetracycline, dilantin, oral contraceptives. The test is positive in 60% to 80% of those having SLE. Antinuclear antibodies (ANA) and anti-DNA are more sensitive tests for lupus and should be used to confirm SLE.

Purposes

- To aid in the diagnosis of SLE
- To compare with ANA and/or anti-DNA tests for diagnosing SLE

Clinical Problems
Increased level: SLE, scleroderma, rheumatoid arthritis, chronic hepatitis
Drugs that may increase LE cells: Hydralazine (Apresoline), procainamide (Pronestyl), quinidine, anticonvulsants (phenytoin [Dilantin], Mesantoin, Tridione), oral contraceptives, methysergide, antibiotics (penicillin, tetracycline, streptomycin, sulfonamides), methyldopa (Aldomet), isoniazid (INH), clofibrate, reserpine, phenylbutazone

Procedure
- No food or fluid restriction is required.
- Collect 3 to 5 ml of venous blood in a red- or green-top tube. Avoid hemolysis.
- On laboratory slip, list drugs taken that might affect test results.

Nursing Implications
- Compare LE test results with serum ANA or serum anti-DNA, or both. LE test should not be the only test used to diagnose SLE.
- Observe for signs and symptoms of SLE (e.g., fatigue, fever, rash [butterfly over nose], leukopenia, thrombocytopenia).
- Be supportive of client and family. Encourage daily rest periods, which help in decreasing symptoms.

Client Teaching
- Instruct the client to have daily rest periods, which help to decrease symptoms.

LECITHIN/SPHINGOMYELIN (L/S) RATIO (AMNIOTIC FLUID)

Reference Values
Before 35 weeks' gestation: 1:1. Lecithin (L): 6–9 mg/dl. Sphingomyelin (S): 4–6 mg/dl
After 35 weeks' gestation: 4:1. Lecithin (L): 15–21 mg/dl. Sphingomyelin (S): 4–6 mg/dl

Description. The L/S ratio can be used to predict neonatal respiratory distress syndrome (also called hyaline membrane disease) before delivery.

Lecithin (L), a phospholipid, is responsible mostly for the formation of alveolar surfactant. Surfactant lubricates the alveolar lining and inhibits alveolar collapse, thus preventing atelectasis. Sphingomyelin (S) is another phospholipid, the value of which remains the same throughout the pregnancy. A marked rise in amniotic lecithin after 35 weeks (to a level three or four times higher than that of sphingomyelin) is considered normal, and so chances for having hyaline membrane disease are small. The L/S ratio is also used to determine fetal maturity in the event that the gestation period is uncertain. In this situation, the L/S ratio is determined at intervals of a period of several weeks.

Purpose
- To check for possible neonatal respiratory distress syndrome (hyaline membrane disease) to the unborn prior to delivery

Clinical Problems
Decreased ratio after 35 weeks: Respiratory distress syndrome, hyaline membrane disease

Procedure
- No food, fluid, or drug restriction is necessary.
- The physician performs an amniocentesis to obtain amniotic fluid. The specimen should be cooled immediately to prevent the destruction of lecithin by certain enzymes in the amniotic fluid. The specimen should be frozen if testing cannot be done at a specified time (check with the laboratory).
- Care should be taken to prevent puncture of the mother's bladder. If urine in the specimen is suspected, then the specimen should be tested for urea and potassium. If these two levels are higher than blood levels, the specimen could be urine and not amniotic fluid.
- Ultrasound is frequently used when obtaining amniotic fluid.

Factors Affecting Laboratory Results
- Maternal vaginal secretions or a bloody tap into the amniotic fluid may cause a falsely increased reading for lecithin.

Nursing Implications

- Check the procedures for amniocentesis. Explain the procedure to the client. Assist the health care provider in obtaining amniotic fluid. Maternal vaginal secretions or a bloody tap into the amniotic fluid may cause a false, increased reading for lecithin.
- Obtain a fetal history of problems occurring during gestation. Also ask for and report information on any previous children born with respiratory distress syndrome.
- Be supportive of the mother and her family before, during, and after the test.
- Assess the newborn at delivery for respiratory complications (substernal retractions, increased respiratory rate, labored breathing, and expiratory grunts).

LEGIONNAIRE'S ANTIBODY TEST (SERUM)

Reference Value

Negative

Description.   Legionnaire's disease, caused by a Gram-negative bacillus, *Legionella pneumophila,* causes acute respiratory infection such as severe, consolidated pneumonia. This organism is in the soil and water (lakes, streams, reservoirs) and is passed by inhalation in aerosol form through plumbing fixtures (shower heads, whirlpool baths) and air conditioning systems (cooling towers and condensers). The bacteria can be isolated from blood, sputum, pleural fluid, and lung-tissue specimen.

A fourfold rise in antibody titer greater than 1:128 during the acute and convalescent phase or a single titer greater than 1:256 is evidence of the disease. Several blood samples and a tissue specimen are useful in confirming Legionnaire's disease.

Purpose

- To diagnose the presence of Legionnaire's disease

Clinical Problems

Increased antibody titer: Legionnaire's disease

Procedure

- No food or fluid restriction is required.
- Collect 3 to 5 ml of venous blood in a red-top tube. Tissue specimen from the lung or bronchiole site may be used.

Nursing Implications

- Obtain a history from the client as to where he or she has been in the last weeks, such as a hotel or institutional site.
- Assess the client's respiratory status by inspection, palpation, percussion, and auscultation.
- Observe the signs and symptoms of Legionnaire's disease, such as malaise, high fever, chills, cough, chest pain, and tachypnea. Fever rises rapidly from 39°C to 41°C, or from 102°F to 105°F.

Client Teaching

- Inform the client that Legionnaire's disease is not transmitted from person to person but through aerosol means such as exhaust vents and fans.

LEUCINE AMINOPEPTIDASE (LAP) (SERUM)

Reference Values

Adult: 8–22 µU/ml, 12–33 international units/l, 75–200 units/ml, 20–50 units/l at 37°C (SI units) (varies according to laboratory method)

Description.   Leucine aminopeptidase (LAP) is an enzyme produced mainly by the liver. This test may be used to differentiate between liver and bone disease. LAP is normal in bone disease, whereas alkaline phosphatase (ALP) may be abnormal in liver and bone disease.

This enzyme test is not frequently ordered but is sometimes used to assist with the evaluation of hepatobiliary disease. Elevated level can indicate biliary obstruction due to liver metastases and choledocholithiasis (calculi in the common bile duct).

Purpose

- To compare with other liver enzyme tests for diagnosing liver disease

Clinical Problems

Increased level: Cancer of the liver, extrahepatic biliary obstruction (stones), acute necrosis of the liver, viral hepatitis, severe preeclampsia, pregnancy (mild)

Drugs that may increase LAP value: Estrogens, progesterone, oral contraceptives

Procedure

- No food or fluid restriction is required.
- Collect 3 to 5 ml of venous blood in a red-top tube. Avoid hemolysis of the blood specimen that may result from rough handling.

Nursing Implications

- Obtain a history of the client's signs and symptoms of the clinical problem.
- Compare LAP with other tests for liver dysfunction, such as alkaline phosphatase (ALP), alanine aminotransferase (ALT or SGPT), gamma-glutamyl transpeptidase (GGT), and/or 5' nucleotidase (5'N). LAP is not considered as sensitive as the other tests, but it may be ordered to verify liver dysfunction.

LEUKOAGGLUTININ TEST (BLOOD, SERUM)

Reference Values

Negative: No dye uptake
Positive: Dye uptake in the lymphocytes

Description.   Leukoagglutinins are antibodies that react with white blood cells (WBCs) and can cause a transfusion reaction. Fever may accompany the transfusion reaction. Usually the leukoagglutinin antibodies develop after the client has received WBCs through transfusions or pregnancies. Normally the client has antibodies to the donor's WBCs; however, the donor could have antibodies to the client's WBCs. The transfusion reaction can occur even though compatible blood has been given. Severe transfusion reactions can lead to pulmonary infiltrates and multiorgan system failure.

To detect leukoagglutinins, the recipients' serum is tested with the donor's lymphocytes. The lymphocytes are examined under the microscope for cell damage. Agglutinating antibodies may be present in the donor or recipient's plasma.

Purpose
- To detect leukoagglutinin antibodies that may be a contributing factor to transfusion reaction

Clinical Problems
Positive test: Pregnancies, numerous transfusions

Procedure
- No food or fluid restriction is required
- Collect 7 ml of venous blood in a red- or lavender-top tube.

Factors Affecting Laboratory Results
- Blood transfusion dextran that has been previously administered
- Previously administered dextran

Nursing Implications
- Obtain a history of past blood transfusions and ascertain whether adverse effects occurred.
- Record baseline vital signs. Vital signs (VS) can be compared with those taken during a transfusion or if a transfusion reaction occurs. Acetaminophen may be prescribed prior to a transfusion to avoid febrile state, as indicated.
- Administer leukocyte-poor blood that has been separated from the donor's blood when necessary to avoid a transfusion reaction.

Client Teaching
- Listen to the client's concerns. Answer questions or contact other health professionals.

LIPASE (SERUM)

Reference Values
Adult: 20–180 international units/l, 14–280 mU/ml, 14–280 units/l (SI units)

Child: Infant: 9–105 international units/l at 37°C; child: 20–136 international units/l at 37°C

Description.   Lipase, an enzyme secreted by the pancreas, aids in digesting fats in the duodenum. Lipase, like amylase, appears in the bloodstream following damage to the pancreas. Lipase and amylase levels increase in 2 to 12 h in acute pancreatitis, but serum lipase can be elevated for up to 14 days after an acute episode, whereas the serum amylase returns to normal after approximately 3 days. Serum lipase is useful for a late diagnosis of acute pancreatitis.

Purpose
- To suggest acute pancreatitis or other pancreatic disorders (see Clinical Problems)

Clinical Problems
Increased level: Acute pancreatitis, chronic pancreatitis, cancer of the pancreas, obstruction of the pancreatic duct, perforated ulcer, acute renal failure (early stage)
Drugs that may increase lipase value: Narcotics, steroids, bethanechol (Urecholine)

Procedure
- Restrict food and fluids except water for 8 to 12 h before test.
- Narcotics should be withheld for 24 h prior to the test. If given, note time on the laboratory slip.
- Collect 3 to 5 ml of venous blood in a red-top tube. Avoid hemolysis.

Factors Affecting Laboratory Results
- Most narcotics elevate the serum lipase level.

Nursing Implication
- Alert health care provider when abdominal pain persists for several days. A serum lipase determination may be ordered, as it is effective for diagnosing latent acute pancreatitis.

LIPOPROTEINS, LIPOPROTEIN ELECTROPHORESIS, LIPIDS (SERUM)

Reference Values

Adult: Total: 400–800 mg/dl, 4–8 g/l (SI units); cholesterol: 150–240 mg/dl (see test on cholesterol); triglycerides: 10–190 mg/dl (see test on triglycerides); phospholipids: 150–380 mg/dl

LDL: 60–160 mg/dl; risk for CHD: high: greater than 160 mg/dl, moderate: 130–159 mg/dl, low: less than 130 mg/dl

HDL: 29–77 mg/dl; risk for CHD: high: less than 35 mg/dl, moderate: 35–45 mg/dl, low: 46–59 mg/dl, very low: greater than 60 mg/dl

Child: See tests on cholesterol and triglycerides

Description.

The three main lipoproteins are cholesterol, triglycerides, and phospholipids. The two fractions of lipoproteins—alpha (α), high-density lipoproteins (HDL) and beta (β), low-density lipoproteins (chylomicrons, VLDL, LDL)—can be separated by electrophoresis. The β groups are the largest contributors of atherosclerosis and coronary artery disease. HDL, called "friendly lipids," are composed of 50% protein and aid in decreasing plaque deposits in blood vessels.

Increased lipoproteins (hyperlipidemia or hyperlipoproteinemia) can be phenotyped into five major types (I, IIA and IIB, III, IV, V).

Purposes

- To identify clients with hyperlipoproteinemia
- To distinguish between the phenotypes of lipidemias
- To monitor lipid counts for clients with hyperlipidemia

LIPOPROTEIN PHENOTYPE: HYPERLIPIDEMIA

Type	Lipid Composition*
I	Increased chylomicrons; increased triglycerides; normal or slightly increased very low-density lipoproteins (VLDLs)

Type	Lipid Composition*
IIA	Increased low-density lipoproteins (LDL); increased cholesterol; slightly increased triglycerides or normal; normal VLDL (common pattern of hyperlipidemia)
IIB	Increased LDL, VLDL; both cholesterol and triglycerides are elevated (common pattern of hyperlipidemia)
III	Moderately increased cholesterol triglycerides; and normal VLDL. Normal or decreased LDL
IV	Increased VLDL; slightly increased cholesterol and markedly increased triglycerides (common pattern of hyperlipidemia)
V	Increased chylomicrons, VLDL, and triglycerides; and slightly increased cholesterol

*Types II and IV are increased in atherosclerosis and coronary artery disease.

Clinical Problems

Increased level: Hyperlipoproteinemia, acute myocardial infarction (AMI), hypothyroidism, diabetes mellitus, nephrotic syndrome, Laënnec's cirrhosis, diet high in saturated fats, eclampsia

Drugs that may increase lipoprotein values: Aspirin, cortisone preparations, oral contraceptives, phenothiazines, sulfonamides

Procedure

- Restrict food and fluids except for water for 12 to 14 h prior to the test. No alcohol intake is allowed for 24 h, and a regular diet is maintained for 3 days before test.
- Collect 5 to 7 ml of venous blood in a red-top tube.

Nursing Implications

- Check the client's serum cholesterol and serum triglyceride levels and compare with the lipoprotein electrophoresis results.

Client Teaching

- Instruct client with hyperlipoproteinemia to avoid foods high in saturated fats and sugar (e.g., bacon, cream, butter, fatty meats, and candy). Limit excess alcohol intake.
- Answer client's questions concerning risk of coronary heart disease related to high LDL and low HDL.

LITHIUM (SERUM)

Reference Values
Adult: Normal: negative; therapeutic: 0.8–1.2 mEq/l; toxic: greater than 1.5 mEq/l; lethal: greater than 4.0 mEq/l
Child: Not usually given to children

Description.   Lithium or lithium salt is used to treat manic-depressive psychosis. This agent is used to correct the mania in manic depression and to prevent depression. Since therapeutic and toxic lithium levels are narrow ranges, serum lithium should be closely monitored.

Purposes
* To identify lithium toxicity
* To monitor lithium levels for therapeutic effect and toxicity

Clinical Problems
Increased level: Lithium toxicity

Procedure
* No food or fluid restriction is required.
* Collect 5 to 7 ml of venous blood in a red-top tube 8 to 12 h after last lithium dose.
* Lithium tolerance test is an alternative. A base blood specimen is obtained, and then the lithium dose is given. Blood specimens are collected 1, 3, and 6 h after the lithium dose.

Nursing Implications
* Observe for signs and symptoms of lithium overdose (e.g., slurred speech, muscle spasm, confusion, and nystagmus). Lithium dosage should be lower in the older adult.

Client Teaching
* Instruct the patient to take prescribed lithium dosage daily, to keep medical appointments, and to have periodic blood specimens drawn to determine lithium levels.

- Encourage adequate fluid and sodium intake while the patient is on lithium. Diuretics should be avoided.
- Instruct nursing mother to consult health care provider. Breast milk can contain high levels of lithium.

LUTEINIZING HORMONE (LH) (SERUM AND URINE)

INTERSTITIAL CELL-STIMULATING HORMONE (ICSH)

Reference Values

Ranges vary among laboratories

Serum: Adult: female: follicular phase: 5–30 mIU/ml; midcycle: 50–150 mIU/ml; luteal phase: 2–25 mIU/ml. Postmenopausal: 40–100 mIU/ml. Male: 5–25 mIU/ml. Child: 6–12 years: less than 10 mIU/ml; 13–18 years: less than 20 mIU/ml

Urine: Adult: female: follicular phase: 5–25 international units/24 h; midcycle: 30–90 international units/24 h; luteal phase: 2–24 international units/24 h; postmenopausal: greater than 40 international units/24 h. Male: 7–25 international units/ml

Description.   Luteinizing hormone (LH), gonadotropic hormone secreted by the anterior pituitary gland, is needed (with follicle-stimulating hormone [FSH]) for ovulation to occur. After ovulation, LH aids in stimulating the corpus luteum in secreting progesterone. FSH values are frequently evaluated with LH values. In men, LH stimulates testosterone production, and with FSH, they influence the development and maturation of spermatozoa.

LH is usually ordered to evaluate infertility in women and men. High serum values are related to gonadal dysfunction, and low serum values are related to hypothalamus or pituitary failure. Women taking oral contraceptives have an absence of midcycle LH peak until the contraceptives are discontinued. This test might be used to evaluate hormonal therapy for inducting ovulation.

Purposes

- To evaluate the serum or urine luteinizing hormone level for determining the cause of hormonal dysfunction

- To identify the gynecological problem related to excess or deficit of LH

Clinical Problems

Decreased level: Hypogonadotropism (defects in pituitary gland or hypothalamus), anovulation, amenorrhea (pituitary failure), hypophysectomy, testicular failure, hypothalamic dysfunction, adrenal hyperplasia or tumors

Drugs that may decrease LH value: Oral contraceptives, estrogen compounds, testosterone administration

Increased level: Amenorrhea (ovarian failure), tumors (pituitary, testicular), precocious puberty, testicular failure, Turner's syndrome, Klinefelter's syndrome, premature menopause, Stein-Leventhal syndrome, polycystic ovary syndrome, liver disease

Procedure

Serum

- No food or fluid restriction is required.
- Withhold medications that could interfere with test results for 24 to 48 h before the test (check with the health care provider).
- Collect 3 to 5 ml of venous blood in a red- or lavender-top tube. Avoid hemolysis. Daily blood samples must be taken at the same time each day to determine if ovulation occurs.
- Note on the laboratory slip the phase of the menstrual cycle, client's age, and if client is postmenopausal.

Urine

- Collect 24-h urine specimen in a container with a preservative, or keep refrigerated if no preservative is added.
- Label the specimen with the client's name, date, and time.

Factors Affecting Laboratory Results

- Hormones (estrogen, progesterone, and testosterone) and oral contraceptives could decrease plasma LH values.
- Collection of the daily specimen at different times of the day may cause inaccurate results.

Nursing Implications

- Obtain a menstrual history from the client. Record the menstrual phase on the laboratory slip.
- Check with the health care provider about withholding medications that could affect test results.

Client Teaching

- Encourage the client to express concerns about infertility or other health problems.
- Be supportive of client and family.

LYME DISEASE ANTIBODY TEST (SERUM)

Reference Values

Adult and Child: Titer: less than 1:256; indirect fluorescent antibody (IFA) titer: ELISA or Western blot: negative for Lyme disease

Description.   *Borrelia burgdorferi* is the spirochete that causes Lyme disease. Several tick vectors, primarily the deer tick, carry the spirochete. The spirochete can be cultivated, with difficulty, from blood, CSF, or skin biopsies. Lyme disease is most prevalent in the northeastern states, upper Midwestern states, and western states.

A reddish, macular lesion usually occurs about 1 week after the tick bite. It can affect the CNS and the peripheral nervous system (PNS), causing a neuritis or aseptic meningitis. It can also affect the heart and joints, causing transient ECG abnormalities, carditis, and problems in one or more joints, mostly the knees, leading to arthritis. It may take a few weeks to 2 years to become symptomatic.

Immunoglobulins (IgM and IgG) aid in diagnosing early, late, or remission stage of Lyme disease. IgM titers occur approximately 2 to 4 weeks after the onset of disease, peaking at 6 to 8 weeks before levels decrease. IgG titers occur 1 to 3 months after onset of Lyme disease and peak at 4 to 6 months. IgG may remain elevated for months or years. Symptoms such as fever with flu-like symptoms may begin 1 week after the spirochete infection. An erythematous, circular rash at the tick site frequently appears. The client may also suffer with malaise, headache, and muscle or joint aches and pain. Testing should be done 4 to 6 weeks after being infected. If the client has symptoms and the test is performed earlier with negative findings, a repeated test should be performed a week or two later. Antibiotic therapy is usually prescribed when symptoms are apparent even if the test result is negative.

Purpose
- To detect the occurrence of Lyme disease

Clinical Problems
Low titers: Infectious mononucleosis, hepatitis B, autoimmune disease (rheumatoid arthritis, SLE), and periodontal disease
Positive titer (fourfold increase): Lyme disease

Procedure
- No food or fluid restriction is required.
- Collect 3 to 5 ml of venous blood in a red-top tube. Avoid hemolysis.
- Repeat the Lyme disease antibody test for symptomatic clients with early negative test results.

Factors Affecting Laboratory Results
- Persons with a high rheumatoid factor could have a false-positive test result.

Nursing Implications
- Obtain a history regarding a tick bite.
- Assess for a macular lesion at the site of the tick bite and elsewhere.
- Check titer level. A fourfold rise in titer is indicative of a recent infection.

Client Teaching
- Instruct the client to wear clothing that covers entirely the extremities when in the woods and areas infested by ticks and deer.
- Instruct the client to see a health care provider immediately if bitten by a tick or if a macular lesion results from a tick bite. Antibiotic therapy is frequently started.

LYMPHOCYTES (T AND B) ASSAY (BLOOD)

(T AND B LYMPHOCYTES; LYMPHOCYTE MARKER STUDIES; LYMPHOCYTE SUBSET TYPING)

Reference Values
Adult: T cells: 60%–80%, 600–2,400 cells/μl. B cells: 4%–16%, 50–250 cells/μl

Description. The two categories of lymphocytes are T lymphocytes and B lymphocytes. The T lymphocytes are associated with cell-mediated immune responses (cellular immunity), such as rejection of transplant and graft, tumor immunity, and microorganism (bacterial and viral) death. If the surface of the host's tissue cell is altered, the T cells might perceive that altered cell as foreign and attack it. This might be helpful if the altered surface is of tumor development; however, this T-cell attack might give rise to autoimmune disease.

The B lymphocytes, derived from bone marrow, are responsible for humoral immunity. The B cells synthesize immunoglobulins to react to specific antigens. An interaction between T and B lymphocytes is necessary for a satisfactory immune response.

Measurement of T and B lymphocytes is valuable for diagnosing autoimmune disease (i.e., immunosuppressive diseases, such as AIDS, lymphoma, and lymphocytic leukemia). T and B cells can be used to monitor changes during the treatment of immunosuppressive diseases.

Purposes
- To detect selected autoimmune diseases, such as lymphoma and lymphocytic leukemia
- To monitor the effects of treatment for immunosuppressive diseases, such as AIDS

Clinical Problems
Decreased level: T lymphocytes: lymphoma, lupus disease (SLE), thymic hypoplasia (DiGeorge's syndrome), acute viral infections. B lymphocytes: IgG, IgA, IgM deficiency, lymphomas, nephrotic syndrome,

sex-linked agammaglobulinemia. T and B lymphocytes: immunodeficiency diseases

Drugs that may decrease T lymphocytes: Immunosuppressive agents

Increased level: T lymphocytes: Autoimmune disorders, such as Graves' disease. B lymphocytes: Acute and chronic lymphocytic leukemias, multiple myeloma, Waldenström's macroglobulinemia

Procedure
- No food or fluid restriction is required.
- Collect 7 ml of venous blood in each of two lavender-top tubes. Refrigerate blood specimens. Check with laboratory procedure in your institution.

Nursing Implications
- Observe for signs and symptoms of lymphocytic leukemias (e.g., fatigue, pallor, vesicular skin lesions, increased WBC).
- Listen to the client's concern. Respond to questions or refer the questions to other health care provider(s) if necessary.

Client Teaching
- Instruct the client to stay away from persons with colds or communicable diseases.

MAGNESIUM (Mg) (SERUM)

Reference Values
Adult: 1.5–2.5 mEq/l; 1.8–3.0 mg/dl
Child: Newborn: 1.4–2.9 mEq/l; child: 1.6–2.6 mEq/l

Description.   Magnesium (Mg) is the second most plentiful cation (positive ion electrolyte) in the cells/intracellular fluid. One third of the magnesium ingested is absorbed through the small intestine, and the remaining unabsorbed magnesium is excreted in the stools. The absorbed magnesium is eventually excreted through the kidneys.

Magnesium influences use of potassium, calcium, and protein. With a magnesium deficit, there is frequently a potassium and calcium deficit.

Magnesium, like potassium, sodium, and calcium, is needed for neuro-muscular activity. This electrolyte activates many enzymes for carbohydrate and protein metabolism. A serum magnesium deficit is known as hypo-magnesemia, and a serum magnesium excess is called hypermagnesemia.

Purposes
- To detect hypomagnesemia or hypermagnesemia
- To monitor magnesium levels when there is a probable magnesium loss

Clinical Problems
Decreased level: Protein malnutrition, malabsorption, cirrhosis of the liver, alcoholism, hypoparathyroidism, hyperaldosteronism, hypokalemia, IV solutions without magnesium, chronic diarrhea, bowel resection complications, dehydration

Drugs that may decrease magnesium value: Diuretics, calcium gluconate, amphotericin B, neomycin, insulin

Increased level: Severe dehydration, renal failure, leukemia (lymphocytic and myelocytic), diabetes mellitus (early phase)

Drugs that may increase magnesium value: Antacids that contain magnesium, such as Maalox, Mylanta, Aludrox, DiGel; laxatives that control magnesium, such as milk of magnesia, magnesium citrate, epsom salts $(MgSO_4)$

Procedure
- No food or fluid restriction is required.
- Collect 3 to 5 ml of venous blood in a red-top tube. Avoid hemolysis.

Nursing Implications
Decreased Level
- Check serum potassium, sodium, calcium, and magnesium levels. Electrolyte deficits may accompany a magnesium deficit. If hypokalemia and hypomagnesemia are present, potassium supplements will not totally correct the potassium deficit until the magnesium deficit is corrected.
- Observe for signs and symptoms of hypomagnesemia, such as tetany symptoms (twitching and tremors, carpopedal spasm, and generalized

spasticity), restlessness, confusion, and dysrhythmias. Neuromuscular irritability can be mistakenly attributed to hypocalcemia.
- Report to the health care provider if the client has been NPO and receiving IV fluids without magnesium salts for several weeks. Hyperalimentation solutions should contain magnesium.
- Check if the client is taking a digitalis preparation, such as digoxin. A magnesium deficit enhances the action of digitalis, causing digitalis toxicity. Signs and symptoms of digitalis toxicity include anorexia, nausea, vomiting, and bradycardia.
- Assess renal function when the client is receiving magnesium supplements. Excess magnesium is excreted by the kidneys.
- Assess ECG changes. A flat or inverted T wave can be indicative of hypomagnesemia. It can also indicate hypokalemia.
- Administer IV magnesium sulfate in solution slowly to prevent a hot or flushed feeling. IV calcium gluconate should be available to reverse hypermagnesemia due to overcorrection. Calcium antagonizes the sedative effect of magnesium.

Client Teaching
- Instruct the client to eat foods rich in magnesium (fish, seafood, meats, green vegetables, whole grains, and nuts).

Increased Level
- Observe for signs and symptoms of hypermagnesemia, such as flushing, a feeling of warmth, increased perspiration (with a serum magnesium level at 3 to 4 mEq/l), muscular weakness, diminished reflex, respiratory distress, hypotension, or a sedative effect (with the magnesium level at 9 to 10 mEq/l).
- Monitor urinary output. Effective urinary output (greater than 750 ml daily) will decrease the serum magnesium level.
- Provide adequate fluids to improve kidney function and restore body fluids. Dehydration can cause hemoconcentration and, as a result, magnesium excess.
- Assess the client's level of sensorium and muscle activity. Severe hypermagnesemia causes sedation, and decreases muscular tone and reflex activity.

- Assess ECG strip for changes. A peaked T wave and wide QRS complex can indicate hypermagnesemia and hyperkalemia. Serum potassium and magnesium levels should be checked.
- Check for digitalis toxicity if the client is taking digoxin and is receiving calcium gluconate for hypermagnesemia. Calcium excess enhances the action of digitalis, and digitalis toxicity can result.

Client Teaching
- Instruct the client to avoid constant use of laxatives and antacids containing magnesium. Suggest that the client increase dietary fiber to avoid constipation and laxative use.

MALARIA (BLOOD)

Reference Values
Adult: Negative
Child: Negative

Description.   Malaria is caused by malarial parasites transmitted by mosquitoes. The parasites rupture the red blood cells (hemolysis), causing the client to have chills and fever.

Malarial parasites can be detected by blood smears (venous or capillary blood). Blood samples are usually taken in the presence of chills and fever daily for 3 days or at specified times—every 6 to 12 h.

Purpose
- To identify the presence of malarial parasites

Clinical Problems
Positive: Malaria (*Plasmodium species*)

Procedure
- There is no food or fluid restriction.
- Venous or capillary blood can be used for the malarial smear.
- Collect 5 ml in a lavender-top tube.

Nursing Implications

- Explain the procedure to the client. The client should inform the nurse when he or she is having chills and fever, because the blood sample is usually requested at that time. The blood sample may also be requested daily for 3 days or at specified times during the day.
- Monitor the client's temperature every 4 h or as ordered. Record temperature changes.
- Report chills and fever to the health care provider.

METHEMOGLOBIN (BLOOD)

HEMOGLOBIN M, HB M

Reference Values

Normal: Less than 1.5% of the total hemoglobin; 0.06–0.24 g/dl; 9.2–37.0 µmol/l (SI units)

Positive: Greater than 20%–70%, complaints of headache, dizziness, fatigue, tachycardia; Greater than 70% death

Description.   Methemoglobin (Hb M) occurs when the deoxygenated heme (iron portion of hemoglobin) is oxidized to a ferric state. In the ferric state, the heme cannot combine with oxygen, thus cyanosis without dyspnea or other cardiovascular problems may result. Methemoglobinemia may be acquired from chemicals, radiation, and such drugs as nitrites, nitrates, certain sulfonamides, antimalarials, local anesthetics, or inherited enzyme deficiency. Poisoning from occupational or environmental contact could cause methemoglobinemia. A deficiency in the glucose-6-phosphate dehydrogenase (G-6-PD) enhances the production of Hb M.

If newborns are cyanotic after oxygen has been given, the methemoglobin level should be checked. Infants are more prone to develop methemoglobinemia.

Purposes

- To detect metheglobin in the blood caused by an acquired chemical or drug condition
- To detect congenital methemoglobinemia

Clinical Problems

Increased level: Acquired or hereditary methemoglobinemia, radiation, carbon monoxide poisoning, smoking

Drugs that may increase the methemoglobin level: Bromo-Seltzer, nitrates (including silver nitrate topical preparation), nitrites, nitrous oxide, nitroglycerin, antimalarials, analgesics, certain sulfonamides, fluoroquinolones, and benzene derivatives such as chlorobenzene, phenacetin, isoniazid, lidocaine, chlorates

Food that may increase the methemoglobin level: Sausage and other foods that contain nitrites.

Procedure

- There is no food or fluid restriction.
- Collect 7 ml of venous blood in a lavender- or green-top tube. Keep blood specimen on ice. Deliver blood specimen to the laboratory within 1 h.

Factors Affecting Laboratory Results

- Certain drugs and food can cause false results (see Clinical Problems).
- Not keeping the blood specimen chilled (on ice) and not delivering the specimen to the laboratory within 1 h.

Nursing Implications

- Obtain a history of the health complaints, drugs, and food the client is consuming. Certain drugs can enhance the production of Hb M (see Clinical Problems). Excessive use of Bromo-Seltzer can increase the Hb M level.
- Check vital signs. Continuously monitor heart rate with a pulse oximetry.
- Check O_2 saturation with the pulse oximetry or arterial blood gases (ABGs).
- Administer oxygen. Blood transfusions may be prescribed.

Client Teaching

- Encourage client to rest if dizziness, fatigue, and headaches occur.

- Explain to the client that the health care provider may discontinue a drug that may be causing an increase in Hb M production.

MUMPS ANTIBODY (SERUM)

Reference Values
Negative: Less than 1:8 titer
Positive or Immunization: Greater than 1:8 (recent infection or immunization undetermined)

Description. Mumps, infectious parotitis, is an acute, contagious viral infection causing an inflammation of the parotid and salivary glands. The mumps virus can be spread by droplets or by direct contact with the saliva of an infected person. Complications of mumps include (1) in adolescent or adult males, unilateral orchitis in approximately 20% of reported cases; (2) in adult women, oophoritis; and (3) in persons of all ages and genders, meningoencephalitis in 1% to 10% of infected cases.

Diagnosis may be made by blood specimen, culture of saliva, or mumps skin test. With a blood specimen two blood samples should be taken, one during the acute phase and one during the convalescent phase. For those persons who are at high risk or who have not had mumps, there is a vaccine to provide immunity.

Purpose
- To detect the presence of the mumps antibody in a person who may be at risk

Clinical Problems
Positive: Mumps virus. *Complications:* Orchitis, oophoritis, meningoencephalitis

Procedure
- No food or fluids are restricted.
- Collect a total of two 3- to 5-ml samples of venous blood in a red-top tube, 1 to 2 weeks apart. The first specimen is drawn during the acute

phase, and the second is taken 1 to 2 weeks later during the convalescent phase. Place ice around specimen tube.
- Label the first specimen "acute."

Nursing Implications
- Assess the client for symptoms of mumps, such as malaise, headache, chills, fever, pain below the ear, and swelling of the parotid glands.
- Assess if the client has been in contact with a person diagnosed as having mumps. Clients who are suspected of having mumps may be isolated up to 9 days after swelling occurs.
- Check if the client had received the mumps vaccine. Those who develop mumps normally have a lifetime immunity.

Client Teaching
- Explain to the client that he/she is to return for a second blood test 1 to 2 weeks later for the convalescent phase of the mumps infection.
- Explain to the client that mumps is contagious and that he/she will be isolated for about 9 days from other persons who have never had mumps or the vaccine. The incubation period for mumps is 16 to 18 days.
- Inform the pregnant female that if mumps occurs during the first trimester of pregnancy, the fetus may have a higher risk of developing congenital anomalies. It is suggested to many young females that if they have not had mumps, they should be tested for mumps antibody; and if the result is negative, they should receive the mumps vaccine.

MYOGLOBIN (SERUM AND URINE)

Reference Values
Serum: Adult: female: 12–75 ng/ml, 12–75 mcg/l (SI units); male: 20–90 ng/ml, 20–90 mcg/l (SI units)
Urine: Negative or less than 20 ng/ml, less than 20 mcg/l (SI units)

Description.   Myoglobin is an oxygen-binding protein, similar to hemoglobin, that is found in skeletal and cardiac muscle cells. Myoglobin is released into circulation after an injury. Increased serum myoglobin occurs about 2 to 6 h following muscle tissue damage, and it reaches its peak following a myocardial infarction (MI) in approximately 8 to 12 h. Elevated serum myoglobin (myoglobinemia) is short-lived; in 50% of persons having an MI, the serum level begins to return to normal range in 12 to 18 h. Urine myoglobin may be detected for 3 to 7 days following muscle injury.

Because serum myoglobin is nonspecific concerning which muscle is damaged, myocardium or skeletal, cardiac enzymes should be ordered and checked. The serum myoglobin is not performed following cardioversion or after an angina attack.

Myoglobin passes rapidly from the blood through the glomeruli in the kidney and is excreted in the urine. Myoglobinuria can appear within 3 h after an MI and may be present in the urine up to 72 h or longer.

Purpose
- To detect myoglobin protein, which is released in high amounts during skeletal or cardiac muscle injury

Clinical Problems
Increased level: Acute MI, skeletal muscle injury, severe burns, trauma, surgical procedure, polymyositis, acute alcohol toxicity (delirium tremens), renal failure, metabolic stress

Procedure
- No food or fluid restriction is required.

Serum: Collect 3 to 5 ml of venous blood in a red-top tube. Avoid hemolysis. The blood sample should be drawn soon after an acute MI or following acute pain.

Urine: Collect 5 to 10 ml of random urine specimen in a sterile plastic container.

Factors Affecting Laboratory Results
- A blood sample taken for a serum myoglobin $1^{1}/_{2}$ to 2 days following acute chest pain

Nursing Implications

- Obtain a history of the current muscle discomfort (skeletal or cardiac). Report findings.
- Assess the client for signs and symptoms of an MI, such as sharp, penetrating pain in the chest, radiating pain in the left arm, diaphoresis, dyspnea, nausea, and vomiting.
- Check vital signs and report abnormal findings.
- Compare elevated serum myoglobin level with positive urine myoglobin. Cardiac enzymes should be ordered.

Client Teaching

- Instruct the client to inform you when pain occurs or recurs. Have the client describe the pain (type, intensity, duration).
- Explain the procedure for urine collection to the client.
- Explain to the client that a blood sample and urine specimen may both be ordered and explain why (see Description).
- Answer client's and family's questions or refer the questions to the appropriate health care professional. Listen to their concerns.

N-TELOPEPTIDE CROSS-LINKS (NTx) (SERUM AND URINE)

Reference Values

Serum: Female: 6.2–19 nM BCE/l (bone collagen equivalents); male: 5.4–24.2 nM BCE/l
Urine: Female: 5–65 mM BCE/mmol creatinine; male: 3–51 mM BCE/mmol creatinine

Description. About 90% of the bone matrix consists of type I collagen that is cross-linked at the N-terminal and C-terminal ends. The N terminals of these proteins are cross-linked to give strength to the bones. The bone resorption by osteoclasts causes a production of cross-linked N-telopeptides of NTx type I collagen. This protein is found both in the serum and urine as an end product of bone degradation. The serum level of NTx correlates with bone resorption and bone density in older women with osteopenia or osteoporosis. It is also used to monitor the effects of the therapy for these conditions.

NTx serum levels correlate well with urine NTx normalized to creatinine.

Purposes
- To correlate with serum NTx and urine NTx to identify bone disease and osteoporosis
- To monitor the effects of antiresorptive therapy with estrogen and/or calcium supplements

Clinical Problems
Decreased level: Hypoparathyroidism, hypothyroidism.
Drug that decreases the NTx: Cortisol therapy.
Increased level: Osteoporosis, osteopenia, Paget's disease, advanced bone tumors, acromegaly, hypoparathyroidism, hypothyroidism.

Procedure
Serum
- There is no food or fluid restriction.
- Collect 3 to 5 ml of venous blood in a red-top tube or serum separator tube.
- Take serum specimen to the laboratory immediately or refrigerate.

Urine
- Collect 20 ml of urine the second void of the morning. A baseline urine specimen should be collected before correction therapy for the bone disease or osteoporosis has been started.
- Refrigerate specimen.

Factors Affecting Laboratory Results
- Hemolysis of the blood specimen
- Unrefrigerated urine

Nursing Implications

- Obtain a health history related to symptoms of osteoporosis and bone disease.
- Compare serum levels with urine levels. Report findings.
- Ask the client when he/she had the last bone density scan. Record answer.
- Provide comfort measures to the client.

Client Teaching

- Explain to the client to collect the second urine sample in the morning.
- Tell the client to take the urine specimen to the laboratory or have it refrigerated. The specimen may be given in the laboratory.

5'NUCLEOTIDASE (5'N OR 5'NT) (SERUM)

Reference Values

Adult: Less than 17 units/l
Pregnancy: Third trimester: slightly above normal value
Child: Values lower than adults, except infants

Description.   Serum 5' nucleotidase (5'N) is a liver enzyme test used to diagnose hepatobiliary disease. 5'N is not elevated in bone disorders; alkaline phosphatase (ALP) may be elevated in bone and liver disorders. Elevated ALP and 5'N indicate liver disorder; elevated ALP and a normal 5'N indicate bone disorder. Usually, several other liver enzyme tests may be used to diagnose liver disorders, such as gamma-glutamyl transferase (GGT) and leucine aminopeptidase (LAP).

Purpose

- To compare test results with other liver enzyme tests for diagnosing a liver disorder

Clinical Problems

Increased level: Cirrhosis of the liver, biliary obstruction from calculi or tumor, and metastasis to the liver

Drugs that may increase 5'N value: Acetaminophen, aspirin, narcotics, phenothiazines, phenytoin

Procedure
- No food or fluid restriction is required.
- Collect 3 to 5 ml of venous blood in a red-top tube. Avoid hemolysis.

Nursing Implications
- Compare 5'N levels with other liver enzyme levels. Elevated ALP, GGT, LAP, and 5'N values indicate that the problem is of liver origin.

Client Teaching
- Instruct the client to maintain effective oral hygiene as bleeding of the gums commonly occurs. With liver disorder, the prothrombin time is usually prolonged.
- Encourage the client to eat well-balanced meals.

OCCULT BLOOD (FECES)

Reference Values
Adult: Negative
Child: Negative
Note: A diet rich in meats, poultry, and fish, as well as certain drugs (i.e., cortisone, aspirin, iron, and potassium preparations) could cause a false-positive occult blood test.

Description.   Occult (nonvisible or hidden) blood in the feces usually indicates GI bleeding. Bright red blood from the rectum can be indicative of bleeding from the lower large intestine (e.g., hemorrhoids), and tarry black stools indicate blood loss of greater than 50 ml from the upper GI tract.

Purpose
- To detect blood in the feces

Clinical Problems

Drugs that may cause false negatives: Large amounts of ascorbic acid
Positive results: Bleeding peptic ulcers, gastritis, gastric carcinoma, bleeding esophageal varices, colitis, intestinal carcinoma, diverticulitis
Drugs that may cause false positives: Aspirin, cortisone, iron, and potassium preparations, NSAIDs drugs (indomethacin [Indocin], ibuprofens), thiazide diuretics, colchicine, reserpine

Procedure

* A variety of blood test reagents may be used. Orthotolidine (Occultest) is considered the most sensitive test.
* Avoid meats, poultry, and fish 2 to 3 days prior to stool specimen.
* On the laboratory slip list drugs the client is taking.
* Obtain a single, random stool specimen (small amount) and send it to the laboratory, or test using a kit to detect occult blood. Stool specimen could be obtained from a rectal examination.

Nursing Implications

* Obtain a history of bleeding episodes, dental hygiene, and/or bleeding gums. Only 2 ml or more blood can cause a positive test result.
* Determine whether the client has had epigastric pain between meals, which could be indicative of a peptic ulcer.
* Be sure the stool is not contaminated with menstrual discharge.

Client Teaching

* Instruct the client not to eat meats, poultry, and fish for 2 to 3 days before the test. Excessive green, leafy vegetables could cause a false-positive result.
* Encourage the client to report abnormally colored stools (e.g., tarry stools). Oral iron preparations can cause the stool to be black.

OPIATES (URINE AND BLOOD)

Reference Values (Urine and Blood)

Negative

Toxic values

Urine: *Codeine:* Greater than 0.005 mg/dl (0.2 µmol/l). *Hydromorphone:* greater than 0.1 mg/dl (5 µmol/l). *Meperidine:* greater than 0.5 mg/dl (20 µmol/l). *Methadone:* greater than 0.2 mg/dl (10 µmol/l). *Morphine:* greater than 0.005 mg/dl (0.2 µmol/l). *Propoxyphene:* greater than 0.5 mg/dl (20 µmol/l)

Blood: *Cocaine:* greater than 1,000 ng/ml (greater than 3,300 µmol/l) (SI units)

Description.   Testing for opiates is primarily done to screen for drug abuse or narcotic toxicity, or to check the progress of opiate detoxification. Specific opiates, such as codeine, morphine, methadone, hydromorphone, and meperidine, can be individually tested. Urine is the preferred specimen for checking for these opiates; however, gastric secretions could be analyzed.

The liver detoxifies opiates, and the urine excretes 90% of the opiates in 24 h. The peak effect of opiates in the body occurs in approximately 1 h.

Cocaine, another narcotic that is frequently abused, is a central nervous system stimulant. It increases blood pressure, respiratory rate, and heart rate and may lead to cardiopulmonary failure. Cocaine has many street names, such as coke, crack, gold dust, stardust, and happy dust.

Purposes

* To detect the presence of opiates
* To check for opiate toxicity
* To monitor the progress of opiate detoxification

Clinical Problems

Increased level: Specific opiate presence or toxicity
Drugs that may increase opiate levels: Use of other opiates

Procedure

* No food or fluid restriction is required.
* List drugs taken by the client in the last 24 h on the laboratory sheet, including over-the-counter (OTC) drugs.
* A signed consent may be necessary.

Urine

- Collect a random urine specimen and send the specimen immediately to the laboratory.
- Refrigerate the urine specimen if the test cannot be done immediately.

Blood

- Collect 5 to 7 ml of venous blood in a lavender- or green-top tube. Place tube on ice and send it to the laboratory immediately.
- If the test is for a legal purpose, have a witness present when obtaining the blood specimen. A signed consent form may be needed; check with hospital or state policy.
- Used for legal evidence, special handling and labeling of the specimen is essential; that is, it should be placed in a sealed container or bag and labeled with the date and time of the drawn blood specimen and the witness's name and signature.

Factors Affecting Laboratory Results

- Blood specimen not tested within an hour after drawing and the tube not placed on ice
- Blood specimen not drawn soon after cocaine use (cocaine has a short action)

Nursing Implications

- Obtain a drug history including OTC drugs. Explain that the information will be given to the health care provider.
- Send the random urine specimen immediately to the laboratory. If the opiate test is for methadone, a 24-h urine specimen is needed. Inform the laboratory that the urine specimen should be tested immediately or refrigerated. Delay in testing can cause false-negative test result.

Client Teaching

- Explain to the client that addictive narcotic drugs can cause withdrawal symptoms when the drug is abruptly stopped.
- Inform the client of the adverse reactions to cocaine, such as lung and kidney problems, heart attacks, suicidal tendency, hallucinations, and others.

OSMOLALITY (SERUM AND URINE)

Reference Values
Adult: Serum: 280–300 mOsm/kg H_2O; urine: 50–1200 mOsm/kg H_2O
Child: Serum: 270–290 mOsm/kg H_2O; urine: child: same as adult; newborn: 100–600 mOsm/kg H_2O
Panic Value: Less than 240 mOsm/kg and greater than 320 mOsm/kg

Description.   Serum osmolality is an indicator of serum concentration. An elevated serum osmolality indicates hemoconcentration and dehydration, and a decreased serum level indicates hemodilution or overhydration. Osmolality measures the number of dissolved particles (electrolytes, sugar, urea) in the serum. Doubling the serum sodium, which accounts for 85% to 95% of the serum osmolality, can give a rough estimate of the serum osmolality. The serum osmolality can be calculated if the sodium, glucose, and urea are known.

$$\text{Serum osmolality} = Na + \frac{BUN}{3} + \frac{glucose}{18}$$

Urine osmolality is more accurate than the specific gravity in determining the concentration, since it is influenced by the number of particles. The state of hydration affects the urine osmolality.

Purposes
* To monitor body fluid balance
* To determine the occurrence of body fluid overload or dehydration

Clinical Problems
Decreased level: Excessive fluid intake, continuous IV D_5W, SIADH (serum only), hyponatremia, acute renal disease, and diabetes insipidus (urine only)
Increased level: Dehydration, hyperglycemia, hypernatremia, diabetes insipidus (serum only), SIADH (urine only), ethanol

Procedure
Serum

* No food or fluid restriction is required.
* Collect 5 to 7 ml of venous blood in a red-top tube. Avoid hemolysis.

Urine

* Give a high-protein diet for 3 days prior to test. Check with your laboratory.
* Restrict fluids for 8 to 12 h.
* Collect a random, morning urine specimen. The first urine specimen in the morning is discarded, and the second specimen, taken 2 h later, is sent to the laboratory. Urine osmolality should be high in the morning.

Nursing Implications
Client Teaching

* Inform client that no food and fluids are restricted with serum osmolality test. Fluids are restricted with urine.

Decreased Level

* Associate a decreased serum osmolality with serum dilution caused by excessive fluid intake (overhydration).
* Observe for signs and symptoms of overhydration (e.g., a constant, irritating cough; dyspnea; neck-and-hand vein engorgement; and chest rales). Instruct to decrease fluid intake.
* Determine whether the decreased urine osmolality could be caused by excessive water intake (greater than 2 quarts daily) or continuous IV administration of D_5W. A urine osmolality less than 200 mOsm/kg after fluids are restricted could be indicative of early kidney impairment.
* Observe for signs and symptoms of water intoxication (e.g., headaches, confusion, irritability, weight gain).

Increased Level

* Determine the hydration status of the client. Dehydration will cause an elevated serum and urine osmolality.
* Assess for signs and symptoms of dehydration (e.g., thirst, dry mucous membranes, poor skin turgor, and shock-like symptoms). Encourage the client to increase fluid intake.

* Check for hyperglycemia and glycosuria. Both could cause an elevation of serum and urine osmolality.
* Compare the serum osmolality with the urine osmolality. If the serum is hypo-osmolar (hypo-osmolality), the problem could be due to the syndrome of inappropriate ADH (SIADH).

OSTEOCALCIN (SERUM)

Oc, BONE Gla PROTEIN (BGP); Gla PROTEIN

Reference Values

Female: Premenopausal: 0.5–7.8 ng/ml; 0.5–7.8 mcg/l (SI units)
            Postmenopausal: 1.2–11 ng/ml; 1.2–11 mcg/l (SI units)
Male: 1.5–11.5 ng/ml; 1.5–11.5 mcg/l (SI units)
            (Check reference values with your institution)

Description.   Osteocalcin or BGP, a biochemical marker, is useful in determining the effectiveness of treatment for bone disease and osteoporosis. This noncollagenous protein in the bone, produced by the osteoblasts, has a function in bone mineralization and bone formation. A small amount of osteocalcin enters the circulation. Osteocalcin synthesis is dependent on vitamin K. A reduced intake of vitamin K is associated with a decrease in the bone Gla protein.

It is an indicator for bone metabolism. Elevated levels occur during osteoporosis and bone disease.

A bone density scan can diagnose osteoporosis. The test cannot identify changes in bone metabolism. A bone density test is also more expensive than laboratory tests for detecting bone disease and osteoporosis.

Purposes

* To determine the effectiveness of bone therapy
* To assess bone metabolism
* To detect bone disease such as osteoporosis

Clinical Problems

Decreased level: Deficiency of growth hormone, hypoparathyroidism, multiple myeloma, cirrhosis of the liver

Drugs that may decrease osteocalcin level: Cortisone drugs, calcitonin, warfarin

Increased level: Fractures, osteoporosis, growth spurt (10–16 years old), acromegaly, bone cancer, Paget's disease, hyperparathyroidism, hyperthyroidism, low estrogen production, low calcium intake, osteomalacia, renal failure with dialysis

Procedure
* No food or fluid restriction is required.
* Collect 7 ml of venous blood in a red-, lavender-, or green-top tube. Check with your institution for the desired color-top tube.

Factors Affecting Laboratory Results
* None known

Nursing Implications
* Obtain a history of health problems, including symptoms of osteoporosis or bone disease.
* Determine if and when the client has had a bone density scan. The scan is useful to identify osteoporosis, but it is not effective for identifying changes in bone metabolism.
* Check the results of previous bone density and osteocalcin (BGP) tests. Compare other bone tests with the current BGP test.

Client Teaching
* Explain to the client that the BGP test is useful in determining the effects of the prescribed medications, for example, estrogen, raloxifene (Evista), alendronate (Fosamax).
* Answer client questions concerning the test and results, or if unknown, refer the question(s) to other health professionals.

OVA AND PARASITES (O & P) (FECES)

Reference Values
Adult: Negative
Child: Negative

Description.   Parasites may be present in various forms in the intestine, including the ova, larvae, cysts, and trophozoites of the protozoa. Some of the organisms identified are amoeba, flagellates, tapeworms, hookworms, and roundworms. A history of recent travel outside the United States should be reported to the laboratory to help in identifying the parasite.

Purpose
* To identify specific ova and parasites in fecal matter

Clinical Problems
Positive result: Protozoa: *Balantidium coli, Chilomastix mesnili, Entamoeba histolytica, Giardia lamblia, Trichomonas hominis;* helminths (adults): *Ascaris lumbricoides* (roundworm), *Diphyllobothrium latum* (fish tapeworm), *Enterobius vermicularis* (pinworm), *Necator americanus* (American hookworm), *Strongyloides stercoralis* (threadworm), *Taenia saginata* (beef tapeworm), *Taenia solium* (pork tapeworm)

Procedure
* Collect stool specimen daily for 3 days or every other day. Take to the laboratory immediately, within 1 h, or refrigerate.
* Mark on the laboratory slip countries the client has visited in the last 1 to 3 years.
* A loose or liquid stool is likely to indicate trophozoites and needs to be kept warm and taken to the laboratory within 30 min.
* If the stool is tested for tapeworm, the entire stool should be sent to the laboratory so that the head (scolex) of the tapeworm can be identified.
* Anal swabs are used to check for pinworm eggs, and the swabbing should be done in the morning before defecation or the morning bath.
* No tissue paper or urine in the fecal collection.
* Avoid taking mineral oil, castor oil, metamucil, barium, antacids, or tetracycline for 1 week before the test with the health care provider's approval.
* Laboratory results are available in 24 to 48 h.

Nursing Implications
* Obtain a history of the client's recent travel, and notify the laboratory and health care provider.

- Handle the stool specimen with care to prevent parasitic contamination of yourself and other clients.
- Check for occult blood in stool. The worm attaches itself to the bowel's lining.

Client Teaching
- Explain that the stool specimen should be collected in the morning.
- Explain that a soap suds enema should not be used, as this may destroy the parasite. The stool specimen should be obtained before treatment is initiated.

PARATHYROID HORMONE (PTH) (SERUM)

Reference Values
Adult: Intact PTH: 11–54 pg/ml; C-terminal PTH: 50–330 pg/ml; N-terminal PTH: 8–24 pg/ml

Description. Parathyroid hormone (PTH), secreted by the parathyroid glands, regulates the concentration of calcium and phosphorus in the extracellular fluid (ECF). The main function of PTH is to promote calcium reabsorption and phosphorus excretion. A low serum calcium level stimulates the secretion of PTH and a high serum calcium level inhibits PTH secretion.

Two forms of PTH, inactive C-terminal PTH and active N-terminal PTH, are used in diagnosing parathyroid disorders. C-terminal assays (PTH-C) are an effective indicator of chronic hyperparathyroidism. N-terminal assays (PTH-N) detect acute changes in the PTH secretion, can differentiate between hypercalcemia due to malignancy or parathyroid disorder, and are useful for monitoring the client's response to PTH therapy. Both assays and serum calcium values are used in diagnosing early and borderline parathyroid disorders.

Purposes
- To identify hypo- or hyperparathyroidism (see Clinical Problems)
- To monitor the client's response to PTH therapy

Clinical Problems

Decreased level: *PTH-C levels:* hypoparathyroidism, nonparathyroid hypercalcemia. *PTH-N levels:* hypoparathyroidism, nonparathyroid hypercalcemia, certain tumors, pseudohyperparathyroidism. *PTH-serum:* hypoparathyroidism, nonparathyroid hypercalcemia, Graves' disease, sarcoidosis

Increased level: *PTH-C levels:* secondary hyperparathyroidism, tumors, hypercalcemia, pseudohypoparathyroidism. *PTH-N levels:* primary and secondary hyperparathyroidism, pseudohypoparathyroidism. *PTH-serum:* primary and secondary hyperparathyroidism, hypercalcemia, chronic renal failure, pseudohyperparathyroidism (defect in renal tubular response)

Procedure

* Restrict food and fluids for 8 h prior to the test.
* Collect 5 to 7 ml of venous blood in a red-top tube in AM. Morning PTH is usually at its lowest point. Avoid hemolysis. N-terminal PTH is unstable and needs to be chilled or frozen if test is not immediately done.
* N-terminal PTH levels decrease during hemodialysis; collect blood specimens before dialysis.

Factors Affecting Laboratory Results

* Food, especially milk products, might lower the PTH level.

Nursing Implications

* Recognize the relationship of serum calcium levels and PTH secretion and serum level.
* Assess for signs and symptoms of hypocalcemia (tetany symptoms), and hypercalcemia (lethargy, muscle flaccidity, weakness, headaches).

Client Teaching

* Instruct the client not to eat until after the blood sample is taken. Foods high in calcium (milk products) may lower PTH level.

PARTIAL THROMBOPLASTIN TIME (PTT); ACTIVATED PARTIAL THROMBOPLASTIN TIME (APTT) (PLASMA)

Reference Values

Adult: PTT: 60–70 seconds; APTT: 20–35 seconds
Anticoagulant therapy: 1.5–2.5 times the control in seconds.
Note: Most laboratories do APTT only.

Description.   The PTT is a screening test used to detect deficiencies in all clotting factors except VII and XIII and to detect platelet variations. The PTT is useful for monitoring heparin therapy.

The APTT is more sensitive in detecting clotting factor defects than the PTT, because the activator added in vitro shortens the clotting time. APTT is also used to monitor heparin therapy and is useful in preoperative screening for bleeding tendencies.

Purposes

* To monitor heparin therapy
* To screen for clotting factor deficiencies

Clinical Problems

Increased (prolonged) levels: Factor deficiencies (V, VIII, IX, X, XI, XII), cirrhosis of the liver, vitamin K deficiency, leukemias, Hodgkin's disease, disseminated intravascular coagulation (DIC), hypofibrinogenemia, von Willebrand's disease (vascular hemophilia)
Drugs that may increase PTT value: Heparin, salicylates

Procedure

* No food or fluid restriction is required.
* APTT test should be drawn 1 h before next heparin dosage.
* Collect 3 to 5 ml of venous blood in a blue-top tube. Blood specimen should be taken to the laboratory *immediately.*

Nursing Implications

* Report APTT or PTT results to the physician.

- Assess the client for signs and symptoms of bleeding (e.g., purpura, hematuria, and nosebleeds).
- Administer heparin subcutaneously (SC) or IV through a heparin lock/IV reservoir. **Do not** aspirate when giving heparin SC, as a hematoma could occur at the injection site.

PARVOVIRUS B 19 ANTIBODY (SERUM)

Reference Values
Negative: No IgG and IgM antibodies to parvovirus B 19

Description.
The parvovirus B 19, a human virus, destroys red blood cells (RBCs) and interferes with RBC production. This virus occurs more frequently in children. Erythema infectiosum causes a low-grade fever and rash, particularly in children; hydrops fetalis and aplastic anemia are associated with the parvovirus B 19.

The presence of IgM antibodies to parvovirus B 19 can indicate an acute infection, and the IgG antibodies can indicate a past infection or immunity. Joint inflammation and purpura are other clinical manifestations of the parvovirus B 19. A positive parvovirus B 19 has been associated with organ transplants; therefore, a serologic assessment should be made on organ donors.

Purposes
- To detect the presence of parvovirus B 19 antibody
- To aid in the diagnosis of erythema infectiosum

Clinical Problems
Positive test: Erythema infectiosum (most common), transient aplastic anemia, joint arthritis, hydrops fetalis, fetal loss, bone marrow failure (aplastic anemia), chronic anemia in immunocompromised clients

Procedure
- There is no food or fluid restriction.

* Collect 5 ml of venous blood in a red-top tube. Avoid hemolysis (shaking tube or rough handling of the blood specimen). Keep blood specimen on ice.
* Take precaution with collection and delivery of the blood specimen to avoid spread of infection.

Factors Affecting Laboratory Results
* Hemolysis of the blood specimen.
* Blood specimen not kept cold or on ice.

Nursing Implications
* Obtain a history of the health complaint from the child, parent, or family member. List symptoms.
* Record vital signs. Report abnormal findings.

Client Teaching
* Explain to organ donors that a blood test may be prescribed to rule out the presence of a virus antibody (parvovirus B 19 antibody) that may affect organ donation. It is for preventive purposes.
* Answer the parent or family members' questions concerning the child or client condition or refer the person(s) to other health professionals for correct answers.

PEPSINOGEN I (SERUM)

Reference Values
Adult: 124–142 ng/ml; 124–142 mcg/l (SI units)
Child: *Premature infant:* 20–24 ng/ml (SEM) × 1:20–24 mcg/l (SI units). Less than *1 year:* 72–82 ng/ml; 72–82 g/l (SI units). *1–2 years:* 90–106 ng/ml; 90–106 mcg/l (SI units). *3–6 years:* 80–104 ng/ml; 80–104 g/l (SI units). *7–10 years:* 77–103 ng/ml; 77–103 mcg/l (SI units). *11–14 years:* 96–118 ng/ml; 96–118 mcg/l (SI units).

Description.   There are seven fractions of pepsinogens in the blood; five are classified as pepsinogen I (PG-I), which are secreted from the lumen of the stomach. The secretion of pepsinogen I is controlled by the hormone gastrin. Pepsinogen I is converted to pepsin when the stomach pH is acidic. Pepsin is needed in the process of digestion of proteins. Low gastrin and pepsinogen I levels are specific for atrophic gastritis. An elevated pepsinogen I level frequently occurs with duodenal ulcer. A high PG-I level can be inherited as an autosomal dominant trait.

Purpose
* To determine the cause of the gastric disorder

Clinical Problems
Decreased level: Atropic gastritis, gastric cancer, achlorhydria, pernicious anemia, Addison's disease, myxedema, hypopituitarism
Increased level: Duodenal ulcer, acute gastritis, Zollinger–Ellison syndrome, hypergastrinemia

Procedure
* NPO 8 to 12 h before the test.
* Collect 5 to 7 ml of venous blood in a red-top tube.

Factors Affecting Laboratory Results
* Poor renal output can cause an elevated serum pepsinogen I level.

Nursing Implications
* Assess the client's renal function, such as adequate urine output and blood urea nitrogen and serum creatinine levels. Poor renal function can cause a false-elevated serum PG-I level.
* Assess the client for complaints of gastric discomfort. Record findings.

Client Teaching
* Instruct the client that the test requires a fasting blood specimen; therefore, the client should take nothing by mouth after midnight.
* Instruct the client to inform you of any abdominal discomfort. The time of gastric or intestinal discomfort should be recorded.

PHENYLKETONURIA (PKU) (URINE); GUTHRIE TEST FOR PKU (BLOOD)

Reference Values

Child: Phenylalanine: 0.5–2.0 mg/dl; PKU: negative, but positive when the phenylalanine is 12–15 mg/dl; Guthrie: negative, but positive when the serum phenylalanine is 4 mg/dl

Description.   The urine PKU and Guthrie tests are two screening tests used for detecting a hepatic enzyme deficiency, phenylalanine hydroxylase, which prevents the conversion of phenylalanine (amino acid) to tyrosine in the infant. Phenylalanine from milk and other protein products accumulates in the blood and tissues and can lead to brain damage and mental retardation.

The Guthrie procedure is the test of choice because a positive test result occurs when the serum phenylalanine reaches 4 mg/dl, 3 to 5 days of life after milk ingestion. If Guthrie test is positive, a specific blood phenylalanine test should be performed. The PKU urine test is done after the infant is 3 to 4 weeks old and should be repeated a week or two later. Significant brain damage usually occurs when the serum phenylalanine level is 15 mg/dl. If either the Guthrie test or the urine PKU is positive, the infant should be maintained on a low phenylalanine diet for 6 to 8 years.

Purposes

* To screen for phenylalanine hydroxylase deficiency
* To repeat phenylketonuria test as indicated

Clinical Problems

Increased level: PKU, low-birth-weight infants, hepatic encephalopathy, septicemia, galactosemia

Drugs that may increase PKU value: Aspirins, ketone bodies

Procedure

Guthrie test (Guthrie bacterial inhibition test):   Phenylalanine promotes bacterial growth (*Bacillus subtilis*) when the serum level is greater than 4 mg/dl.

- Cleanse the infant's heel, and prick it with a sterile lancet. Obtain several drops of blood on a filter paper streaked with *B subtilis.* If the bacillus grows, the test is positive.
- Test should be performed on the fourth day after 2 to 4 days of milk ingestion (either cow's milk or breast milk).
- Note on the laboratory slip the date of birth and the date of the first milk ingested.

Urine PKU: Phenylalanine is converted to phenylpyruvic acid and is excreted in the urine when the serum level is 12 to 15 mg/dl.

- Dip Phenistix (dipstick with ferric salt) in fresh urine, or press against a fresh wet diaper. If positive, the dipstick will turn green.
- Perform PKU urine test 3 to 6 weeks after birth, preferably at 4 weeks, and repeat if necessary.

Factors Affecting Laboratory Results
- Urine that is not fresh can cause an inaccurate result.
- Vomiting and/or decreased milk intake may cause a normal serum phenylalanine level in the infant with PKU.
- Aspirins and salicylate compounds can cause a false-positive result.
- Early PKU testing before the infant is 3 days old may cause a false-negative test result.

Nursing Implications
- Determine if the infant has had at least 3 days of milk intake before performing the Guthrie test. Vomiting and refusing to eat are common problems of PKU infants. This may cause a normal serum phenylalanine level.
- Compare the Guthrie test with serum phenylalanine.
- Obtain history if mother was a "PKU baby." If so, the mother should be on a low phenylalanine diet before and during pregnancy.

Client Teaching
- Explain to the mother the screening tests used to detect PKU. The Guthrie test is normally done while in the hospital. Many pediatricians want the urine PKU done 4 weeks after birth as a follow-up test.

* Teach the mother how to perform a urine PKU test accurately. Fresh urine on diaper or urine specimen should be used.
* Instruct that the baby should receive Tylenol and not aspirin or salicylate compounds for 24 h before testing the urine to prevent a false-positive test. Check with the health care provider.
* Tell the mother which foods the baby should and should not have. The preferred milk substitute is Lofenalac (Mead Johnson) with vitamins and minerals. Other low-phenylalanine foods are fruits, fruit juices, vegetables, cereals, and breads. Avoid high-protein foods, such as milk, ice cream, and cheese.

PHENYTOIN (*SEE* DILANTIN)

PHOSPHORUS (P) (SERUM)

PHOSPHATE (PO$_4$)

Reference Values
Adult: 1.7–2.6 mEq/l, 2.5–4.5 mg/dl, 0.78–1.52 mmol/l (SI units)
Child: Newborn: 3.5–8.6 mg/dl; infant: 4.5–6.7 mg/dl; child: 4.5–5.5 mg/dl
Elderly: Slightly lower than adult

Description.   Phosphorus is the principal intracellular anion, and most exists in the blood as phosphate. From 80% to 85% of the total phosphates in the body are combined with calcium in the teeth and bones. Phosphates also regulate enzymatic activity for energy transfer.

Phosphorus and calcium concentrations are controlled by the parathyroid hormone. Usually there is a reciprocal relationship between calcium and phosphorus (i.e., when serum phosphorus levels increase, serum calcium levels decrease, and vice versa).

Purposes
* To check phosphorus level
* To monitor phosphorus levels during renal insufficiency or failure

- To compare phosphorus level with other electrolytes (e.g., potassium, calcium)

Clinical Problems

Decreased level: Starvation, malabsorption syndrome, hyperparathyroidism, hypercalcemia, hypomagnesemia, chronic alcoholism, vitamin D deficiency, diabetic acidosis, myxedema, continuous IV fluids with glucose, nasogastric (NG) suctioning, and vomiting

Drugs that may decrease phosphorus value: Antacids (aluminum hydroxide [Amphojel]); epinephrine (adrenalin); insulin, mannitol

Increased level: Renal insufficiency, renal failure, hypoparathyroidism, hypocalcemia, hypervitaminosis D, bone tumors, acromegaly, healing fractures, sarcoidosis, Cushing's syndrome

Drugs that may increase phosphorus value: Methicillin, phenytoin (Dilantin), heparin, Lipomul, laxatives with phosphate

Procedure

- Restrict food and fluids except for water 4 to 8 h. Carbohydrate lowers serum phosphorus levels.
- Hold IV fluids with glucose for 4 to 8 h with health care provider's approval.
- Collect 3 to 5 ml of venous blood in a red-top tube. Avoid hemolysis. Take to the laboratory *immediately.*

Factors Affecting Laboratory Results

- A high-carbohydrate diet and IV fluids with glucose can lower the serum phosphorus level; hence a fasting specimen is needed.
- Hemolysis of the blood sample can increase the serum phosphorus level. When RBCs rupture, they release intracellular phosphate into the serum.
- Late delivery of the blood sample (greater than 30 min) may cause the release of phosphorus from the blood cells into the serum. The serum should be separated from the blood clot within 30 min.
- Amphojel can lower the serum phosphorus level.

Nursing Implications

Decreased level: Hypophosphatemia

* Check the serum phosphorus, calcium, and magnesium levels. An elevated calcium level causes a decreased phosphorus level.
* Observe for signs and symptoms of hypophosphatemia (e.g., anorexia, pain in the muscles and bone).

Client Teaching

* Instruct the client to eat foods rich in phosphorus (e.g., meats [beef, pork, turkey], milk, whole-grain cereals, and almonds) if the decrease is caused by malnutrition. Most carbonated drinks are high in phosphates.
* Instruct *not* to take antacids that contain aluminum hydroxide (Amphojel). Phosphorus binds with aluminum hydroxide; a low serum phosphorus level results.

Increased level: Hyperphosphatemia

* Check serum calcium level; if low, observe for tetany symptoms.
* Monitor urinary output. A decreased urine output, less than 25 ml/h or less than 600 ml/d, can increase the serum phosphorus level.

Client Teaching

* Instruct the client to eat foods that are low in phosphorus (e.g., vegetables). Avoid drinking carbonated sodas that contain phosphates.

PLATELET AGGREGATION AND ADHESIONS (BLOOD)

Reference Values

Adult: Aggregation in 3 to 5 min

Description.   *Platelet aggregation test* measures the ability of platelets to adhere to each other when mixed with an aggregating agent such as collagen, ADP, or ristocetin (an antibiotic). This test is performed to detect abnormality in platelet function and to aid in diagnosing hereditary and acquired platelet deficiencies such as von Willebrand's disease. Increased bleeding tendencies result from a decrease in platelet aggregation time.

Platelet adhesion test, like platelet aggregation, evaluates platelet function and helps to confirm hereditary diseases such as von Willebrand's disease. This test is also performed on clients taking large doses of aspirin for several weeks and on persons having a prolonged bleeding time. It is not performed in many laboratories because of the difficulty in standardizing the technique.

Purposes
* To evaluate platelet function
* To detect platelet bleeding disorders

Clinical Problems
Decreased platelet aggregation: Von Willebrand's disease (ristocetin test), Bernard-Soulier syndrome (ristocetin test), cirrhosis of the liver, afibrinogenemia, Glanzmann's disease (thrombasthenia) (ADP, epinephrine, or collagen test), idiopathic thrombocytopenic purpura, platelet release defects, uremia

Drugs that may decrease platelet aggregation: Aspirin and aspirin compounds, anti-inflammatory agents such as NSAIDS (ibuprofen and others), 5-fluorouracil, phenothiazines, tricyclic antidepressants, diazepam (Valium), antihistamines, dipyridamole (Persantine), cortisone preparations, theophylline, marijuana, cocaine, heparin, furosemide (Lasix), penicillins, Vitamin E, volatile general anesthetics, theophylline, propranolol, pyrimidine compounds, and others

Increased platelet aggregation: Diabetes mellitus, hyperlipemia, hyper coagulability, polycythemia vera

Procedure
* Collect 5 to 7 ml of venous blood in a blue-top tube. Avoid hemolysis. Test of blood should be completed within 2 h after collection. Do not refrigerate.
* NPO, including medications, except for water, with the physician's approval.
* No aspirin or aspirin compounds for 7 to 10 days prior to the test, with the physician's approval. List drugs the client is taking on the laboratory slip.

Factors Affecting Laboratory Results
* Foods high in fat content eaten before the test (hyperlipemia increases platelet aggregation)

Nursing Implications
- Obtain a drug history from the client.
- Check for bleeding tendencies, petechiae, purpura.

Client Teaching
- Instruct the client about the importance of not taking aspirin or aspirin compounds 7 to 10 days before the test (check with the health care provider). Aspirin inhibits clotting time.
- Inform the client that medications, food, and fluids (except water) should not be taken after midnight. It may be necessary to take some medications.

PLATELET ANTIBODY TEST (BLOOD)

PLATELET ANTIBODY DETECTION TEST, ANTIPLATELET ANTIBODY DETECTION

Reference Values
Negative

Description.   When client becomes sensitized to platelet antigen of transfused blood, platelet antibodies (autoantibodies or isoantibodies) develop, thus causing thrombocytopenia because of destruction to the platelets. The platelet autoantibodies are IgG immunoglobulins of autoimmune origin. With idiopathic thrombocytopenic purpura (ITP), platelet autoantibodies are present.

Drug-induced thrombocytopenia is caused by platelet-associated IgG autoantibodies because of hypersensitivity to certain drugs. Some of the drugs that may cause drug-induced immunologic thrombocytopenia include salicylates, acetaminophen, antibiotics (sulfonamides, penicillin, cephalosporins), quinidine and quinidine-like drugs, gold, cimetidine, oral hypoglycemic agents, heparin, digoxin.

Maternal–fetal platelet antigen incompatibility can occur if the mother has ITP autoantibodies that are passed to the fetus. Neonatal thrombocytopenia may result.

Purpose
* To detect the presence of platelet antibodies

Clinical Problems
Positive test: Thrombocytopenia because of platelet autoantibodies or isoantibodies, idiopathic thrombocytopenic purpura, post-transfusion purpura, drug-induced thrombocytopenia
Drugs that may cause drug-induced thrombocytopenia: See Description

Procedure
* No food or fluid restriction is required.
* Collect two (2) 10 ml of venous blood in a blue-top tube. Deliver to the laboratory immediately with the time of collection written on the requisition form.

Nursing Implications
* Obtain a drug history from the client.
* Check platelet count. If thrombocytopenia is present, a platelet antibody test may be ordered.
* Check for sites of petechiae, purpura.

Client Teaching
* Instruct the client to report any abnormal bleeding.
* Listen to client's and family's concerns.

PLATELET (THROMBOCYTE) COUNT (BLOOD)

Reference Values
Adult: 150,000–400,000 µl (mean, 250,000 µl); 0.15–0.4 × 10^{12}/l (SI units)
Child: Premature: 100,000–300,000 µl; newborn: 150,000–300,000 µl; infant: 200,000–475,000 µl

Description.   Platelets (thrombocytes) are basic elements in the blood that promote coagulation. A low platelet count (thrombocytopenia) is associated with bleeding, and an elevated platelet count (thrombocytosis) may cause increased clotting. With a platelet count of 100,000 µl, bleeding is likely to occur, and with a platelet count less than 50,000 µl, hemorrhage is apt to occur.

Purposes
* To check platelet count
* To monitor platelet count during cancer chemotherapy

Clinical Problems
Decreased level: Idiopathic thrombocytopenic purpura, cancer (bone, GI, and brain), leukemias, aplastic anemia, liver disease, kidney disease, disseminated intravascular coagulation (DIC), SLE
Drugs that can decrease platelet count: Aspirin, chloromycetin, sulfonamides, quinidine, thiazide diuretics, phenylbutazone (Butazolidin), chemotherapeutic agents, tolbutamide (Orinase)
Increased level: Infections, acute blood loss, splenectomy, polycythemia vera, myeloproliferative disorders

Procedure
* No food or fluid restriction is required.

Venous
* Collect 3 to 5 ml of venous blood in a lavender-top tube.

Capillary Blood
* Discard the first few drops of blood, and collect the next drops of blood from a finger puncture. Dilute with appropriate solution.

Factors Affecting Laboratory Results
* Chemotherapy and X-ray therapy can cause a decreased platelet count.

Nursing Implications
* Check the platelet count, especially with bleeding episodes, and report abnormal levels to the health care provider.

- Observe for signs and symptoms of bleeding (e.g., purpura, petechiae, hematemesis, rectal bleeding), and report to the health care provider.
- Monitor the platelet count, especially when the client is receiving chemotherapy or radiation therapy.

Client Teaching
- Teach the client to avoid injury.

POTASSIUM (K) (SERUM AND URINE)

Reference Values
Serum: Adult: 3.5–5.3 mEq/l, 3.5–5.3 mmol/l (SI units)
Child: 3.5–5.5 mEq/l; infant: 3.6–5.8 mq/l
Panic values: Less than 2.5 mEq/l and greater than 7.0 mEq/l
Urine: Adult: Broad range: 25–120 mEq/24 h; average range: 40–80 mEq/24 h, 40–80 mmol/24 h (SI units)

Description.   Serum potassium (K) has a narrow range; therefore, potassium values should be closely monitored; death could occur if serum levels are less than 2.5 mEq/l or greater than 7.0 mEq/l. Eighty to 90% of the body's potassium is excreted in the urine. When there is tissue breakdown, potassium leaves the cells and enters the extracellular fluid. With adequate kidney function, the potassium in the vascular fluid will be excreted, and if renal shutdown or insufficiency occurs, then potassium will continue to increase in the vascular fluid.

The body does not conserve potassium, and the kidneys excrete an average of 40 mEq/l daily (the range is 25 to 120 mEq/24 h), even with a low dietary potassium intake. A decrease in urinary potassium can indicate hyperkalemia (elevated serum potassium), and an increase in urinary potassium can indicate hypokalemia (low serum potassium).

Purposes
- To check potassium level
- To detect the presence of hypo- or hyperkalemia

- To monitor potassium levels during health problems (i.e., renal insufficiency, debilitating illness, cancer) and with certain drugs (e.g., thiazide diuretics)

Clinical Problems

Decreased level: (Hypokalemia)

Serum: Vomiting/diarrhea, laxative abuse, dehydration, malnutrition/ starvation, crash diet, stress, trauma, injury and surgery (with renal function), gastric suction, diabetic acidosis, burns, hyperaldosteronism, excessive ingestion of licorice, metabolic alkalosis

Drugs that may decrease potassium value: Diuretics (potassium wasting), cortisone, estrogen, insulin, laxatives, lithium carbonate, sodium polystyrene sulfonate (Kayexalate), and aspirin

Urine: Elevated serum potassium level, acute renal failure

Increased level: (Hyperkalemia)

Serum: Oliguria and anuria, acute renal failure, IV potassium in fluids, Addison's disease, severe tissue injury or burns (with kidney shutdown), metabolic acidosis

Drugs that may increase potassium value: Diuretics (potassium sparing— spironolactone), antibiotics (penicillin, cephalosporins, heparin, epinephrine, histamine, isoniazid)

Urine: Decreased serum potassium level, dehydration, starvation, vomiting, and diarrhea

Procedure

Serum

- No food, fluid, or drug restrictions are necessary.
- Collect 3 to 5 ml of venous blood in a red-top tube. Avoid leaving tourniquet on for greater than 2 min if possible. Avoid hemolysis.

Urine

- The 24-h urine specimen should be kept on ice or refrigerated.
- Potassium supplements given as salt replacement should be eliminated for 48 h.

Factors Affecting Laboratory Results

* The use of a tourniquet can cause an increase in the serum potassium level.

Nursing Implications

* Compare serum potassium levels with urine potassium levels. When serum potassium level is decreased, urine potassium level is frequently increased and vice versa.

Decreased Serum Level

* Observe for signs and symptoms of hypokalemia (e.g., vertigo, hypotension, cardiac dysrhythmias, nausea, vomiting, diarrhea, abdominal distention, decreased peristalsis, muscle weakness, and leg cramps).
* Record intake and output. Polyuria can cause an excessive loss of potassium.
* Determine the client's hydration status when hypokalemia is present. Overhydration can dilute the serum potassium level.
* Recognize behavioral changes as a sign of hypokalemia. Low potassium levels can cause confusion, irritability, and mental depression.
* Report ECG changes. A prolonged and depressed S-T segment and a flat or inverted T wave is indicative of hypokalemia.
* Dilute oral potassium supplements in at least 6 ounces of water or juice to reduce irritation to the gastric mucosa.
* Monitor the serum potassium level in clients receiving potassium-wasting diuretics and steroids. Cortisone steroids cause sodium retention and potassium excretion.
* Assess for signs and symptoms of digitalis toxicity when the client is receiving a digitalis preparation and a potassium-wasting diuretic or steroid. A lower serum potassium level enhances the action of digitalis. Signs and symptoms of digitalis toxicity are nausea and vomiting, anorexia, bradycardia, dysrhythmia, and visual disturbances.
* Administer IV KCl in a liter of IV fluids. *Never* give an IV or bolus push of KCl, as cardiac arrest can occur. KCl can be administered IV only when it is diluted (20 to 40 mEq/l of KCl) and should never be given SC or IM. Concentrated IV KCl is irritating to the heart muscle and to the veins, causing phlebitis.

Client Teaching

* Teach the client and family to eat foods high in potassium (e.g., fruits, fruit juices, dry fruits, vegetables, meats, nuts, coffee, tea, and cola).

Increased Serum Level

* Observe for signs and symptoms of hyperkalemia (e.g., bradycardia, abdominal cramps, oliguria or anuria, tingling, and twitching or numbness of the extremities).
* Assess urine output to determine renal function; urine output should be at least 25 ml/h or 600 ml daily, and a urine output of less than 600 ml/d may cause hyperkalemia.
* Report serum potassium levels greater than 5.0 mEq/l. Restriction of potassium intake may be necessary, and if serum level is higher, Kayexalate (ion exchange resin) may be needed. High serum potassium levels, greater than 7.0 mEq/l, could cause cardiac arrest.
* Regulate the rate of IV fluids so that no more than 10 mEq KCl/h are administered.
* Check the age of whole blood before administering it to a client with hyperkalemia. Blood 3 to 4 weeks old or older has an elevated serum potassium level, which could be five times the normal serum potassium level.
* Monitor the ECG for QRS spread and peaked T waves, a sign of hyperkalemia. The pulse may be rapid, but if hyperkalemia persists, bradycardia can occur.
* Observe for signs and symptoms of hypokalemia when administering Kayexalate for a prolonged period (2 or more days).

PREALBUMIN (PA, PAB) ANTIBODY ASSAY (SERUM)

TRANSTHYRETIN (TTR), TRYPTOPHAN-RICH PREALBUMIN, THYROXINE BINDING PREALBUMIN (TBPA)

Reference Values

Adult: 17–40 mg/dl, 170–400 mg/l (SI units); Female (average): 18 mg/dl, 180 mg/l (SI units); Male (average): 21.6 mg/dl, 216 mg/l (SI units)
Child: Newborn: 10–11.5 mg/dl, 100–115 mg/l (SI units); 2 to 3 years: 16–28 mg/dl, 160–280 mg/l (SI units)

Description.   Prealbumin, also known as thyroxin-binding protein, thyroxin-binding prealbumin (TBPA) or transthyretin, is a test used primarily for nutritional assessment. Transthyretin, a transport protein, is a precursor of albumin. Prealbumin has a shorter half-life (2 to 4 days) than albumin (20 to 24 days); it can readily indicate any change affecting protein synthesis and catabolism.

This test is more sensitive for determining nutritional status and liver dysfunction than an albumin test. It is also useful in monitoring the effectiveness of total parenteral nutrition (TPN) and evaluating the nutritional needs in critically ill clients. Prealbumin transports protein for triiodothyronine and thyroxine. Prealbumin is also needed for the metabolism and transporting of vitamin A. Prealbumin is greatly reduced in hepatobiliary disease and chronic malignancy disease. A prealbumin value of less than 5 mg/dl indicates severe protein depletion, and a value less than 10 mg/dl indicates severe nutritional deficiency.

Purposes

- To assess the client's nutritional status
- To evaluate the client's nutritional needs on admission to the hospital, or following a surgical procedure, or during a critical illness

Clinical Problems

Decreased level: Protein-wasting diseases, malnutrition, malignancies, cirrhosis of the liver, zinc deficiency (zinc is required for synthesis of prealbumin), chronic illness

Drugs that decrease prealbumin value: Estrogen, oral contraceptives

Increased level: Hodgkin's disease, chronic kidney disease, adrenal hyperfunction

Drugs that increase prealbumin value: Steroids (high doses), nonsteroidal anti-inflammatory drugs (NSAIDs) (high doses)

Procedure

- No food or fluid restriction; some institutions request NPO 8 to 12 h prior to the test.
- Collect 2 to 5 ml of venous blood in a red-top tube. Avoid hemolysis.

Nursing Implications

* Obtain a history of the client's nutritional intake. Record findings.
* Check vital signs and weight.
* Listen to the client's concerns; answer questions or refer them to other health care providers.

Client Teaching

* Inform the client of ways in which nutritional status can be improved.

PREGNANEDIOL (URINE)

Reference Values

Adult: Female: 0.5–1.5 mg/24 h (proliferative phase), 2–7 mg/24 h (luteal phase), 0.1–1.0 mg/24 h (postmenopausal); male: 0.1–1.5 mg/24 h
Pregnancy: 10–19 gestation weeks: 5–25 mg/24 h; 20–28 gestation weeks: 15–42 mg/24 h; 28–32 gestation weeks: 25–49 mg/24 h
Child: 0.4–1.0 mg/24 h

Description. Pregnanediol is the major metabolite of progesterone produced by the ovary during the luteal phase of the menstrual cycle and by the placenta. Progesterone is responsible for uterine changes after ovulation and for maintaining pregnancy after fertilization. A steady rise in urine pregnanediol levels occurs during pregnancy, and a decrease in these levels indicates placental, not fetal, dysfunction and the possibility of an abortion.

Urine pregnanediol levels may be used to determine menstrual disturbances and are used to verify ovulation in those who have not been able to become pregnant.

Purposes

* To determine the occurrence of placental dysfunction
* To compare test results with other laboratory tests for determining cause of menstrual disorder

Clinical Problems

Decreased level: Menstrual disorders (amenorrhea), ovarian hypofunction, threatened abortion, fetal death, placental failure, preeclampsia, benign neoplasms of the ovary and breast

Increased level: Pregnancy, ovarian cyst, choriocarcinoma of the ovary, adrenal cortex hyperplasia

Procedure

* No food or fluid restriction is required.
* Collect urine over a 24-h period in a large refrigerated container with preservative.
* Label the bottle with the client's name, date, and exact times of collection (e.g., 11/7/09, 8 AM to 11/8/09, 8 AM).
* Record on the laboratory slip the date of the last menstrual period or weeks of gestation.
* Post urine collection time and procedure at appropriate places.

Nursing Implications
Decreased Level

* Obtain a history of menstrual changes (patterns, frequency, length of period, flow, and discomfort).
* Obtain a history of pregnancy complications or problems. Record when the client had her last menstrual period.
* Give support to the client and family.
* Monitor the urine pregnanediol levels if sequential tests have been ordered. Progesterone therapy may be needed.

Increased Level

* Recognize clinical problems that can cause an elevated pregnanediol level, such as pregnancy and an ovarian cyst. After 20 to 28 weeks of pregnancy, the pregnanediol level should be 15 to 42 mg/24 h, and after 28 to 32 weeks, the level should be 25 to 49 mg/24 h. In the last 2 weeks of pregnancy, the urine pregnanediol level decreases.

PREGNANETRIOL (URINE)

Reference Values
Adult: Male: 0.4–2.4 mg/24 h; female: 0.5–2.0 mg/24 h
Child: Infant: 0–0.2 mg/24 h; child: 0–1.0 mg/24 h

Description.   Pregnanetriol comes from adrenal corticoid synthesis. It should not be mistaken for pregnanediol. The pregnanetriol test is useful in diagnosing congenital adrenocortical hyperplasia.

Purpose
* To detect anterior pituitary hypofunction or adrenocortical hyperfunction (see Clinical Problems)

Clinical Problems
Decreased level: Anterior pituitary hypofunction
Increased level: Adrenogenital syndrome, congenital adrenocortical hyperplasia, adrenocortical hyperfunction, malignant neoplasm of the adrenal gland

Procedure
* No food or fluid restriction is required.
* Collect urine for 24 h in a large, refrigerated container.
* Label the bottle with the client's name, date, and exact times of collection.

Nursing Implications
* Assess for changes in external genitalia.
* Monitor urine pregnanetriol levels with cortisone replacement.
* Be supportive of client and family.

PROGESTERONE (SERUM)

Reference Values
Adult: Female: Follicular phase: 0.1–1.5 ng/ml; 20–150 ng/dl

Luteal phase: 2–28 ng/ml; 250–2,800 ng/dl
Postmenopausal: Less than 1.0 ng/ml; less than 100 ng/dl
Pregnancy: First trimester: 9–50 ng/ml
Second trimester: 18–150 ng/ml
Third trimester: 60–260 ng/ml
Male: Less than 1.0 ng/ml; less than 100 ng/dl

Description.   Progesterone, a hormone produced primarily by the corpus luteum of the ovaries and a small amount by the adrenal cortex, peaks during the luteal phase of the menstrual cycle for 4 to 5 days and during pregnancy. It prepares the endometrium for implantation of the fertilized egg. This hormone remains elevated during early pregnancy. Higher levels of progesterone occur when there are twins or more than a single fetus. Placenta secretes about ten times the normal amount (luteal phase). Only a small amount of progesterone is detected in the blood, since most is metabolized in the liver to pregnanediol, a progesterone metabolite.

Serum progesterone is useful in evaluating infertility problems, confirming ovulation, assessing placental functions in pregnancy, and determining the risk of a possible threatened abortion. A urine pregnanediol might be ordered to verify serum progesterone results.

Purposes

- To aid in the diagnosis of ovarian or adrenal tumor
- To assist in the diagnosis of placental failure
- To evaluate infertility problems resulting from a decreased progesterone level

Clinical Problems

Decreased levels: Gonadal dysfunction, luteum deficiency, threatened abortion, toxemia of pregnancy, placental failure, fetal death
Drugs that may decrease progesterone value: Oral contraceptives
Increased levels: Ovulation, pregnancy, ovarian cysts, tumors of the ovary or adrenal gland
Drugs that may increase progesterone value: ACTH, progesterone preparations

Procedure
- No food or fluid restriction is required.
- Collect 5 to 7 ml of venous blood in a red- (preferred) or green-top tube. Avoid hemolysis. Invert the green-top tube several times to mix with the anticoagulant in the tube.
- Note on the laboratory slip the phase of the client's menstrual cycle, or weeks of gestation if pregnant.

Nursing Implications
- Obtain a history from the client of her menstrual phase or weeks or months of gestation.
- Listen to the client's concerns and fears. Refer client's questions to health professionals when appropriate.

Client Teaching
- Inform the client that the blood test may be repeated or that a urine test may be ordered. Repeated tests may be indicated to obtain complete information concerning progesterone secretion.

PROLACTIN (PRL) (SERUM)

LACTOGENIC HORMONE, LACTOGEN

Reference Values
Female: Follicular phase: 0–23 ng/ml
Luteal phase: 0–40 ng/ml
Postmenopausal: Less than 12 ng/ml
Pregnancy: First trimester: Less than 80 ng/ml
Second trimester: Less than 160 ng/ml
Third trimester: Less than 400 ng/ml
Male: 0.1–20 ng/ml
Pituitary adenoma: Greater than 100–300 ng/ml

Description.   Prolactin is a hormone secreted by the adenohypophysis (anterior pituitary gland) and is necessary for developing the mammary glands for lactation. If breastfeeding after delivery, prolactin levels remain elevated for maintaining lactation. Impotence in the male might be attributed to excess prolactin secretion that suppresses gonad function.

Serum prolactin levels greater than 100–300 ng/ml in nonpregnant females and in males may indicate a pituitary adenoma (tumor). Bromocriptine (Parlodel) decreases the serum prolactin level and tumor growth until the pituitary tumor can be removed.

Purposes
- To detect various health problems related to an increased prolactin level (see Clinical Problems)
- To check drugs that the client is taking which influence increased prolactin levels

Clinical Problems
Decreased level: Postpartum pituitary infarction

Drugs that may decrease prolactin value: Bromocriptine, levodopa, ergot derivatives, apomorphine

Increased level: Pregnancy, breastfeeding, pituitary tumor, amenorrhea, galactorrhea, ectopic prolactin-secreting tumors (such as the lung), primary hypothyroidism, hypothalamic disorder, endometriosis, chronic renal failure, polycystic ovary, Addison's disease, stress, sleep, coitus, exercise

Drugs that may increase prolactin value: Amphetamines, estrogens, antihistamines, oral contraceptives, phenothiazines, tricyclic antidepressants, monoamine oxidase inhibitors (MAO inhibitors), methyldopa (Aldomet), haloperidol (Haldol), cimetidine (Tagamet), procainamide derivatives, reserpine (Serpasil), isoniazid (INH), verapamil

Procedure
- Withhold medications that interfere with the test.
- Fasting specimen is preferred.
- Collect 3 to 5 ml of venous blood in a red- or lavender-top tube. Avoid hemolysis. Client should be awake for 1 to 2 h before blood test; sleep elevates the serum prolactin level.

Factors Affecting Laboratory Results
- Exercise, stress, pain, surgical trauma, and sleep may affect test results.

Nursing Implications
- List drugs the client is taking that may affect test results on the laboratory slip.
- Listen to the client's concerns.

Client Teaching
- Instruct the client about the test procedure, such as blood specimen to be drawn 1 to 2 h after awakening.
- Instruct the client to avoid stress and exercise prior to the test. Note the presence of stress or pain on the laboratory slip.

PROSTATE-SPECIFIC ANTIGEN (PSA) (SERUM)

Reference Values
PSA: Normal: less than 4.0 ng/ml; benign prostatic hypertrophy (BPH): 4.0–10 ng/ml;

Prostate cancer: 10–120 ng/ml (depends on the stage of prostatic cancer)

Total PSA: Normal: 2.5–4.0 ng/ml

Free PSA: Normal: greater than 1.0 ng/ml

% Free PSA: Normal: greater than 25%

% Free PSA	Probability of Cancer
0–10	56%
11–15	28%
16–20	20%
21–25	15%
Greater than 26	8%

Description.   Before the 1970s, prostatic cancer was screened by only digital rectal examination and serum prostate acid phosphatase (PAP). By the time the PAP was elevated and the prostate gland was enlarged, metastasis occurred. After the prostate-specific antigen (PSA) test was developed, fewer men were diagnosed with metastatic cancer.

Prostate-specific antigen (PSA), a glycoprotein from the prostatic tissues, is increased in both benign prostatic hypertrophy (BPH), and prostatic cancer; however, it is markedly increased in prostatic cancer. The PSA value may also be increased after a rectal examination and prostate surgery. An annual PSA test should be started at the age of 50. It should be started at the age of 40 if the male has a familial history of prostate cancer or is an African American. A digital rectal examination (DRE) is usually done along with a PSA test. With an abnormal DRE, a biopsy of the prostate gland may be performed regardless of whether the PSA test is normal or elevated.

With serum PSA, there can be a false-positive or a false-negative result. However, this test gives an indication of the risk of prostate cancer. If the PSA is less than 4.0 ng/ml, the chance of prostate cancer is very small, but not zero. If the PSA is over 10 ng/ml, there is a 70% chance that the prostate gland is malignant. Doubling time of PSA results in 12 months is a concern, for example, an elevation from 2.0 to 4.0 ng/ml. Also, an elevated PSA could be due to an enlarged prostate gland such as BPH or prostatitis, which is inflammation of the prostate gland from a bacterial infection or other causes.

The serum PSA may be used to monitor the effect of prostatic cancer treatment with chemotherapy or radiation, determine disease process and prognosis, and detect a recurrence of the tumor. Repeating the PSA test may be necessary.

Today, the PSA assays are composed of three tests; serum PSA, total PSA, and percent free PSA. If the serum PSA is slightly elevated or its previous result is doubled, the total PSA (tPSA) and percent free PSA (%FPSA) are prescribed.

Total PSA (tPSA):   The PSA is comprised of a free portion and complexed (bound) PSA. The total PSA value is used for obtaining the % PSA.

% Free PSA (%FPSA):   If %FPSA is greater than 25%, the chance of having prostate cancer is very low, less than 8%. If the %FPSA is less than 25%, the chances of prostate cancer increases. The %FPSA can be determined by dividing the free PSA by the total PSA. If the total PSA of a person is 2.4 ng/ml and the free PSA is 0.3 ng/ml, the percent of free PSA (%FPSA) would be 13%. This person would have a 28% chance of having prostate cancer (see Reference Values). A prostate gland biopsy would be suggested.

It has been suggested that the norm for serum PSA should be lower than 4.0 ng/ml. This may be true for men 50 years old or younger, but not for older men. If reference values need to be changed, then the normal serum PSA for men who are 50 years old or younger would be less than 2.5 ng/ml and the serum PSA value for men 50 years old or older would remain as 4.0 ng/ml.

Purpose
- To aid in the diagnosis of prostatic cancer.

Clinical Problems
Increased level: Prostatic cancer, benign prostatic hypertrophy (BPH), prostatitis, prostatic tissue biopsy, prostatic surgery.

Procedure
- No food or fluid restriction is required.
- Collect blood specimen before rectal and prostate examination.
- Collect 3 to 5 ml of venous blood in a red-top tube.

Factors Affecting Laboratory Results
- Rectal and prostate examinations can increase serum PSA levels.

Nursing Implications
- Ascertain if there is a family history of prostate cancer.
- Obtain a history regarding changes in urinary pattern, such as interrupted urine flow; frequent urination, especially at night; difficulty in starting and stopping the urine flow; hematuria; and/or pain in the back during urination.
- Explain to the client that a blood sample will be obtained and the test results would be available within 24 h.

Client Teaching
- Instruct the client that a manual rectal examination is usually part of the test regimen to determine prostatic changes. The prostatic palpation should be done *after* the blood sample is drawn.

- Be supportive to the client. Provide an atmosphere in which the client feels comfortable expressing his concerns.

PROSTATIC ACID PHOSPHATASE (PAP) (*SEE* ACID PHOSPHATASE [ACP])

PROTEIN (TOTAL); PROTEIN ELECTROPHORESIS (SERUM)

Reference Values
Adult: Total protein: 6.0–8.0 g/dl

Protein Fraction	Weight (g/dl)	% of Total Protein
Albumin	3.5–5.0	52–68
Globulin	1.5–3.5	32–48
Alpha-1	0.1–0.4	2–5
Alpha-2	0.4–1.0	7–13
Beta	0.5–1.1	8–14
Gamma	0.5–1.7	12–22

Child: Total protein: premature: 4.2–7.6 g/dl; newborn: 4.6–7.4 g/dl; infant: 6.0–6.7 g/dl; child: 6.2–8.0 g/dl

	Albumin (g/dl)		Globulins (g/dl)		
	(g/dl)	Alpha-1	Alpha-2	Beta	Gamma
Premature	3.0–4.2	0.1–0.5	0.3–0.7	0.3–1.2	0.3–1.4
Newborn	3.5–5.4	0.1–0.3	0.3–0.5	0.2–0.6	0.2–1.2
Infant	4.4–5.4	0.2–0.4	0.5–0.8	0.5–0.9	0.3–0.8
Child	4.0–5.8	0.1–0.4	0.4–1.0	0.5–1.0	0.3–1.0

Description.   The total protein is composed mostly of albumin and globulins. The use of the total serum protein test is limited unless the protein electrophoresis test is performed.

Serum protein electrophoresis is a process that separates various protein fractions into albumin and alpha-1, alpha-2, beta, and gamma globulins.

Albumin plays an important role in maintaining serum colloid osmotic pressure. The gamma globulin is the body's antibodies, which contribute to immunity.

Purposes
- To associate and differentiate between albumin and globulin
- To monitor protein levels
- To identify selected health problems associated with protein deficit

Clinical Problems

Globulins	Decreased Level	Increased Level
Total Protein	Malnutrition, starvation	Dehydration
	Malabsorption syndrome	Vomiting, diarrhea
	Severe liver disease	Multiple myeloma
	Cancer of GI tract	Sarcoidosis
	Severe burns	Respiratory distress
	Hodgkin's disease	syndrome
	Ulcerative colitis	
	Chronic renal failure	
Albumin	Chronic liver disease	Dehydration
	Malnutrition, starvation	Exercise
	Malabsorption syndrome	
	Leukemia, malignancies	
	Chronic renal failure	
	SLE	
	Severe burns	
	Nephrotic syndrome	
	Toxemia of pregnancy	
	CHF	

Globulins	Decreased Level	Increased Level
Alpha-1	Emphysema due to alpha-1 antitrypsin deficiency, nephrosis	Pregnancy
		Neoplasm
		Acute and chronic infection
		Tissue necrosis

(continued)

Globulins	Decreased Level	Increased Level
Alpha-2	Hemolytic anemia Severe liver disease	Acute infection Injury, trauma Severe burns Extensive neoplasm Rheumatic fever Rheumatoid arthritis AMI Nephrotic syndrome Biliary cirrhosis Obstructive jaundice
Beta	Hypocholesterolemia	Hypothyroidism Biliary cirrhosis Kidney nephrosis Nephrotic syndrome Diabetes mellitus Cushing's disease Malignant hypertension

Gamma	Nephrotic syndrome
	Lymphocytic leukemia
	Lymphosarcoma
	Hypogammaglobulinemia or
	  agammaglobulinemia
		Collagen disease
		Rheumatoid arthritis
		Lupus erythematosus
		Malignant lymphoma
		Hodgkin's disease
		Chronic lymphocytic
		  leukemia
		Multiple myeloma
		Liver disease
		Chronic infections

Procedure
- No food or fluid restriction is required. Check with your laboratory.
- Collect 5 to 7 ml of venous blood in a red-top tube. Avoid hemolysis.

Factors Affecting Laboratory Results
- A high-fat diet before the test

Nursing Implications

- Assess client's dietary intake. Suggest foods high in protein (e.g., beans, eggs, meats, milk).
- Assess for peripheral edema in the lower extremities when the albumin level is decreased.
- Assess urinary output. Urinary output should be 25 ml/h or 600 ml/24 h.
- Check for albumin/protein in the urine.

PROTEIN (URINE)

Reference Values
Random specimen: Negative: 0–5 mg/dl; positive: 6–2,000 mg/dl (trace to +2)
24-h specimen: 25–150 mg/24 h

Description.   Proteinuria is usually caused by renal disease due to glomerular damage or impaired renal tubular reabsorption, or both. With a random urine specimen, protein can be detected by using a reagent strip or dipstick, such as Combistix. If a random specimen is positive for proteinuria, a 24-h urine specimen is usually ordered for protein. The amount of protein is an indicator of severity of renal involvement. Emotions and physiologic stress may cause transient proteinuria. Newborns may have an increased proteinuria during the first 3 days of life.

Purposes
- To compare urine protein with serum protein level in relation to health problems (see Clinical Problems)
- To identify renal dysfunction with increased protein level in the urine

Clinical Problems
Increased level: *Heavy proteinuria:* acute or chronic glomerulonephritis, nephrotic syndrome, lupus nephritis, amyloid disease; *Moderate proteinuria:* drug toxicities (aminoglycosides), cardiac disease, acute infectious

disease, multiple myeloma, chemical toxicities; *Mild proteinuria:* chronic pyelonephritis, polycystic kidney disease, renal tubular disease

Drugs that may increase urine protein: Penicillin, gentamicin, sulfonamides, cephalosporins, contrast media, tolbutamide (Orinase), acetazolamide (Diamox)

Procedure
- No food or fluid restriction is required.
- List drugs client is taking that could affect test results.

Qualitative Test: Random Urine Specimen
- Collect clean-caught or midstream urine specimen.
- Place the reagent strip/dipstick in the urine specimen. Match the dipstick with the color chart on the bottle for results.

Quantitative Analysis Test: 24-h Specimen
- Discard first urine specimen. Then save all urine for 24 h in a refrigerated urine-collection bottle.
- Label the urine bottle with client's name, date, exact time of collection (e.g., 7/12/09, 8:01 AM to 7/13/09, 8:02 AM).

Nursing Implications
- Explain the test procedure to the client.
- Assess for signs and symptoms of renal dysfunction (e.g., fatigue, decreased urine output, peripheral edema, increased serum creatinine).
- Notify the health care provider if the urine output is less than 25 ml/h.

PROTHROMBIN TIME (PT) (PLASMA)

PRO-TIME, INR (INTERNATIONAL NORMALIZED RATIO)

Reference Values
Adult: 10–13 seconds (depending on the method and reagents used); anticoagulant therapy: PT: 1.5–2.0 times the control in seconds; *INR (international normalized ratio)* for anticoagulant (warfarin) therapy: 2.0–3.0
Child: Same as adult

Description.   Prothrombin, synthesized by the liver, is an inactive precursor in the clotting process. The PT test measures the clotting ability of factors I (fibrinogen), II (prothrombin), V, VII, and X. The major use of the PT test is to monitor oral anticoagulant therapy (e.g., warfarin sodium [Coumadin]). If PT is greater than 2.5 times the control value, bleeding is likely to occur.

  International Normalized Ratio (INR): It has been recommended that the PT be reported as an international normalized ratio (INR). The INR was devised to improve the monitoring process for warfarin (Coumadin) anticoagulant therapy. A client's response to the same dose of warfarin varies, thus the INR is used because of it being an international standardized test for PT. The INR is designed for long-term warfarin therapy and should only be used after the client has been stabilized on warfarin. Stabilization takes at least 1 week. The target INR range for a client having heart valve replacement is 2.5–3.5 (see International Normalized Ratio [INR]).

Purpose
- To monitor oral anticoagulant (warfarin) therapy

Clinical Problems
Decreased level: Thrombophlebitis, myocardial infarction, pulmonary embolism
Drugs that may decrease PT time and INR: Barbiturates, oral contraceptives, diphenhydramine (Benadryl), rifampin, metaproterenol (Alupent), vitamin K, digitalis, diuretics
Increased (prolonged) level: Liver diseases; afibrinogenemia; factor deficiencies II, V, VII, X; leukemias; erythroblastosis fetalis; CHF
Drugs that may increase PT time and INR: Oral anticoagulants (Coumadin, Dicumarol), antibiotics, salicylates (aspirin), sulfonamides, phenytoin (Dilantin), chlorpromazine (Thorazine), chlordiazepoxide (Librium), methyldopa (Aldomet), mithramycin, reserpine (Serpasil)

Procedure
- No food or fluid restriction is required.
- Collect 3 to 5 ml of venous blood in a blue- or black-top tube. The blood must be tested within 2 h. Fill tube to capacity.

- Control values are given with the client's PT and INR values.
- List drugs on the laboratory slip that can affect test results.

Factors Affecting Laboratory Results
- A high-fat diet (decreases PT) and alcohol use (increases PT)

Nursing Implications
- Monitor the plasma PT and/or INR when the client is receiving oral anticoagulant therapy.
- Inform the health care provider of the client's PT daily or as ordered. The health care provider may want the anticoagulant held or the dose adjusted.
- Observe for signs and symptoms of bleeding (e.g., purpura, nose-bleeds, hematemesis, hematuria). Report and record symptoms.
- Administer vitamin K as ordered when the PT is over 40 seconds or when bleeding is occurring.
- Assess the alcohol consumption and diet. Alcohol intake can increase PT, INR; and a high-fat diet may decrease PT, INR.

Client Teaching
- Instruct the client not to self-medicate when receiving anticoagulant therapy. Over-the-counter (OTC) drugs may either increase or decrease the effects of the anticoagulant.
- Instruct the client to take the prescribed anticoagulant as ordered by the health care provider and not to miss a dose.

RABIES ANTIBODY TEST (SERUM)

FLUORESCENT RABIES ANTIBODY (FRA)

Reference Values
Indirect fluorescent antibody (IFA): Less than 1:16

Description. The rabies rhabdovirus affecting the central nervous system may be present in the saliva, brain, spinal cord, urine, and feces of rabid animals. The virus can be transmitted to the human by an infected dog, bat, skunk, squirrel, or other animal and is nearly 100% fatal if the person does not receive treatment before the symptoms occur.

This rabies antibody test is performed to diagnose rabies both in animals and in humans that have been bitten by a rabid animal. Also, it is useful to test the effects of rabies immunization on employees working in animal shelters. Both the rabies antibody test and the animal's brain tissue are preferred to positively diagnose rabies that was transmitted to the human. If the animal suspected of having rabies survives longer than 10 days, it is unlikely that the animal is rabid.

Purpose
- To aid in the diagnosis of rabies in animals and humans

Clinical Problems
Increased titer count: Rabies transmission

Procedure
- No food or fluid restriction is required.
- Collect 5 to 7 ml of venous blood in a red-top tube. The animal brain should be sent along with the blood sample to the laboratory if possible.

Nursing Implications
- Obtain a history of the animal bite. Rabies immunoglobulin (RIG) may be given soon after the exposure to neutralize the virus.
- The animal responsible for the bite should be captured. If the animal's rabies vaccination is not current, the animal is usually destroyed in order to test the brain tissue. A wait of 10 days to determine the survival of a "wild" animal is not suggested.

Client Teaching
- Suggest to persons working with animals, such as those working in veterinary practices, kennels, wildlife areas, and research laboratories, that they receive a preexposure rabies vaccine such as HDVC (human diploid cell rabies vaccine) to protect them from rabies exposure.

- Instruct the person who was bitten or the family to seek medical care immediately. Encourage the family to notify the humane society concerning the animal bite. The animal should be captured.
- Inform the client and/or family that if the animal is not located, then a series of rabies vaccinations is necessary and should be taken.
- Answer the client's questions or refer the questions to appropriate health professionals.

RAPID PLASMA REAGIN (RPR) (SERUM)

Reference Values
Adult: Nonreactive
Child: Nonreactive

Description.   The RPR test is a rapid-screening test for syphilis. A nontreponemal antibody test like VDRL, the RPR test detects reagin antibodies in the serum and is more sensitive but less specific than VDRL. Frequently it is used on donor's blood as a syphilis detection test. As with other nonspecific reagin tests, false positives can occur as the result of acute and chronic diseases. A positive RPR should be verified by VDRL and/or FTA-ABS tests.

Purpose
- To compare test results with other laboratory tests for diagnosing syphilis

Clinical Problems
Reactive (positive):   Syphilis. False positives: tuberculosis, pneumonia, infectious mononucleosis, chickenpox, smallpox vaccination (recent), rheumatoid arthritis, lupus erythematosus, hepatitis, pregnancy

Procedure
- Follow the directions on the RPR kit. Positive test: Flocculation occurs on the plastic card.

Nursing Implications

- If test result is positive, explain to the client that further testing will be done to verify test results.
- If repeat result is positive, sexual contacts need to be notified for treatment.

RBC INDICES (RED BLOOD CELL COUNT, MCV, MCH, MCHC) (BLOOD)

ERYTHROCYTE INDICES

Reference Values

	Adult	*Newborn*	*Child*
RBC count (million)/ μL or × 10^{12}/l	Male: 4.6–6.0 Female: 4.0–5.0	4.8–7.2	3.8–5.5
[SI units])	4.6–6.0 × 10^{12}	4.8–7.2 × 10^{12}	3.8–5.5 × 10^{12}
MCV (cuμ [conventional] or fl [SI units])	80–98	96–108	82–92
MCH (pg [conventional and SI units])	27–31	32–34	27–31
MCHC (% or g/dl [conventional] or SI units)	32%–36% 0.32–0.36	32%–33% 0.32–0.33	32%–36% 0.32–0.36
RDW (coulter S)	11.5–14.5		

Description.   RBC indices provide information about the size (MCV, mean corpuscular volume); weight (mean corpuscular hemoglobin [MCH]); and hemoglobin concentration (mean corpuscular hemoglobin concentration [MCHC]) of RBCs. A decreased MCV or microcytes, small-sized RBCs, is indicative of iron deficiency anemia and thalassemia. An increased MCV or macrocytes, large-sized RBCs, is indicative of pernicious anemia and folic acid anemia. In macrocytic anemias, the MCH is elevated, and it is decreased in hypochromic anemia. The MCHC can be calculated from MCH and MCV as follows:

$$MCHC = \frac{MCH}{MCV} \times 100 \quad \text{or} \quad MCHC - \frac{Hb}{Hct} \times 100$$

A decreased MCHC can indicate hypochromic anemia.

The RBC distribution width (RDW) is the size (width) differences of RBCs. RDW is the measurement of the width of the size distribution curve on a histogram. It is useful in predicting anemias early, before MCV changes and before signs and symptoms occur. An elevated RDW can indicate iron deficiency, folic acid deficiency, or vitamin B_{12} deficiency anemias.

Purposes
- To monitor red blood cell count
- To differentiate between the components of RBC indices for determining health problem (see Clinical Problems)

Clinical Problems

Indices	Decreased Level	Increased Level
RBC count	Hemorrhage (blood loss)	Polycythemia vera
	Anemias	Hemoconcentration/
	Chronic infections	dehydration
	Leukemias	High altitude
	Multiple myeloma	Cor pulmonale
	Excessive IV fluids	Cardiovascular disease
	Chronic renal failure	
	Pregnancy	
	Overhydration	
MCV	Microcytic anemia:	Macrocytic anemia;
	iron deficiency	aplastic, hemolytic,
	Malignancy	pernicious, folic acid
	Rheumatoid arthritis	deficiency
		Chronic liver disease
	Hemoglobinopathies;	Hypothyroidism
	thalassemia, sickle cell	(myxedema)
	anemia, hemoglobin C	Drugs affect vitamin B12
	Lead poisoning	anticonvulsants,
	Radiation	antimetabolics
MCH	Microcytic, hypochromic	Macrocytic anemias
	anemia	

Indices	Decreased Level	Increased Level
MCHC	Hypochromic anemia Iron deficiency anemia Thalassemia	
RDW		Iron-deficiency anemia, folic acid deficiency, pernicious anemia, homozygous hemoglobinopathies (S, C, H)

Procedure

- No food or fluid restriction is required.
- Collect 3 to 5 ml of venous blood in a lavender-top tube. Avoid hemolysis.
- Usually a particle counter is used, which will provide all CBC results along with all the indices.

Nursing Implications

- Assess for the cause(s) of a decreased RBC count. Check for blood loss, and obtain a history of anemias, renal insufficiency, chronic infection, or leukemia. Determine whether the client is overhydrated.
- Observe for signs and symptoms of advanced iron deficiency anemia (e.g., fatigue, pallor, dyspnea on exertion, tachycardia, and headache). Chronic symptoms include cracked corners of the mouth, smooth tongue, dysphagia, and numbness and tingling of the extremities.
- Assess for signs and symptoms of hemoconcentration. Dehydration, shock, and severe diarrhea can elevate the RBC level.

Client Teaching

- Instruct the client to eat foods rich in iron (e.g., liver, red meats, green vegetables, and iron-fortified bread).
- Explain to the client who is taking iron supplements that the stools usually appear dark in color (tarry). Tell the client to take iron medication with meals. Milk and antacids can interfere with iron absorption.

RENIN (PLASMA)

PLASMA RENIN ACTIVITY (PRA)

Reference Values

Adult: Thirty minutes supine: 0.2–2.3 ng/ml; upright: 1.6–4.3 ng/ml; restricted salt diet: 4.1–10.8 ng/ml.

Child: 1–3 years old: 1.7–11.0 ng/ml; 3–5 years old: 1.0–6.5 ng/ml; 5–10 years old: 0.5–6.0 ng/ml

Description.   Renin is an enzyme secreted by the juxtaglomerular cells of the kidneys. This enzyme activates the renin–angiotensin system, which causes the release of aldosterone and causes vasoconstriction. Aldosterone promotes sodium reabsorption from the kidneys, thus sodium and water retention. Vasoconstriction and aldosterone can cause hypertension. Elevated plasma renin rarely occurs in essential hypertension, but its value is frequently elevated in renovascular and malignant hypertension.

Postural changes (from a recumbent to an upright position) and a decreased sodium (salt) intake will stimulate renin secretion. Plasma renin levels are usually higher from 8 AM to 12 noon and lower from noon to 6 PM.

Purpose

- To identify a possible cause of hypertension

Clinical Problems

Decreased level: Essential hypertension, Cushing's syndrome, diabetes mellitus, hypothyroidism, high-sodium diet

Drugs that may decrease renin value: Antihypertensives, levodopa, propranolol (Inderal)

Increased level: Hypertension (malignant, renovascular), hyperaldosteronism, cancer of the kidney, acute renal failure, Addison's disease, cirrhosis, chronic obstructive pulmonary disease (COPD), manic-depressive disorder, pregnancy (first trimester), preeclampsia and eclampsia, hyperthyroidism, low-sodium diet, hypokalemia

Drugs that may increase renin value: Estrogens, diuretics, certain antihypertensives, oral contraceptives

Procedure
- Keep the syringe and collecting tube cold in an ice bath before collection.
- The tourniquet should be released before the blood is drawn.
- Collect 5 to 7 ml of venous blood in a lavender-top tube.
- Note on the laboratory slip if the client is in a supine or upright position. Note also if the client is on a normal or low-salt diet.
- Take the blood specimen (in ice) to the laboratory immediately.

Nursing Implications
- Check with the laboratory on procedural changes or modifications.
- Monitor the client's blood pressure every 4 to 6 h or as indicated.
- Assess kidney function by recording urinary output. Urine output should be at least 600 ml/day.

RETICULOCYTE COUNT (BLOOD)

Reference Values
Adult: 0.5%–1.5% of all RBCs, 25,000–75,000 µl
Reticulocyte count = reticulocytes (%) × RBC count
Child: Newborn: 2.5%–6.5% of all RBCs; infant: 0.5%–3.5% of all RBCs; child: 0.5%–2.0% of all RBCs

Description.   The reticulocyte count is an indicator of bone marrow activity and is used in diagnosing anemias. Reticulocytes are immature, non-nucleated RBCs that are formed in the bone marrow, pass into circulation, and in 1 to 2 days are matured RBCs. If the reticulocyte percent or count is abnormal, the test should be repeated, since the results can be different according to the time when the blood was tested. Both the RBC count and the reticulocyte count should be reported.

Purpose
- To aid in the diagnosis of anemias (pernicious, folic acid deficiency, hemolytic, sickle cell) (see Clinical Problems)

Clinical Problems

Decreased level: Anemias (pernicious, folic acid deficiency, aplastic), radiation therapy, X-ray irradiation, adrenocortical hypofunction, anterior pituitary hypofunction, cirrhosis of the liver (alcohol suppresses reticulocytes)

Increased level: Anemias (hemolytic, sickle cell), treatment for anemias (iron deficiency, vitamin B_{12}, folic acid), thalassemia major, leukemias, posthemorrhage (3 to 4 days), erythroblastosis fetalis, hemoglobin C and D diseases, pregnancy

Procedure

Venous Blood

- No food or fluid restriction is required.
- Collect 3 to 5 ml of venous blood in a lavender-top tube.

Capillary Blood

- Cleanse the finger, and puncture the skin with a sterile lancet. Wipe the first drop of blood away.
- Collect blood by using a micropipette.

Nursing Implications

- Obtain a history regarding radiation exposure.
- Check the reticulocyte count and the RBC count. If the reticulocyte count is given as a percentage, convert the percentage to the count (see Reference Values).
- Monitor the reticulocyte count when the client is taking iron supplements for iron deficiency anemia or is being treated for pernicious anemia or folic acid anemia. An increased count suggests that the marrow is responding.

RHEUMATOID FACTOR (RF); RHEUMATOID ARTHRITIS (RA) FACTOR (SERUM)

RA LATEX FIXATION

Reference Values

Adult: Less than 1:20 titer; 1:20–1:80 positive for rheumatoid and other conditions; greater than 1:80 positive for rheumatoid arthritis

Child: Not usually done
Elderly: Slightly increased

Description.   The rheumatoid factor (RF), or rheumatoid arthritis (RA) factor, test is a screening test to detect antibodies (IgM, IgG, or IgA) found in the serum of clients with rheumatoid arthritis. The RF occurs in 53% to 94% of clients with rheumatoid arthritis, and if the test is negative, it should be repeated.

The RF tests should not be used for monitoring follow-up or treatment stages of rheumatoid arthritis (RA), because RF tests often remain positive when clinical remissions have been achieved. It also takes approximately 6 months for a significant elevation of titer. For diagnosing and evaluating RA, the ANA and the C-reactive protein agglutination tests are frequently used.

Purposes
- To screen for IgM, IgG, or IgA antibodies present in clients with possible rheumatoid arthritis
- To aid in the diagnosis of rheumatoid arthritis
- To compare test results in relation to other laboratory tests for diagnosing rheumatoid arthritis

Clinical Problems
Increased level: Rheumatoid arthritis, lupus erythematosus, dermatomyositis, scleroderma, infectious mononucleosis, tuberculosis, leukemia, sarcoidosis, cirrhosis of the liver, hepatitis, syphilis, chronic infections, myocardial infarction, renal disease

Procedure
- No food or fluid restriction is required.
- Collect 3 to 5 ml of venous blood in a red-top tube.

Factors Affecting Laboratory Results
- A positive RF test result frequently remains positive regardless of clinical improvement.

- The RF test result can be positive in various clinical problems, such as collagen diseases, cancer, and liver cirrhosis.
- The older adult may have an increased RF titer without the disease.

Nursing Implications
- Consider the age of the client when the RF is slightly increased. Elderly may have slightly increased RF titers without clinical symptoms of RA. With juvenile rheumatoid arthritis, only 10% of the children have a positive RF titer.
- Assess for pain in the small joints of the hands and feet, which could be indicative of early-stage rheumatoid arthritis.
- Compare RF test results with C-reactive protein test. With RF test it may take 6 months for a significant elevation of the RF titer.

RH TYPING (BLOOD)

Reference Values
Adult: Rh$^+$ (positive), Rh$^-$ (negative)
Child: Same as adult

Description.   Rh typing is performed when typing donor/recipient blood and for crossmatching blood for transfusion. Rh positive (most common Rh factor) indicates the presence of antigen on RBCs, and Rh negative indicates an absence of the antigen. An Rh-negative woman carrying a fetus with an Rh-positive blood group can cause Rh-positive antigens from the fetus to seep into the mother's blood, causing Rh antibody formation. To prevent Rh antibodies, the Rh-negative woman is given Rho(D) immune globulin, such as RhoGAM, within 3 days after delivery with the first child or after a miscarriage to neutralize any anti-Rh antibodies.

Purpose
- To identify client's Rh factor during pregnancy or for blood transfusion

Clinical Problems
Increased anti-Rh antibodies
Infant: Erythroblastosis fetalis

Procedure
- No food or fluid restriction is required.
- Collect 5 ml of venous blood in a red-top tube or 7 ml in a lavender-top tube.

Nursing Implications
- Obtain a history of previous blood transfusions. If pregnant, determine whether she has been pregnant before and whether the child was born jaundiced.
- Compare the tested Rh factor with the client's stated Rh factor.

Client Teaching
- Inform the pregnant woman with Rh-negative blood that her blood will be tested at intervals during pregnancy to determine if antibodies are produced. Rh-negative women usually receive RhoGAM after delivery to prevent anti-Rh antibody production.

ROTAVIRUS ANTIGEN (BLOOD AND FECES)

Reference Values
Blood and stool: Negative

Description.   Rotavirus is an RNA virus that frequently causes infectious diarrhea in infants and young children, usually between 2 months and 2 years old. Rotavirus is a significant cause of enteritis in infants and gastroenteritis in very young children. It is more prevalent in the winter months in the United States; it is year-round in the tropical areas. Adults can also become infected with this virus. Clinical symptoms include vomiting (usually precedes diarrhea), diarrhea, fever, and abdominal pain. This virus is frequently transmitted to infants and children in day-care centers, group homes, and preschools, and to the elderly in nursing homes. Symptoms in adults are normally mild.

The rotavirus is mainly transmitted by the fecal–oral route. It can be detected in the stool using electron microscopy or preferably ELISA screening. Kits are available for testing the stool specimen.

Purpose

- To identify the rotavirus that is causing gastroenteritis in infants and young children

Clinical Problems

Positive test result: Gastroenteritis caused by the rotavirus

Procedure

- Food and fluid are not restricted.

Blood

- Collect 3 to 5 ml of venous blood in a red-top tube. Avoid hemolysis.
- Test results are available in 24 h.

Stool

- Obtain liquid stool and place the specimen in a closed container. The container should be placed on ice. A freshly soiled diaper may be used. Take immediately to the laboratory.
- A cotton-tip swab may be used to swab the rectum in a rotating motion. Leave the swab in the rectum for a few seconds for absorption. Place the swab in a tube or container, pack in ice, and send it immediately to the laboratory.
- No preservatives or metal container should be used. It interferes with ELISA testing.
- Test results are available in approximately 24 h.

Nursing Implications

- Obtain a history of diarrhea, vomiting, and fever occurring in the child. Record the frequency of the symptoms and the color of the stool and vomitus.
- Take vital signs. Keep a chart of body temperatures.
- Collect stool according to the procedure. Have the specimen container iced and taken immediately to the laboratory.
- Answer the family's questions. Be supportive of the child and family members.

Client Teaching

- Demonstrate to the parent collection of the stool specimen. The stool specimen should be collected during the acute stage.
- Instruct the family member that the stool can be infectious and that the rotavirus could be transmitted to others if precautions are not taken. Hands should be thoroughly washed after changing soiled diapers. Diapers should be carefully placed in plastic bags and properly discarded.
- Instruct the parent to check the child's body temperature at specified intervals.
- Encourage the parent to increase the child's fluid intake, particularly electrolyte-based fluids.
- Inform the parent that the rotavirus is easily transmitted and that there is a higher risk of transmission in nurseries, day-care centers, group homes, and nursing homes.

RUBELLA ANTIBODY DETECTION (SERUM)

HEMAGGLUTINATION INHIBITION TEST (HAI OR HI) FOR RUBELLA

Reference Values

Adult: Titer less than 1:8. Susceptibility to rubella: titer 1:8–1:32. Past rubella exposure and immunity: titer 1:32–1:64; definite immunity: greater than 1:64

Description.   Rubella (German measles) is a mild viral disease of short duration causing a fever and a transient rash. The rubella virus produces antibodies against future rubella infections, but the exact antibody titer is unknown. Hemagglutination inhibition (HI or HAI) measures rubella antibody titers and is considered to be a sensitive and reliable test. Women should be immune to rubella or should receive the rubella vaccine before marriage and definitely before pregnancy. When women contract rubella during the first trimester of pregnancy, serious congenital deformities in the fetus could result.

Purpose
- To identify clients who are susceptible to rubella or have immunity to the rubella virus

Clinical Problems
Decreased level: Less than 1:8: susceptible to rubella
Increased level: Greater than 1:32: immunity; greater than 1:64: definite immunity

Procedure
- No food or fluid restriction is required.
- Collect 3 to 5 ml of venous blood in a red-top tube.

Nursing Implications
- Obtain a history of having rubella and recent exposure to rubella virus.

Client Teaching
- Teach women the need to have their blood checked for rubella immunity before marriage and pregnancy. If the titer is less than 1:8, rubella vaccine should be received.
- Instruct pregnant women who are susceptible to German measles to avoid exposure to the disease. If exposed, the obstetrician should be notified immediately so that an HAI antibody titer test can be done.
- Explain to interested persons that fetal abnormalities can occur if the woman develops German measles during the first trimester of pregnancy. Professional help may be needed.
- Be supportive of individual and family.

RUBEOLA ANTIBODIES (SERUM)

Reference Values
Negative: 0 to fourfold titer
Positive: A rise greater than fourfold titer indicates a current infection

Description.   Rubeola, "old fashion" measles (not German measles) is a contagious, viral communicable disease that is caused by the RNA paramyxovirus. It is transmitted via respiratory secretions. Since the 1970s, rubeola vaccine has been available for prevention of the disease. Symptoms of rubeola include a rash that develops into red-colored maculopapular skin eruptions, fever, Koplik's spots in the mouth, cough, conjunctivitis, and lymphadenopathy. An elevated immunoglobulin M (IgM) suggests an acute infection and an elevated immunoglobulin G (IgG) suggests a current or past infection. IgM and IgG rubeola antibodies are tested to differentiate between an acute or a past infection. Immunity to rubeola can be obtained from past infection of the measles virus or from the vaccine.

Groups of people frequently tested are college students, women contemplating on becoming pregnant, and pregnant women. If a pregnant woman contracts the measles infection, spontaneous abortion or preterm delivery might occur.

One or 2 weeks after the measles test, a retest may be suggested to determine the acute versus the convalescent period of the measles infection.

Purposes
- To determine the presence of the rubeola (measles) infection
- To differentiate between the acute phase of the measles infection and the immunity phase according to IgM and IgG

Clinical Problems
Increased level: Measles infection, immunity to the measles virus

Procedure
- No food or fluid restriction is required.
- Collect 5 ml of venous blood in a red-top tube.

Factors Affecting Test Results
- Hemolysis of the blood specimen

Nursing Implications
- Obtain a history of symptoms related to measles infection.
- Ask the client if she has been exposed to a person having measles.

- Determine if the client has had a previous measles vaccination or a previous measles infection.
- Ask if the female client is pregnant.
- Explain to the client that test results are usually available in 24 h.

Client Teaching
- Inform the client to return for a retest if indicated.
- Suggest to the woman of childbearing age, who has not been infected or vaccinated during childhood years, to receive the rubeola (measles) vaccine before pregnancy.
- Be available to provide support to the client and family if the client has been infected with the measles virus.

SALICYLATE (SERUM)

Reference Values
Adult: Normal: negative; therapeutic: 5 mg/dl (headache), 10–30 mg/dl (rheumatoid arthritis); mild toxic: greater than 30 mg/dl; severe toxic: greater than 50 mg/dl; lethal: greater than 60 mg/dl
Child: Toxic: greater than 25 mg/dl
Elderly: Mild toxic: greater than 25 mg/dl

Description.   Salicylate levels are measured to check the therapeutic level, as in the treatment of rheumatic fever, and to check the levels caused by an accidental or deliberate overdose. Blood salicylate reaches its peak in 2 to 3 h, and the blood level can be elevated for as long as 18 h. Prolonged use of salicylates (aspirins) can cause bleeding tendencies, since it inhibits platelet aggregation. It can increase the risk of Reye's syndrome in children having a viral infection.

Purposes
- To monitor salicylate level for daily therapeutic range
- To check for salicylate toxicity

Clinical Problems
Increased level: Greater than 30 mg/dl: overdose or large, continuous doses of aspirin or drugs containing aspirin

Procedure
- No food or fluid restriction is required.
- Collect 5 to 7 ml of venous blood in a red- or green-top tube.
- A urine test may also be done as a screening test.

Nursing Implications
- Observe for signs and symptoms of early aspirin overdose (e.g., hyperventilation, flushed skin, and ringing in the ears).
- Obtain a history from the child or parent concerning the approximate number of aspirins taken. A toxic dose for a small child is 3.33 grains/kg, or 299 mg/kg. Salicylates are not the choice agent for children with virus because of the possibility of developing Reye's syndrome.

Client Teaching
- Instruct the client who takes aspirins regularly that before any surgery the surgeon should be informed of the number of aspirins taken daily.

SARS (SEVERE ACUTE RESPIRATORY SYNDROME)

Reference Values
Normal WBC; no coronavirus antibodies

Description. Severe acute respiratory syndrome, known as SARS, is an infectious disease believed to be caused by a coronavirus. SARS may have started in China in November 2002. By the first of June 2003, 6 months later, 31 countries had reported 8,300 cases of SARS and 750 deaths. Some people have mild cases of SARS, whereas others have become critically ill and died from SARS; the severity of the illness is unpredictable. The Centers for Disease Control (CDC) has developed recommendations and information regarding SARS. The CDC suggests for those persons caring for or in contact with SARS patients to use strict hand hygiene, wear a surgical mask, and, if available, an N–95 filtering disposable respirator. Isolation technique is essential.

The incubation period for SARS is 2 to 10 days. The symptoms of SARS include fever, chills, headache, malaise, myalgia and may progress to a dry cough, dyspnea, and hypoxemia. Abnormal laboratory findings include leukopenia, lymphopenia, thrombocytopenia, elevated LDH, CK, and AST levels. Antibodies to the virus may take more than 21 days to occur after the illness. During the acute stage of illness, the antibodies to the virus may not be isolated. In the early stage of the illness, the lungs can look normal; however, later the chest X-ray may show patchy infiltrates and even areas of consolidation. Some persons diagnosed as having SARS do not have the viral illness. It has been difficult to determine this illness.

Treatment includes supportive care, steroids, and antiviral agents such as oseltamivir, ribavirin. To identify and isolate suspected SARS cases, the CDC provides a Web site for case definition, www.cdc.gov/ncidod/sars/casedefinition.htm.

Purposes
- To prevent the spread of SARS
- To provide effective care for patients with SARS

Clinical Problems
Acute respiratory distress, severe acute respiratory syndrome

Procedure
- Provide isolation for persons with acute respiratory distress symptoms if SARS is suspected unless respiratory problem is known or until SARS is ruled out.
- Utilize mask and strict handwashing technique when in contact with SARS clients or if a client is suspected of having SARS.

Nursing Implications
- Obtain a history of patient's travel to areas where SARS is prevalent, fever, symptoms of respiratory problems, and contact with other persons having SARS.

- Obtain the blood specimens, such as WBC, CK, LHD, AST, or others as ordered.
- Monitor vital signs, especially the client's temperature.
- Use mask and strict isolation technique as indicated by the institution when caring for SARS clients or clients suspected of having SARS.

Client Teaching
- Give support to the client and family. Answer questions if known or have other health professionals answer their questions.

SEMEN EXAMINATION/ANALYSIS

Reference Values
Male adult: Volume: 1.5–5.0 ml; count: 50–150 million/ml (20 million/ml–low, low normal); morphology: greater than 75% mature spermatozoa; motility: greater than 60% actively mobile spermatozoa
Child: Not usually done
Antisperm antibody test: Adult: Negative to 1:32

Description. Semen examination is one test that may determine the cause of infertility. The sperm count, volume of fluid, percent of normal mature spermatozoa (sperms), and the percent of actively mobile spermatozoa are studied when analyzing the semen content. Sexual abstinence is usually required for 3 days before the test. Masturbation is the usual method for obtaining a specimen; however, for religious reasons, intercourse with a condom is sometimes preferred.

Sperm count can be used to monitor the effectiveness of sterilization after a vasectomy. In cases of rape, a forensic or medicolegal analysis is done to detect semen in vaginal secretions or on clothes.

The ***antisperm antibody test*** could be ordered to identify a possible cause of infertility. Autoantibodies to sperm might result from a blocking of the efferent ducts in the testes.

Purposes
- To check the sperm count
- To determine if the decreased sperm count could be the cause of infertility

Clinical Problems
Decreased level: Infertility (0–2 million/ml), vasectomy
Drugs that may cause a low count: Antineoplastic agents, estrogen

Procedure
- Avoid alcoholic beverages for several days (at least 24 h) before the test. No other food or fluid restrictions are required.
- Instruct client to abstain from intercourse for 3 days before collection of semen.
- Collect semen by
  - Masturbation: collect in a clean container.
  - Coitus interruptus: collect in a clean glass container.
  - Intercourse with a clean, washed condom: place the condom in a clean container.
- Keep the semen specimen from chilling, and take it to the laboratory within 30 min.

Factors Affecting Laboratory Results
- Recent intercourse (within 3 days) could have an effect on the sperm count.

Nursing Implications
- Be available to discuss methods of semen collection with the client and his spouse/partner.
- Be supportive of the client and his spouse/partner. Be a good listener, and give them time to express their concerns.
- Answer their questions or refer the questions to the appropriate person (e.g., health care provider, clergy).
- Avoid giving your moral convictions about the test or the surgical procedure (vasectomy).

SEROTONIN (PLASMA)

5-HYDROXYTRYPTAMINE

Reference Values
Adult: 50–175 ng/ml; 10–30 mcg/dl, 0.29–1.15 µmol/1 (SI units)

Description.   Serotonin is produced by the argentaffin cells of the intestinal mucosa. It is transmitted in the body by platelets and acts as a vasoconstrictor to small arterioles after tissue injury. It can also be found in the tissues of the central nervous system and has been classified as one of the neurotransmitters. Other functions of serotonin include contraction of smooth muscle such as in peristalsis, release of the growth hormone, and release of prolactin; it can cause hemocoagulation.

The primary purpose of this test is to confirm the diagnosis of carcinoid tumors of the argentaffin cells in the gastrointestinal tract. Most of the serotonin is excreted as the metabolite 5-hydroxyindole-acetic acid (5-HIAA) in the urine. The 5-HIAA urine test should be ordered with the plasma serotonin test. Ectopic production of serotonin can result from oat cell carcinoma of the lung, pancreatic tumors, and thyroid cancer.

Purpose

- To aid in the diagnosis of carcinoid tumors

Clinical Problems

Decreased level: Parkinson's disease, Down syndrome, depression, renal insufficiency, phenylketonuria

Increased level: Carcinoid tumors: Ectopic production due to oat cell carcinoma of the lung, pancreatic tumor, thyroid medullary cancer; myocardial infarction; endocarditis; chronic pain; cystic fibrosis

Drugs that may increase serotonin level: Monoamine oxidase (MAO) inhibitors, methyldopa, imipramine, reserpine

Procedure

- There is no food or fluid restriction.
- Collect 7 to 10 ml of venous blood in a lavender-top tube. The blood specimen should be placed on ice immediately and sent promptly to the laboratory.
- Withhold MAO inhibitors for a week prior to the test with the health care provider's approval. MAO inhibitors taken prior to the test should be noted on the laboratory slip.

Factors Affecting Laboratory Results
- Blood specimen that has not been cooled and not taken immediately to the laboratory. Blood serotonin samples are unstable.
- Certain drugs can increase the plasma serotonin level, especially MAO inhibitors (see Drugs that may increase serotonin level).
- The drug lithium may decrease or elevate the serotonin in the brain.
- A radioactive scan performed on the client 7 days before the serotonin blood sample is taken.

Nursing Implications
- Obtain a list of drugs the client is taking. Notify the health care provider if the client is taking a drug that could elevate the plasma serotonin level, especially MAO inhibitors.
- Check if a urine 5-HIAA has been ordered. This urine test is usually ordered if a carcinoid tumor is suspected.
- Note if the client has chronic pain, which may increase the plasma serotonin level, or depression, which could decrease the plasma level.

SICKLE CELL (SCREENING) TEST (BLOOD)

Reference Values
Adult: 0
Child: 0

Description.   Hemoglobin S (sickle cell), an abnormal hemoglobin, causes RBCs to form a crescent or sickle shape when deprived of oxygen. With adequate oxygen, the red cells with hemoglobin S will maintain a normal shape.

If a sickle cell screening test is positive for hemoglobin S, hemoglobin electrophoresis should be ordered to differentiate between sickle cell anemia caused by hemoglobin S/S and sickle cell trait caused by hemoglobin A/S. If the client's hemoglobin level is less than 10 g/dl or the hematocrit is less than 30%, test results could be falsely negative.

Purpose
- To screen for sickle cell anemia

Clinical Problems
Positive results: Sickle cell anemia, sickle cell trait

Procedure
- No food or fluid restriction is required.
- Collect 3 to 7 ml of venous blood in a lavender-top tube.
- Note on the laboratory slip if blood transfusion was given 3 to 4 months before the screening test. If so, inaccurate results could result.
- If a commercial test kit (e.g., Sickledex) is used, follow the directions given on the kit.

Factors Affecting Laboratory Results
- A blood transfusion given within 3 to 4 months could cause inaccurate results.
- Hemoglobin less than 10 g/dl or hematocrit less than 30% could cause false-negative test results.

Nursing Implications
- Observe for signs and symptoms of sickle cell anemia. Early symptoms are fatigue and weakness. Chronic symptoms are dyspnea on exertion, swollen joints, "aching bones," and chest pains.

Client Teaching
- Instruct the client to avoid people with infections and colds.
- Encourage the client to seek genetic counseling if he or she has sickle cell anemia or the sickle cell trait.
- Instruct the client with sickle cell anemia to minimize strenuous activity and to avoid high altitudes and extreme cold. Encourage the client to take rest periods.

SODIUM (Na) (SERUM AND URINE)

Reference Values
Serum: Adult: 135–145 mEq/l; 135–145 mmol/l (SI units)
Infant: 134–150 mEq/l
Child: 135–145 mEq/l
Panic value: Less than 115 mEq/l
Urine: Adult: 40–220 mEq/l/24 h
Child: Same as adult

Description.   Sodium (Na) is the major cation in the extracellular fluid (ECF), and it has a water-retaining effect. Sodium has many functions: it helps to maintain body fluids, it is responsible for conduction of neuromuscular impulses via the sodium pump; and it is involved in enzyme activity.

The urine sodium level should be monitored when edema is present and the serum sodium level is low or normal. In congestive heart failure (CHF) the urine sodium level is usually low, and the serum sodium level is low-normal or normal due to hemodilution, or it is elevated.

Purposes
- To monitor sodium level
- To detect sodium imbalance (hypo- or hypernatremia)
- To compare sodium level with other electrolytes (e.g., calcium, potassium, sodium, chloride)

Clinical Problems
Serum sodium and urine sodium have many different clinical and drug problems.

Serum
Decreased level: Vomiting, diarrhea, gastric suction, syndrome of inappropriate antidiuretic hormone (SIADH), continuous IV D_5W, tissue injury, low-sodium diet, burns, salt-wasting renal disease, water intoxication/fluid overload, seizure precaution

Drugs that may decrease sodium value: Diuretics (furosemide [Lasix], ethacrynic acid [Edecrin], thiazides, mannitol)

Increased level: Dehydration, severe vomiting and diarrhea, CHF, adrenal hyperfunction, high-sodium diet, hepatic failure

Drugs that may increase sodium value: Cortisone preparations, antibiotics, laxatives, cough medicines

Urine

Decreased level: Adrenal hyperfunction, CHF, hepatic failure, renal failure, low-sodium diet

Drugs that may decrease urine sodium: Cortisone preparations

Increased level: Adrenal hypofunction, dehydration, essential hypertension, anterior pituitary hypofunction, high-sodium diet

Drugs that may increase urine sodium: Loop or high-ceiling diuretics

Procedure
Serum
- No food or fluid restriction is required. If the client has eaten large quantities of foods high in salt content in the last 24 to 48 h, this should be noted on the laboratory slip.
- Collect 3 to 5 ml of venous blood in a red- or green-top tube.

Urine
- Collect a 24-h urine specimen, place all urine in a large container, and refrigerate. Label the container with the exact times the urine collection started and ended. First-voided specimen should be discarded.

Factors Affecting Laboratory Results
- A diet high in sodium

Nursing Implications
Decreased level: Hyponatremia
- Assess for signs and symptoms of hyponatremia (e.g., apprehension, anxiety, muscular twitching, muscular weakness, headaches, tachycardia, and hypotension).

- Recognize that hyponatremia may occur after surgery as the result of SIADH.
- Monitor the medical regimen for correcting hyponatremia (e.g., water restriction, normal saline solution to correct a serum sodium level of 120 to 130 mEq/l, and 3% saline to correct a serum sodium level of less than 115 mEq/l).
- Check the specific gravity of urine. A specific gravity of less than 1.010 could indicate hyponatremia.
- Irrigate NG tubes and wound sites with normal saline instead of sterile water.
- Compare the serum sodium level with the urine sodium level. A low or normal serum sodium and a low urine sodium could indicate sodium retention or a decrease in sodium intake.

Client Teaching

- Suggest that the client drink fluids with solutes, such as broth and juices; the client should avoid drinking only plain water.

Increased level: Hypernatremia

- Observe for signs and symptoms of hypernatremia (e.g., restlessness; thirst; flushed skin; dry, sticky mucous membranes; a rough, dry tongue; and tachycardia).
- Check for body fluid loss by keeping an accurate intake and output record and by weighing the client daily.
- Check the specific gravity of the urine. A specific gravity over 1.030 could indicate hypernatremia.
- Observe for edema and overhydration resulting from an elevated serum sodium level. Signs and symptoms of overhydration are a constant, irritating cough; dyspnea; neck-and-hand vein engorgement; and chest rales.

Client Teaching

- Instruct the client to avoid foods that are high in sodium (e.g., corned beef, bacon, ham, canned or smoked fish, cheese, celery, catsup, pickles, olives, potato chips, and Pepsi Cola). Also, avoid using salt when cooking or at mealtime.

TESTOSTERONE (SERUM OR PLASMA)

Reference Values
Adult: Male: 0.3–1.0 mcg/dl, 300–1,000 ng/dl; female: 0.03–0.1 mcg/dl, 30–100 ng/dl
Child: Male: 12–14 years: greater than 0.1 mcg/dl, greater than 100 ng/dl

Description.
Testosterone, a male sex hormone, is produced by the testes and adrenal glands in the male and by the ovaries and adrenal glands in the female. It is useful in diagnosing male sexual precocity before the age of 10 years and male infertility. The highest serum testosterone levels occur in the morning.

Purposes
- To assess testosterone value
- To detect testicular hypofunction
- To aid in the diagnosis of male sexual precocity

Clinical Problems
Decreased level: Testicular hypofunction, primary hypogonadism (Klinefelter's syndrome), alcoholism, anterior pituitary hypofunction, estrogen therapy
Increased level: Male sexual precocity, adrenal hyperplasia, adrenogenital syndrome in women, polycystic ovaries

Procedure
- No food or fluid restriction is required.
- Collect 5 to 7 ml of venous blood in a red- or green-top tube. Avoid hemolysis.

Nursing Implications
- Be supportive of the male patient and his family concerning physical changes caused by hormonal deficiency.

- Observe for signs and symptoms of excess testosterone secretion (e.g., hirsutism, masculine voice, and increased muscle mass).

THEOPHYLLINE (SERUM)

AMINOPHYLLINE, THEO-DUR, THEOLAIR, SLO-PHYLLIN

Reference Values
Therapeutic range: Adult: 5–20 mcg/ml, 28–112 μmol/l (SI units); Elderly: 5–18 mcg/ml; **premature** infants: 7–14 mcg/ml; **neonate:** 3–12 mcg/ml; child: same as adult
Toxic level: Adult: greater than 20 mcg/ml, greater than 112 μmol/l (SI units); elderly: same as adult; child: premature infants: greater than 14 mcg/ml; neonate: greater than 13 mcg/ml; child: same as adult

Description.   Theophylline, a xanthine derivative, relaxes smooth muscle of the bronchi and pulmonary blood vessels; stimulates the CNS; stimulates myocardium; increases renal blood flow, causing diuresis; and relaxes smooth muscles of the GI tract. Usually, theophylline products are given to control asthmatic attacks and to treat acute attack. Theophylline has a shorter half-life in smokers and children, so dosage may need to be increased. It has a narrow therapeutic range, and serum levels should be monitored. If severe theophylline toxicity occurs, greater than 30 mcg/ml, cardiac dysrhythmias, seizures, respiratory arrest, and/or cardiac arrest might result. Toxicity could develop quickly in persons with heart failure or liver disease or who are either very young or elderly.

Purpose
- To monitor theophylline levels

Clinical Problems
Decreased level: Smoking
Drugs that may decrease serum theophylline: Phenytoin (Dilantin), barbiturates
Increased level: Theophylline overdose, CHF, liver disease, lung disease, renal disease

Drugs that may increase serum theophylline: Cimetidine (Tagamet), propranolol (Inderal), erythromycin, allopurinol

Procedure
- No food or fluid restriction is required, except no coffee, tea, colas, or chocolates 8 h prior to test.
- Collect 3 to 5 ml of venous blood in a red-top tube. Avoid hemolysis.
- Record the name of the drug, dose, route, and last dose administered on the laboratory requisition slip.
- List drugs the client is taking that could affect test results on the laboratory slip.

Factors Affecting Laboratory Tests
- Chocolate, coffee, tea, and colas could increase serum theophylline level.

Nursing Implications
- Check theophylline level, and report nontherapeutic levels to the health care provider immediately.
- Recognize that smoking and the drug phenytoin (Dilantin) shorten half-life and promote a faster theophylline clearance.
- Observe for signs and symptoms of theophylline toxicity (e.g., anorexia, nausea, vomiting, abdominal discomfort, nervousness, jitters, irritability, tachycardia, and cardiac dysrhythmias).
- Monitor pulse rate, and report signs of tachycardia and skipped beats.
- Monitor intake and output. Report if client's output has greatly increased due to the theophylline effect.

THYROID ANTIBODIES (TA) (SERUM)

THYROID AUTOANTIBODIES; ANTITHYROGLOBULIN ANTIBODY AND ANTIMICROSOMAL ANTIBODY

Reference Values
Antithyroglobulin: negative to titer less than 1:20; antimicrosomal: negative to titer less than 1:100

Description. Thyroid autoimmune disease produces thyroid antibodies (antithyroglobulin antibodies and antimicrosomal antibodies). If thyroglobulin breaks away from thyroxine and enters the circulation, antithyroglobulin antibodies usually form. Antimicrosomal antibodies form if the microsomes of the thyroid epithelial cells are attacked. An increase in these thyroid antibodies damage the thyroid gland. Usually, serum titers are ordered to detect the presence of one or both of the thyroid antibodies.

With thyrotoxicosis, a positive titer of 1:1600 may occur and with Hashimoto's thyroiditis, the titer may be greater than 1:5000. Antibodies to thyroglobulin may be detected in 40% to 70% of clients with chronic thyroiditis, 40% of clients with Graves' disease (thyrotoxicosis), and 70% of clients having hypothyroidism (low to moderate titer elevation). Antibodies to thyroid microsomes occur in 70% to 90% of clients with chronic thyroiditis.

Purposes
- To aid in the diagnosis of Graves' disease
- To detect the presence of thyroid antibodies which may cause a thyroid autoimmune disease

Clinical Problems
Increased titer: Chronic thyroiditis, Hashimoto's thyroiditis, Graves' disease (thyrotoxicosis), pernicious anemia, lupus erythematosus, rheumatoid arthritis

Procedure
- No food or fluid restriction is required.
- Collect 5 ml of venous blood in a red-top tube. Avoid hemolysis.

Nursing Implications
- Obtain a family history of thyroid disease. Determine whether the client has had a viral infection in the last few weeks or months. It is believed that viral infections can trigger autoimmune disease.
- Check the serum thyroglobulin antibody and serum microsomal antibody results. An extremely high serum thyroglobulin test can indicate Hashimoto's thyroiditis.
- Be supportive to the client and family.

THYROID-STIMULATING HORMONE (TSH) (SERUM)

Reference Values
Values differ according to laboratory method used.
Adult: 0.35–5.5 µIU/ml, less than 10 µU/ml, less than 10^3 IU/l (SI units), less than 3 ng/ml
Child: Newborn: less than 25 µIU/ml by the third day

Description.   The anterior pituitary gland secretes thyroid-stimulating hormone (TSH) in response to thyroid-releasing hormone (TRH) from the hypothalamus. TSH stimulates the secretion of thyroxine (T_4) produced in the thyroid gland. TSH and T_4 levels are frequently measured to differentiate pituitary from thyroid dysfunctions. A decreased T_4 level and a normal or elevated TSH level can indicate a thyroid disorder. A decreased T_4 level with a decreased TSH level can indicate a pituitary disorder.

Purposes
- To suggest secondary hypothyroidism due to pituitary involvement
- To compare test results with T_4 level to differentiate between pituitary and thyroid dysfunction

Clinical Problems
Decreased level: Secondary hypothyroidism (pituitary involvement), hyperthyroidism, anterior pituitary hypofunction
Drugs that may decrease TSH value: Aspirin, steroids, dopamine, and heparin
Increased level: Primary hypothyroidism (thyroid involvement), thyroiditis (Hashimoto's autoimmune disease), antithyroid therapy for hyperthyroidism
Drugs that may increase TSH value: Lithium, potassium iodide

Procedure
- No food or fluid restriction is required. Avoid shellfish for several days prior to test.

- Collect 5 ml of venous blood in a red- or green-top tube. Avoid hemolysis.
- Neonate measurement: see Thyroxine.

Nursing Implications

- Recognize the cause of hypothyroidism by comparing the TSH level with the T_4 level. Decreased TSH and T_4 levels could be due to anterior pituitary dysfunction causing secondary hypothyroidism. A normal or elevated TSH and a decreased T_4 could be due to thyroid dysfunction.
- Observe for signs and symptoms of hypothyroidism (e.g., anorexia; fatigue; weight gain; dry and flaky skin; puffy face, hands, and feet; abdominal distention; bradycardia; infertility; and ataxia).
- Monitor vital signs before and during treatment for hypothyroidism. Report if tachycardia occurs.

THYROXINE (T₄) (SERUM)

Reference Values

Adult: Reported as serum thyroxine: T_4 by column: 4.5–11.5 mcg/dl. T_4 RIA: 5–12 mcg/dl; free T_4: 1.0–2.3 ng/dl; reported as thyroxine iodine: T_4 by column: 3.2–7.2 mcg/dl

Child: Newborn: 11–23 mcg/dl; 1–4 months; 7.5–16.5 mcg/dl; 4–12 months; 5.5–14.5 mcg/dl; 1–6 years; 5.5–13.5 mcg/dl; 6–10 years; 5–12.5 g/dl

Description.   Thyroxine (T_4) is the major hormone secreted by the thyroid gland and is at least 25 times more concentrated than triiodothyronine (T_3). The serum T_4 levels are commonly used to measure thyroid hormone concentration and to determine thyroid function. Other thyroid laboratory tests should be performed to verify and confirm thyroid gland disorders.

In some institutions the T_4 test is required for all newborns to detect a decreased thyroxine secretion, which could lead to irreversible mental retardation.

Purposes
- To determine thyroid function
- To aid in the diagnosis of hypo- or hyperthyroidism
- To compare test results with other laboratory thyroid tests

Clinical Problems
Decreased level: Hypothyroidism (cretinism, myxedema), protein mal-nutrition, anterior pituitary hypofunction, strenuous exercise, renal failure
Drugs that may decrease T$_4$ value: Cortisone, chlorpromazine (Thorazine), phenytoin (Dilantin), heparin, lithium, sulfonamides, reserpine (Serpasil), testosterone, propranolol (Inderal), tolbutamide (Orinase), salicylates (high doses)
Increased level: Hyperthyroidism, acute thyroiditis, viral hepatitis, myasthenia gravis, pregnancy, preeclampsia
Drugs that may increase T$_4$ value: Oral contraceptives, estrogen, clofibrate, perphenazine (Trilafon)

Procedure
- No food or fluid restriction is required.
- Collect 5 to 7 ml of venous blood in a red-top tube. Prevent hemolysis.
- List drugs that may affect test results on the laboratory slip.
- Neonate measurement: Warm or massage heel of neonate; clean area; wipe alcohol from site; wipe off first drop of blood; touch special filter paper with drops of blood. Test is usually performed after third day.

Nursing Implications
Decreased Level
- Observe for signs and symptoms of hypothyroidism (e.g., fatigue, forgetfulness, weight gain, dry skin with poor turgor, dry and thin hair, bradycardia, decreased peripheral circulation, depressed libido, infertility, and constipation).

Elevated Level
- Observe for signs and symptoms of hyperthyroidism (e.g., nervousness, tremors, emotional instability, increased appetite, weight loss, palpitations, tachycardia, diarrhea, decreased fertility, and exophthalmos).

- Monitor the pulse rate. Tachycardia is common and, if severe, could cause heart failure and cardiac arrest.

TORCH SCREEN TEST (SERUM)

TORCH BATTERY, TORCH TITER

Reference Values
Maternal: IgG titer antibodies: negative
IgM titer antibodies: negative
Infant: Same as mother; infant should be tested under 2 months of age

Description.   TORCH stands for toxoplasmosis, rubella, cytomegalovirus (CMV), and herpes simplex. It is a screen test to detect the presence of these organisms in the mother and newborn infant. The two common viruses that affect the infant most are CMV and rubella. During pregnancy, TORCH infections can cross the placenta and could result in mild or severe congenital malformation, abortion, or stillbirth. The severe effect from these organisms occurs during the first trimester. If the fetus is infected, the organism remains throughout the pregnancy.

TORCH screening test is more frequently performed when congenital infection in the newborn is suspected. The IgG titers are compared with both the mother and newborn serum. If the IgG titer level is higher in the fetus than the mother, congenital TORCH infection is likely. The test may be repeated in several weeks. Individual testing may be necessary along with a clinical examination and history taking to identify the TORCH infection.

Purpose
- To detect TORCH infection in newborns and mothers

Clinical Problems
Positive IgG, IgM titers: Toxoplasmosis, rubella, CMV, herpes simplex

Procedure

- No food or fluid restriction is required.
- Collect 7 ml of venous blood in a red-top tube.
- TORCH kits: Follow directions on the kit.

Nursing Implications

- Obtain a history from the client about any previous infection.
- Be supportive to the client and family regarding their concerns and fear.

Client Teaching

- Inform the client that several tests may be necessary to confirm a diagnosis.

TOXOPLASMOSIS ANTIBODY TEST (SERUM)

Reference Values

Titer: Less than 1:4, no previous infection from *Toxoplasma gondii*
Titer: 1:4 to 1:64, past exposure, many persist for life
Titer: Greater than 1:256, recent infection
Titer: Greater than 1:424, acute infection

Description. *Toxoplasma gondii (T gondii)* is a protozoan organism that causes the parasitic disease, toxoplasmosis. In the United States 25% to 40% of the population have antibodies to *T gondii.* Half of these persons are asymptomatic. This organism can remain in body muscle and be dormant for years or for life. This organism is transmitted in raw or poorly cooked meat or by ingesting oocysts from feces of infected cats. Transmission from the latter may occur when changing the cat litter.

Congenital form of toxoplasmosis occurs to the fetus when the mother is acutely infected with the *T gondii* during pregnancy and passed the organism via placenta to the unborn child. Congenital toxoplasmosis may cause mental retardation, hydrocephalus, microcephalus, and chronic retinitis, or could lead to fetal death. The Centers for Disease Control recommends a serological test for *T gondii* antibody titer for all pregnant women before the 20th week. Toxoplasmosis is not communicable between individuals except for maternal–fetal transfer.

The IgM antibody titer begins to rise 1 week after infection and peaks in 1 to 3 weeks. The IgG antibody titer rises in approximately 4 to 7 days after the IgM antibody, peaks 1 to 3 weeks later, and falls slowly within 6 months. Sulfonamides may be used to treat toxoplasmosis.

Purposes
- To identify the *T gondii* organism
- To detect the *T gondii* organism in pregnant woman before the 20th week

Clinical Problems
Increased titers: Toxoplasmosis. Low-positive titer: Past infection of *T gondii*. High positive titer: Current active infection of *T gondii*.

Procedure
- No food or fluid restriction is required.
- Collect 5 to 7 ml of venous blood in a red-top tube during early weeks of pregnancy or if suggestive symptoms are present. Test may be repeated in 2 weeks to determine if there is a rise in antibody titer.

Nursing Implications
- Obtain a history of meat ingested that was raw or poorly cooked or of contact with a cat and cat litter. Ask whether the cat roams the street or is completely housebound.
- Check if the client is pregnant and has a cat. Ascertain if the pregnant woman handles the cat litter.
- Check if the client has ever been serologically tested for toxoplasmosis. Chronic toxoplasmosis has a low-positive titer.

Client Teaching
- Instruct the client to cook all meat thoroughly. Raw or poorly cooked meat may have the *T gondii* organism.
- Inform cat owners that meticulous handwashing is essential after changing the cat litter.

- Instruct the pregnant woman not to handle the cat litter. Cats that are allowed to roam the streets may have acquired the *T gondii* organism.
- Instruct the pregnant woman with an outdoor cat to inform her obstetrician so that a titer level could be taken and monitored.
- Answer client's questions or refer them to appropriate personnel.

TRANSFERRIN (SERUM)

SIDEROPHILIN

Reference Values
Adult: 200–430 mg/dl; 2–4.3 g/l (SI units)
Pregnancy (full term): 300 mg/dl; 3.0 g/l (SI units)
Newborn: 125–275 mg/dl
Transferrin saturation: 20%–50%

Description.   Transferrin is a β-globulin protein that is formed in the liver. Iron from the diet is absorbed from the intestinal mucosa and is transported by transferrin to the bone marrow for utilization in hemoglobin (hemoglobin synthesis) and to iron-storage sites such as the muscle. When protein malnutrition is present, serum transferrin levels decrease quickly, even faster than serum albumin levels. Another purpose for transferrin is for stimulation of body growth.

The iron saturation of transferrin, called *transferrin saturation,* is calculated by percent using the following formula:

$$\% \text{ of transferrin saturation} = \frac{\text{serum iron level}}{\text{TIBC}} \times 100\%$$

A transferrin saturation of less than 15% can indicate chronic iron deficiency anemia and other chronic illnesses.

Additional information concerning iron, total iron-binding capacity (TIBC), and transferrin is discussed under Iron (Fe), Total Iron-binding Capacity (TIBC), Transferrin, Transferrin Saturation (Serum).

Purposes
- To detect a serum transferrin deficit
- To aid in the diagnosis of chronic iron deficiency anemia and iron overload

Clinical Problems
Decreased level: Chronic iron deficiency anemia (% saturation), protein malnutrition, hepatic damage, renal disease, chronic infection or inflammation, cancer, rheumatoid arthritis, proteinuria, hemolytic states, iron overload
Increased level: Severe iron deficiency, pregnancy, polycythemia, acute hepatitis
Drugs that may increase the transferrin level: Oral contraceptives

Procedure
- NPO for 12 h before the test. Water is permitted.
- Collect 3 to 5 ml of venous blood in a red-top tube. Avoid hemolysis. The blood specimen should be taken in the morning if the transferrin saturation test is to be performed.

Factors Affecting Laboratory Test
- Hemolysis of the blood sample.
- Pregnancy or use of oral contraceptives may increase the serum transferrin level.

Nursing Implications
- Compare serum transferrin level with serum iron level and the TIBC if these tests were ordered. To determine transferrin saturation (%), serum iron and TIBC values are needed.

Client Teaching
- Instruct the client to eat foods rich in protein, such as meats, beans, and fish.
- Answer questions the client may have or refer the questions to other health professionals.

TRIGLYCERIDES (SERUM)

Reference Values

Adult: 12–29 years; 10–140 mg/dl; 30–39 years; 20–150 mg/dl; 40–49 years; 30–160 mg/dl; greater than 50 years; 40–190 mg/dl, 0.44–2.09 mmol/l (SI units)

Child: Infant: 5–40 mg/dl; 5–11 years; 10–135 mg/dl

Risk Values of Cardiovascular Disease: *Low risk:* less than 100 mg/dl; *normal risk:* 149 mg/dl; *borderline high risk:* 150–199 mg/dl; *high risk:* 200–499 mg/dl; *very high risk:* greater than 500 mg/dl

Description.

Triglycerides are a blood lipid carried by the serum lipoproteins. Triglycerides are a major contributor to arterial diseases and are frequently compared with cholesterol with the use of lipoprotein electrophoresis. As the concentration of triglycerides increases, so will the very low-density lipoproteins (VLDL) increase, leading to hyperlipoproteinemia. Alcohol intake can cause a transient elevation of serum triglyceride levels.

Persons who are at highest risk of elevated triglyceride levels are those who drink alcohol, are obese, consume foods high in simple sugars, take certain medications (Thiazides, hormone therapy), have a familial history of high triglycerides, and have medical conditions such as type 2 diabetes mellitus; hypothyroidism; cardiac, kidney, and liver disease. The statins drugs for lowering cholesterol have less effect on lowering the triglycerides.

Purposes

- To monitor triglyceride levels
- To compare test results with lipoprotein groups (VLDL) that indicate hyperlipemia

Clinical Problems

Decreased level: Congenital β-lipoproteinemia, hyperthyroidism, protein malnutrition, exercise

Drugs that may decrease triglyceride value: Ascorbic acid, clofibrate (Atromid-S), phenformin, metformin

Increased level: Hyperlipoproteinemia, acute myocardial infarction (AMI), hypertension, hypothyroidism, nephrotic syndrome, cerebral thrombosis, alcoholic cirrhosis, uncontrolled diabetes mellitus, Down syndrome, stress, high-carbohydrate diet, pregnancy

Drugs that may increase triglyceride value: Estrogen, oral contraceptives

Procedure
- Restrict food, fluids, and medications after 6 PM the night before the test, except for water. Hold medications until blood is drawn. Maintain a normal diet for 2 or more days before the test.
- No alcohol is allowed for 24 h before the test.
- Collect 3 to 5 ml of venous blood in a red-top tube.
- Note on laboratory slip if client's weight has increased or decreased in the last 2 weeks.

Factors Affecting Laboratory Results
- A high-carbohydrate diet and alcohol can elevate the serum triglyceride level.

Nursing Implications
- Check to see if a lipoprotein electrophoresis has been ordered, which is frequently done when the triglycerides are elevated.

Client Teaching
- Instruct the client with a high serum triglyceride level to avoid eating excessive amounts of sugars and carbohydrates as well as dietary fats. The client should be encouraged to eat fruits.

TRIIODOTHYRONINE (T$_3$) (SERUM)

T$_3$ RIA

Reference Values
Adult: 80–200 ng/dl
Child: Newborn: 40–215 ng/dl; 5 to 10 years: 95–240 ng/dl; 10 to 15 years: 80–210 ng/dl

Description.   Triiodothyronine (T$_3$), one of the thyroid hormones, is present in small amounts in blood and is more short acting and more potent than thyroxine (T$_4$). Both T$_3$ and T$_4$ have similar actions in the body. Serum T$_3$ radioimmunoassay (RIA) measures both bound and free T$_3$. It is effective for diagnosing hyperthyroidism, especially T$_3$ thyrotoxicosis, in which T$_3$ is increased and T$_4$ is in normal range. It is not as reliable for diagnosing hypothyroidism, for T$_3$ remains in normal range. T$_3$ RIA and T$_3$ update are two different tests.

Purposes
- To aid in the diagnosis of hyperthyroidism
- To compare T$_3$ with T$_4$ for determining thyroid disorder

Clinical Problems
Decreased level: Severe illness and trauma, malnutrition
Drugs that may decrease T$_3$ value: Propylthiouracil, methylthiouracil, methimazole (Tapazole), lithium, phenytoin (Dilantin), propranolol (Inderal), reserpine (Serpasil), aspirin (large doses), steroids, sulfonamides
Increased level: Hyperthyroidism, T$_3$ thyrotoxicosis, toxic adenoma, Hashimoto's thyroiditis
Drugs that may increase T$_3$ value: Estrogen, progestins, oral contraceptives, liothyronine (T$_3$), methadone

Procedure
- No food or fluid restriction is required.
- Withhold drugs that affect test results for 24 h with health care provider's approval.
- Collect 5 to 7 ml of venous blood in a red-top tube. Avoid hemolysis.

Nursing Implications
Increased Level
- Observe for signs and symptoms of hyperthyroidism (e.g., nervousness, tremors, emotional instability, increased appetite, weight loss, palpitations, tachycardia, diarrhea, decreased fertility, and exophthalmos).
- Monitor pulse rate. Tachycardia is common and, if severe, could cause heart failure.

TRIIODOTHYRONINE RESIN UPTAKE (T$_3$ RU) (SERUM)

T$_3$ UPTAKE

Reference Value
Adult: 25%–35% uptake

Description. T$_3$ resin uptake is an indirect measure of free thyroxine (T$_4$), whereas serum T$_3$ RIA is a direct measurement of T$_3$. This is an in vitro test in which the client's blood is mixed with radioactive T$_3$ and synthetic resin material in a test tube. The radioactive T$_3$ will bind at available thyroid-binding globulin (protein) sites. The unbound radioactive T$_3$ is added to resin for T$_3$ uptake. In hyperthyroidism there are few binding sites left, so more T$_3$ is taken up by the resin, thus causing a high T$_3$ resin uptake. In hypothyroidism there is less T$_3$ resin uptake.

This test is performed when clients receive drugs, diagnostic agents, inorganic or organic iodine. It should not be used as the only test to determine thyroid dysfunction.

Purposes
- To differentiate between hypo- or hyperthyroidism
- To compare test result with T$_3$ for determining thyroid disorder

Clinical Problems
Decreased level: Hypothyroidism (cretinism, myxedema), pregnancy, Hashimoto's thyroiditis, menstruation, acute hepatitis
Drugs that may decrease T$_3$ RU: Corticosteroids, estrogen, oral contraceptives, antithyroid agents (methimazole, propylthiouracil), thiazides, chlordiazepoxide (Librium), tolbutamide (Orinase), clofibrate
Increased level: Hyperthyroidism, protein malnutrition, metastatic carcinoma, myasthenia gravis, nephrotic syndrome, threatened abortion, renal failure, malnutrition
Drugs that may increase T$_3$ RU: Corticosteroids, warfarin (Coumadin), heparin, phenytoin (Dilantin), phenylbutazone (Butazolidin), aspirin (high doses), thyroid agents, salicylates (high doses)

Procedure

- No food or fluid restriction is required.
- Collect 5 to 7 ml of venous blood in a red-top tube. Prevent hemolysis.
- List drugs that may affect test results on the laboratory slip.

Nursing Implications

Decreased level: See Thyroxine (T_4) (serum)
Elevated level: See Thyroxine (T_4) (serum)

TROPONINS (SERUM, BLOOD)

CARDIAC-SPECIFIC TROPONIN 1 (cTn1), CARDIAC-SPECIFIC TROPONIN T (cTnT)

Reference Values

Cardiac Troponin 1:   0.1–0.5 ng/ml; 0.1–0.5 mcg/l (SI units)
Suspicious myocardium injury: 0.5–2.0 ng/ml
Positive myocardium injury: Greater than 2.0 ng/ml; greater than 2.0 mcg/l (SI units)
Cardiac Troponin T: Less than 0.2 ng/ml; less than 0.2 mcg/l (SI units)

Description.   Troponins are biochemical markers for cardiac diseases especially for the diagnosis of acute myocardial infarction (AMI). The troponins are proteins, present in both the heart muscle and skeletal muscles; the enzyme-linked immunosorbent assay (ELISA) test can identify the muscle that is involved. The cardiac-specific troponin 1 (cTn1) and the cardiac-specific troponin T (cTnT) are released from the heart into the bloodstream 1 to 3 h after the onset of symptoms of AMI. Thrombolytic treatment (clot busters) may be available for early onset of AMI. The troponins are also useful in detecting silent myocardial infarction (MI) and microinfarctions accompanied with chest pain. The electrocardiogram may not have changed.

Troponins are more specific for cardiac muscle injury than creatine phosphokinase MB (CPK-MB). The cardiac troponins are usually within normal range in noncardiac muscle diseases, whereas CPK-MB can be elevated with severe skeletal muscle injury.

Following post infarction, the CTnl remains elevated for 5 to 9 days and the cTnT remains elevated for 10–14 days. A new qualitative immunoassay testing for troponins may be performed at the bedside. The new test takes about 20 min and is read much like a glucometer.

Purposes
- To differentiate between cardiac and noncardiac chest pain
- To evaluate clients with unstable angina pectoris as to whether myocardial damage has occurred
- To assist in the diagnosis of AMI

Clinical Problems
Increased level: AMI, cardiac chest pain, myocardial damage.

Procedure
- No food or fluid restriction is required.
- Collect 5 ml of venous blood in a red-top tube or a heparinized green-top tube.
- Record on the laboratory slip the time the blood specimen was obtained.
- For qualitative immunoassay testing done at the bedside, a micropipette is used to obtain whole blood and is placed in the testing device.

Factors Affecting Laboratory Results
- Elevation of cTnT may occur with severe skeletal muscle injury.

Nursing Implications
- Obtain a history of the chest pain and its severity.
- Check other cardiac enzyme levels (e.g., CPK-MB) with cardiac troponins.
- Record baseline vital signs. Keep a record of the vital signs taken periodically.
- Provide comfort measures for the client.

Client Teaching
- Instruct the client to notify the health professional immediately when chest pain occurs.
- Explain the bedside troponin test and how it will be done (if ordered).

URIC ACID (SERUM AND URINE)

Reference Values
Values may differ among laboratories.

Serum
Adult: Male: 3.5–8.0 mg/dl; female: 2.8–6.8 mg/dl. *Panic values:* greater than 12 mg/dl
Child: 2.5–5.5 mg/dl
Elderly: 3.5–8.5 mg/dl

Urine
Adult: 250–500 mg/24 h (low-purine diet); 250–750 mg/dl (normal diet)
Child: Same as adult

Description.   Uric acid is a by-product of purine metabolism. An elevated urine and serum uric acid (hyperuricemia) depend on renal function, purine metabolism rate, and dietary intake of purine foods. Excess quantities of uric acid are excreted in the urine. Uric acid can crystallize in the urinary tract in acidic urine; therefore, effective renal function and alkaline urine are necessary with hyperuricemia. The most common problem associated with hyperuricemia is gout. Uric acid levels frequently change day by day; thus, uric acid levels may be repeated for several days or weeks.

Purposes
- To monitor serum uric acid during treatment for gout
- To aid in the diagnosis of health problems (see Clinical Problems)

Clinical Problems
Serum
Decreased level: Wilson's disease, proximal renal tubular acidosis, folic acid anemia, burns, pregnancy

Drugs that may decrease uric acid value: Allopurinol, azathioprine (Imuran), warfarin (Coumadin), probenecid (Benemid), sulfinpyrazone

Increased level: Gout, alcoholism, leukemias, metastatic cancer, multiple myeloma, severe eclampsia, hyperlipoproteinemia, diabetes mellitus (severe), renal failure, glomerulonephritis, stress, congestive heart failure, lead poisoning, strenuous exercise, malnutrition, lymphoma, hemolytic anemia, megaloblastic anemia, infectious mononucleosis, polycythemia vera

Drugs that may increase uric acid value: Acetaminophen, ascorbic acid, diuretics (thiazides, acetazolamide [Diamox], furosemide [Lasix]), levodopa, methyldopa (Aldomet), phenothiazine, prolonged use of aspirin, theophylline, 6-mercaptopurine

Urine
Decreased level: Renal diseases (glomerulonephritis [chronic], urinary obstruction, uremia), eclampsia, lead toxicity

Increased level: Gout, high-purine-diet leukemias, neurologic disorders, manic-depressive disease, ulcerative colitis

Procedure
Serum
- No food or fluid restriction is necessary, unless purine diet is restricted.
- Collect 3 to 5 ml of venous blood in a red-top tube.
- List drugs the client is taking that can affect test results on the laboratory slip.

Urine
- Collect a 24-h urine specimen in a large container and refrigerate. A preservative in the container may be necessary.
- Label the container with the client's name, dates of collection, and times (e.g., 9/23/09, 7:11 AM to 9/24/09, 7:15 AM).
- Note on the laboratory slip if the client is on a low, high, or normal purine diet.

Nursing Implications

- Request the dietitian to visit the client to discuss food preferences and to plan a low-purine diet.
- Observe for signs and symptoms of gout (e.g., tophi [crystallized uric acid deposits] of the ear lobe and joints, joint pain, and edema in the "big toe").
- Monitor urinary output. Poor urine output could indicate inadequate fluid intake or poor kidney function.
- Check urine pH, especially if hyperuremia is present. Uric acid stone can occur when the urine pH is low (acidic). Alkaline urine helps to prevent stones in urinary tract.
- Compare the serum uric acid level with the urine uric acid level. An elevated serum uric acid level (hyperuricemia) and a decreased urine uric acid level can indicate kidney dysfunction. Increased serum and urine uric acid levels are frequently seen in gout.

Client Teaching

- Teach the client to avoid eating foods that have moderate or high amounts of purines, such as:

  High (100–1,000 mg purine nitrogen): brains, heart, kidney, liver, sweetbreads, roe, sardines, scallops, mackerel, anchovies, broth, consommé, mincemeat

  Moderate (9–100 mg purine nitrogen): meat, poultry, fish, shellfish, asparagus, beans, mushrooms, peas, spinach
- Instruct the client to decrease alcoholic intake, since alcohol can cause renal retention of urate.

URINALYSIS (ROUTINE)

Reference Values

	Adult	*Newborn*	*Child*
Color	Light straw to dark amber		Light straw to dark yellow
Appearance	Clear	Clear	Clear
Odor	Aromatic		Aromatic

(continued)

	Adult	Newborn	Child
pH	4.5–8.0	5.0–7.0	4.5–8.0
Specific gravity	1.005–1.030	1.001–1.020	1.005–1.030
Protein	2–8 mg/dl; negative reagent strip test		
Glucose	Negative		Negative
Ketones	Negative		Negative
Microscopic examination	1–2 per low-power field		
RBC			Rare
WBC	3–4		0–4
Casts	Occas hyaline		Rare

Description. Urinalysis is useful for diagnosing renal disease and urinary tract infection and for detecting metabolic disease not related to the kidneys. Many routine urinalyses are done in the health care provider's office.

Purposes
- To detect normal versus abnormal urine components
- To detect glycosuria
- To aid in the diagnosis of renal disorder

Clinical Problems
Color: **Colorless or pale:** large fluid intake, diabetes insipidus, chronic kidney disease, alcohol ingestion; **Red or red-brown:** hemoglobinuria, porphyrins, menstrual contamination; Drugs: sulfisoxazole–phenazopyridine (Azo Gantrisin), phenytoin (Dilantin), cascara, chlorpromazine (Thorazine), docusate calcium and phenolphthalein (Doxidan), phenolphthalein; Foods: beets, rhubarb, food color; **Orange:** restricted fluid intake, concentrated urine, urobilin, fever; Drugs: amidopyrine, nitrofurantoin, phenazopyridine (Pyridium), sulfonamides; Foods: carrots, rhubarb, food color; **Blue or green:** *Pseudomonas* toxemia; Drugs: amitriptyline (Elavil), methylene blue, methocarbanol (Robaxin), yeast concentrate; **Brown or black:** Lysol poisoning, melanin, bilirubin, methemoglobin, porphyrin; Drugs: cascara, iron injectable

Appearance: **Hazy or cloudy:** bacteria, pus, RBC, WBC, phosphates, prostatic fluid spermatozoa, urates; **Milky:** fat, pyuria

Odor: **Ammonia:** urea breakdown by bacteria; **Foul or putrid:** bacteria (urinary tract infection); **Mousey:** phenylketonuria; **Sweet or fruity:** diabetic ketoacidosis, starvation

Foam: **Yellow:** severe cirrhosis of the liver, bilirubin, or bile

pH: **Less than 4.5:** Metabolic acidosis, respiratory acidosis, starvation diarrhea, diet high in meat protein; Drugs: ammonium chloride, mandelic acid; **Greater than 8.0:** bacteriuria, urinary tract infection; Drugs: antibiotics (neomycin, kanamycin), sulfonamides, sodium bicarbonate, acetazolamide (Diamox), potassium citrate

Specific gravity: **Less than 1.005:** diabetes insipidus, excess fluid intake, overhydration, renal disease, severe potassium deficit; **greater than 1.026:** decreased fluid intake, fever, diabetes mellitus, vomiting, diarrhea, dehydration. Contrast media

Protein: **Greater than 8 mg/dl or greater than 80 mg/24 h:** proteinuria, exercise, severe stress, fever, acute infectious diseases, renal diseases, lupus erythematosus, leukemia, multiple myeloma, cardiac disease, toxemia of pregnancy, septicemia, lead, mercury; Drugs: barbiturates, neomycin, sulfonamides

Glucose: **Greater than 15 mg/dl or +4:** diabetes mellitus, CNS disorders (stroke), Cushing's syndrome, anesthesia, glucose infusions, severe stress, infections; Drugs: ascorbic acid, aspirin, cephalosporins, epinephrine

Ketones: **+1 to +3:** ketoacidosis, starvation, diet high in proteins

RBCs: **Greater than 2 per low-power field:** trauma to the kidneys, renal diseases, renal calculi, cystitis, lupus nephritis, excess aspirin, anticoagulants, sulfonamides, menstrual contamination

WBCs: **Greater than 4 per low-power field:** urinary tract infection, fever, strenuous exercise, lupus nephritis, renal diseases

Casts: fever, renal diseases, heart failure

Procedure

- No food or fluid restriction is required, unless NPO for an early morning specimen is ordered by the health care provider.
- Collect a freshly voided urine specimen (50 ml) in a clean, dry container and take it to the laboratory within 30 min. An early morning

urine specimen collected before breakfast is preferred. The urine specimen could be refrigerated for 6 to 8 h.
- A clean-caught or midstream urine specimen may be requested if bacteria or WBCs are suspected. Follow directions on the clean-caught urine container.
- Make sure there are no feces or toilet paper in the urine specimen.

Factors Affecting Laboratory Results
- A urine specimen that has been sitting for an hour or longer without refrigeration.

Nursing Implications
- Assist the client with the urine collection as needed.
- Obtain a history of any drugs the client is currently taking.
- Obtain a history of foods taken in excess amounts that could affect test results.
- Assess the fluid status of the client. Early morning urine specimen, dehydration, and decreased fluid intake usually result in concentrated urine.

Client Teaching
- Instruct client that the urine specimen should be taken to the laboratory within 30 min or else refrigerated.

UROBILINOGEN (URINE)

Reference Values
Adult: Random: negative or less than 1.0 Ehrlich units; 2-h specimen: 0.3–1.0 Ehrlich units; 24 h: 0.5–4.0 mg/24 h, 0.5–4.0 Ehrlich units/24 h, 0.09–4.23 µmol/24 h (SI units)
Child: Similar to adult

Description.   Urobilinogen test is one of the most sensitive tests for determining liver damage, hemolytic disease, and severe infections. In early hepatitis, mild liver cell damage, or mild toxic injury, the urine urobilinogen level will increase despite an unchanged serum bilirubin level. The urobilinogen level will frequently decrease in severe liver damage, since less bile will be produced. The urobilinogen test may be one of the tests performed during urinalysis.

Purpose

- To aid in determining liver damage

Clinical Problems

Decreased level: Biliary obstruction, severe liver disease, cancer of the pancreas, severe inflammatory disease

Drugs that may decrease urine urobilinogen: Antibiotics, ammonium chloride, ascorbic acid

Increased level: Cirrhosis of the liver (early), infectious hepatitis, toxic hepatitis, hemolytic and pernicious anemia, erythroblastosis fetalis, infectious mononucleosis

Drugs that may increase urine urobilinogen: Sulfonamides, phenothiazines, cascara, phenazopyridine (Pyridium), methenamine mandelate (Mandelamine), sodium bicarbonate

Procedure

- No food or fluid restriction is required.

2-h Urine Specimen

- Collect 2-h specimen between 1 and 3 PM or 2 and 4 PM, as urobilinogen peaks in the afternoon. Urine should be kept refrigerated or in a dark container. Urine should be tested within 0.5 h, as urine urobilinogen oxidizes to urobilin (orange substance).

24-h Urine Specimen

- Collect 24-h urine specimen, place in a large container, and keep refrigerated. A preservative may be added to the container.
- Label the container with the client's name, date, and time of urine collection.
- List drugs that affect test results on the laboratory slip.

Nursing Implications

- Check for an elevated urobilinogen level in freshly voided urine with a reagent color dipstick. Record the results of the single test.
- Assess for signs and symptoms of jaundice (e.g., yellow sclera, skin on the forearm is yellow).

Client Teaching

- Explain the procedure to the client for the 2- or 24-h test.

VIRAL CULTURE (BLOOD, BIOPSY, CEREBROSPINAL FLUID, PHARYNX, RECTUM, SPUTUM, STOOL, URINE)

Reference Value

Negative culture result

Description. The virus culture is performed to confirm a suspected viral infection. A blood sample, sputum, and a pharyngeal swab are the most common specimens to obtain for identifying a virus. The specimen is placed on a special viral culture medium of growing cells; it will not grow on nonliving media.

Purpose

- To identify a viral infection

Clinical Problems

Positive: Pneumonia (viral), meningitis (viral), rhinovirus, sinusitis, conjunctivitis, shingles, varicella-zoster virus, herpes simplex, enteroviruses, influenza, cytomegalovirus (CMV)

Procedure

- No food or fluid restriction is required.
- Collect 5 ml of venous blood in a green-top tube. Tube should be chilled. A repeated test is suggested in 14 to 28 days as a convalescent specimen.

- A culturette swab may be used to obtain a specimen from the conjunctiva, lesion, throat, and rectum. The swab should be placed in a chilled viral transport medium.
- Obtain 5 ml of cerebrospinal fluid and place in a chilled sterile vial.
- Obtain a midstream, clean-caught urine specimen in a sterile container.
- Deliver the specimen immediately to the laboratory.

Nursing Implications
- Obtain a history regarding the possibility of a viral infection. Note the severity of the infection.
- Record symptoms that the client is having in relation to the suspected virus.

Client Teaching
- Explain the procedure for collecting the specimen to the client.
- Inform the client that a second blood sample may be needed in 2 to 4 weeks. Check with the health care provider.
- Listen to the client's concerns.

VITAMIN A (SERUM)

RETINOL

Reference Values
Adult: 30–95 mcg/dl, 1.05–3.0 μmol/l (SI units); 125–150 international units/dl
Child: 1–6 years: 20–43 mcg/dl, 0.7–1.5 μmol/l (SI units); 7–12 years: 20–50 mcg/dl, 0.91–1.75 μmol/l (SI units); 13–19 years: 26–72 mcg/dl, 0.91–2.5 μmol/l (SI units)

Description. Vitamin A is a fat-soluble vitamin that is absorbed from the intestine in the presence of lipase and bile. Vitamin A moves to the liver and is stored there as retinyl ester and in the body as retinol. It binds to the serum protein prealbumin.

The functions of vitamin A include the mucous membrane epithelial cell integrity of the eyes, cornea, and the respiratory, gastrointestinal, and genitourinary tracts; body growth; night vision; and skin integrity. Vitamin A has played a major role for years in treating acne; however, high doses of vitamin A can be toxic because it is a fat-soluble vitamin and accumulates in the body tissues.

Purposes
- To detect a vitamin A deficit
- To check for vitamin A toxicity

Clinical Problems
Decreased level: Night-blindness; liver, intestinal, or pancreatic diseases; chronic infections; carcinoid syndrome; cystic fibrosis; protein malnutrition; malabsorption; celiac disease
Drugs that may decrease vitamin A level: Mineral oil, neomycin, cholestyramine
Increased level: Hypervitaminosis, chronic kidney disease
Drugs that may increase vitamin A level: Glucocorticoids, oral contraceptives

Procedure
- NPO for 8 to 12 h before the test except for water.
- Collect 5 to 7 ml of venous blood in a red-top tube. Avoid hemolysis and protect the specimen from light. The blood specimen may be placed in a paper bag.

Nursing Implications
- Obtain a history of the client's nutrient intake and supplementary vitamin intake. Note if the client avoids foods that are rich in vitamin A, such as green leafy and yellow vegetables; yellow fruits such as apricots and cantaloupe; eggs, whole milk, liver. Individuals with a well-balanced dietary intake normally do not need vitamin supplements.

Client Teaching
Decreased Level
- Encourage the client to eat foods rich in vitamin A.

- Inform the client that vitamin supplements can be helpful in preventing vitamin deficiency. The client may wish to contact the health care provider concerning vitamin supplements.

Elevated Level

- Instruct the client that megadoses of vitamin A for treating acne can be toxic. The health care provider should be contacted before taking megadoses of vitamin A.
- Instruct pregnant women that vitamins are usually prescribed during pregnancy; however, megadoses of vitamin A should be avoided because it may cause a birth defect in the newborn.

VITAMIN B$_{12}$ (SERUM)

Reference Values
Adult: 200–900 pg/ml
Child: Newborn: 160–1,200 pg/ml

Description.   Vitamin B$_{12}$ is essential for RBC maturation. The extrinsic factor of vitamin B$_{12}$ is obtained from foods and is absorbed in the small intestines when the intrinsic factor is present. The intrinsic factor is produced by the gastric mucosa, and when this factor is missing, pernicious anemia, a megaloblastic anemia, develops.

Purposes
- To detect pernicious anemia as determined by a decreased vitamin B$_{12}$
- To suggest other health problems (see Clinical Problems)

Clinical Problems
Decreased level: Pernicious anemia, malabsorption syndrome, inadequate intake, liver diseases, hypothyroidism, sprue, pancreatic insufficiency, gastrectomy, Crohn's disease
Drugs that may decrease vitamin B$_{12}$ value: Neomycin, metformin, ethanol, anticonvulsants

Increased level: Acute hepatitis, acute and chronic myelocytic leukemia, polycythemia vera

Drugs that may increase vitamin B$_{12}$ value: Oral contraceptives

Procedure
- No food or fluid restriction is required.
- Collect 3 to 5 ml of venous blood in a red-top tube. Prevent hemolysis.

Nursing Implications
- Assess for signs and symptoms of pernicious anemia (e.g., pallor, fatigue, dyspnea, sore mouth, smooth beefy-red tongue, indigestion, tingling numbness in the hands and feet, and behavioral changes).

Client Teaching
- Inform the client of foods high in vitamin B$_{12}$, such as milk, eggs, meat, and liver. Contact the dietitian to assist the client in meal planning. IM vitamin B$_{12}$ may be ordered.

VITAMIN C (*SEE ASCORBIC ACID*)

WEST NILE VIRUS ANTIBODIES (SERUM, CSF)

Reference Values
Negative for IgM antibodies to flaviviruses (10 days after flu-like symptoms)

Description.   West Nile virus is a flavivirus commonly found in Africa, West Asia, and the Middle East. West Nile first occurred in the United States in 1999. Since this time, almost every state has reported occurrences of the West Nile virus. It can infect human, birds, mosquitoes, horses, and some other mammals. In people it is normally a mild disease, characterized by flu-like symptoms, such as fever, headaches, lethargy, body aches, and possible skin rash, lasting only a few days. When it is severe, it may cause encephalitis, meningitis, or meningoencephalitis. This virus mainly occurs in late summer or early fall. The main route of infection is through the bite of an infected mosquito.

Purpose
- To aid in the diagnosis of West Nile viral infection

Clinical Problems
Positive test: West Nile disease, flavivirus

Procedure
- No food or fluid restriction is required
- Collect 5 ml of venous blood in a red-top tube.
- Perform a spinal tap to obtain spinal fluid from the spinal cord. The CSF is evaluated for the presence of flavivirus.

Factors Affecting Laboratory Results
- None known

Nursing Implications
- Obtain a history from the client of a mosquito bite. Ascertain if the client has flu-like symptoms.
- Check the vital signs (VS). Continue to monitor VS.
- Note if the client has a severe headache, is confused, has difficulty in turning his/her head, or has any symptoms that may be due to meningitis or encephalitis.
- Provide comfort measures for the client.

Client Teaching
- Encourage the client to express to the health professionals all symptoms that he/she has.
- Tell the client to rest for several days after the flu-like symptoms have ceased. Temperature should be monitored.
- Inform the client that the test results of having West Nile virus may take up to 2 weeks.

WHITE BLOOD CELLS (WBCs): TOTAL (WBC) (BLOOD)

LEUKOCYTES

Reference Values
Adult: Total WBC count: 4,500–10,000 μl (mm³)
Child: Newborn: 9,000–30,000 μl; 2 years: 6,000–17,000 μl; 10 years: 4,500–13,500 μl

Description. (See White Blood Cell Differential.) WBCs (leukocytes) are divided into two groups, the polymorphonuclear leukocytes (neutrophils, eosinophils, and basophils) and the mononuclear leukocytes (monocytes and lymphocytes). Leukocytes are a part of the body's defense system; they respond immediately to foreign invaders by going to the site of involvement. An increase in WBCs is called leukocytosis, and a decrease in WBCs is called leukopenia.

Purposes
* To assess WBCs as a part of a complete blood count (CBC)
* To determine the presence of an infection
* To check WBC values for diagnosing health problems (see Clinical Problems)

Clinical Problems
Decreased level: Hematopoietic diseases (aplastic anemia, pernicious anemia, hypersplenism, Gaucher's disease), viral infections, malaria, agranulocytosis, alcoholism, SLE, RA
Drugs that may decrease WBC value: Antibiotics (penicillins, cephalothins, chloramphenicol), acetaminophen (Tylenol), sulfonamides, propylthiouracil, barbiturates, cancer chemotherapy agents, diazepam (Valium), diuretics (furosemide [Lasix], ethacrynic acid [Edecrin]), chlordiazepoxide (Librium), oral hypoglycemic agents, indomethacin (Indocin), methyldopa (Aldomet), rifampin, phenothiazine
Increased level: Acute infection (pneumonia, meningitis, appendicitis, colitis, peritonitis, pancreatitis, pyelonephritis, tuberculosis, tonsillitis,

diverticulitis, septicemia, rheumatic fever), tissue necrosis (myocardial infarction, cirrhosis of the liver, burns, cancer of the organs, emphysema, peptic ulcer), leukemias, collagen diseases, hemolytic and sickle cell anemia, parasitic diseases, stress (surgery, fever, emotional upset [long lasting]), histamine

Drugs that may increase WBC value: Aspirin, antibiotics (ampicillin, erythromycin, kanamycin, methicillin, tetracyclines, vancomycin, streptomycin), gold compounds, procainamide (Pronestyl), triamterene (Dyrenium), allopurinol, potassium iodide, hydantoin derivatives, sulfonamides (long acting), heparin, digitalis, epinephrine, lithium

Procedure
Venous Blood
- No food or fluid restriction is required.
- Collect 7 ml of venous blood in a lavender-top tube. Avoid hemolysis.

Capillary Blood
- Collect blood from a finger puncture with a micropipette. Dilute immediately with the proper reagent.

Factors Affecting Laboratory Results
- The age of the individual. Children can have a high WBC count, especially during the first 5 years of life.

Nursing Implications
- Check the vital signs and signs and symptoms of inflammation and infection.
- Notify the health care provider of changes in the client's condition (e.g., fever, increased pulse and respiration rate, and leukocytosis).

Client Teaching
- Teach the client to check the side effects of patent medicines such as cold medications, which could cause agranulocytosis or severe leukopenia.
- Instruct clients with leukopenia to avoid persons with any contagious condition. Their body resistances are reduced, and they are prime candidates for severe colds or infections.

WHITE BLOOD CELL DIFFERENTIAL (BLOOD)

DIFFERENTIAL WBC

Reference Values

DIFFERENTIAL WBC VALUES

	Adult		*Child*
WBC Type	*%*	*μl (mm³)*	*Same as Adult Except*
Neutrophils (total)	50–70	2,500–7,000	Newborn: 61%; 1 year; 32%
Segments	50–65	2,500–6,500	
Bands	0–5	0–500	
Eosinophils	1–3	100–300	
Basophils	0.4–1.0	40–100	
Monocytes	4–6	200–600	1–12 years 4%–9%
Lymphocytes	25–35	1,700–3,500	Newborn: 34%; 1 year 60%; 6 years 42%; 12 years: 38%

Description.   Differential WBC count, part of the complete blood count (CBC), is composed of five types of WBC (leukocytes): neutrophils, eosinophils, basophils, monocytes, and lymphocytes. The differential WBC count is expressed as cubic millimeters (μl, mm³) and percent of the total number of WBCs. Neutrophils and lymphocytes make up 80% to 90% of the total WBCs. Differential WBC count provides more specific information related to infections and disease process.

Neutrophils: Neutrophils are the most numerous circulating WBCs, and they respond more rapidly to the inflammatory and tissue injury sites than other types of WBC. During an *acute* infection, the body's first line of defense is the neutrophils. The segments are mature neutrophils, and the bands are immature ones that multiply quickly during an acute infection.

Eosinophils: Eosinophils increase during allergic and parasitic conditions. With an increase in steroids, either produced by the adrenal glands during stress or administered orally or by injection, eosinophils decrease in number.

Basophils: Basophils increase during the healing process. With an increase in steroids, the basophil count will decrease.

Monocytes: Monocytes are the second line of defense against bacterial infections and foreign substances. They are slower to react to infections and inflammatory diseases, but they are stronger than neutrophils and can ingest larger particles of debris.

Lymphocytes: Increased lymphocytes (lymphocytosis) occur in chronic and viral infections. Severe lymphocytosis is commonly caused by chronic lymphocytic leukemia. Lymphocytes play a major role in the immune response system with B lymphocytes and T lymphocytes.

Purpose

- To differentiate between the various types of WBCs for diagnosing health problems (see Description)

Clinical Problems

Decreased Level

Neutrophils: Viral diseases, leukemias, agranulocytosis, aplastic and iron deficiency anemias

Eosinophils: Stress (burns, shock), adrenocortical hyperfunction

Basophils: Stress, hypersensitivity reaction, pregnancy

Monocytes: Lymphocytic leukemia, aplastic anemia

Lymphocytes: Cancer, leukemia, adrenocortical hyperfunction, agranulocytosis, aplastic anemia, multiple sclerosis, renal failure, nephrotic syndrome, SLE

Increased Level

Neutrophils: Acute infections, inflammatory diseases, tissue damage (AMI), Hodgkin's disease, hemolytic disease of newborns, acute appendicitis, acute pancreatitis

Eosinophils: Allergies; parasitic disease; cancer of bone, ovary, testes, brain; phlebitis and thrombophlebitis

Basophils: Inflammatory process, leukemia, healing stage of infection or inflammation

Monocytes: Viral diseases, parasitic diseases, monocytic leukemia, cancer, collagen diseases

Lymphocytes: Lymphocytic leukemia, viral infections, chronic infections, Hodgkin's disease, multiple myeloma, adrenocortical hypofunction

Procedure
- No food or fluid restriction is required.
- Collect 7 ml of venous blood in a lavender-top tube. Prevent hemolysis.

Factors Affecting Laboratory Results
- Steroids could decrease eosinophil and lymphocyte values.

Nursing Implications
- Check the WBC count and the differential WBC count. Elevated neutrophils may be indicative of an acute infection. Elevated eosinophils may be a sign of allergy. Increased basophils can be caused by the healing process. Increased monocytes occur during infection, and increased lymphocytes occur in chronic or viral infections.
- Assess the client for signs and symptoms of an infection (e.g., elevated temperature, increased pulse rate, edema, redness, and exudate [wound drainage]).
- Assess the client for signs and symptoms of allergies, such as tearing, runny nose, rash, and more severe reactions.
- Assess for signs and symptoms of healing (e.g., ability to increase movement at the injured site, decreased edema, and exudate).

ZINC (PLASMA AND URINE)

Reference Values
Plasma: Adult: 60–150 mcg/dl, 11–23 μmol/l (SI units)
Urine: 150–1,250 mcg/24 h

Description.   Zinc (Zn), a heavy metal, is an element found in the body and is required for body growth and metabolism. Approximately 80% of zinc is in the blood cells. About 30% of the zinc ingested is absorbed from the small intestine. Most of the body's excretion of zinc is in the stool, but a small amount is excreted in the urine.

Zinc is a component of many enzymes, such as carbonic anhydrase, DNA and RNA polymerases, lactic dehydrogenase, and alkaline phosphatase, and it plays an important role in enzyme catalytic reactions. Zinc deficiency is not apparent until it becomes severe, when it is manifested by growth retardation, delayed sexual development, severe dermatitis, alopecia, or poor wound healing. Zinc toxicity is rare but it can be related to workers' inhaling zinc oxide during industry exposure.

Purposes
- To detect a zinc deficiency
- To determine the cause of diarrhea, malnutrition, growth retardation, delayed sexual development, alopecia, and poor healing
- To detect zinc toxicity due to industry exposure (inhaling zinc oxide)

Clinical Problems
Decreased level: Malnutrition, malabsorption, diarrhea, anemia, alcoholism, myocardial infarction, hereditary deficiency, cirrhosis of the liver, chronic renal failure, gallbladder disease
Drugs that decrease zinc levels: Corticosteroids, estrogens, penicillamine, anticancer agents, antimetabolites, cisplatin, diuretics
Increased level: Ingestion of acidic food or beverages from galvanized containers, industrial exposure

Procedure
- No food or fluid restriction is required.
- Collect 3 to 5 ml of venous blood in a metal-free, navy blue–top tube. Avoid hemolysis.
- Send the blood specimen to the laboratory immediately.

Factors Affecting Laboratory Results
- Use of a tube or needle containing metal

Nursing Implications
- Obtain a history of the client's nutritional intake. Zinc is present in many foods. Malnutrition, cirrhosis of the liver, alcoholism, or severe diarrhea contributes to a zinc deficit. Zinc is required for the synthesis of prealbumin.

- Monitor intravenous therapy including total parenteral nutrition (TPN); continuous use can cause a zinc deficit.
- Check the history for anemia. With sickle cell anemia, the zinc level is decreased because abnormal red blood cells cause excess loss of zinc.

Client Teaching

- Instruct the pregnant client that vitamins prescribed should contain zinc. An increase in zinc requirement is needed during pregnancy and for lactation.
- Instruct the client who has poor nutrition to take vitamins. Tell the client to check the label on vitamin containers to determine that zinc is one of the elements.

ZINC PROTOPORPHYRIN (ZPP) (BLOOD)

FREE ERYTHROCYTE PROTOPORPHYRIN (FEP)

Reference Values

Adult and child: 15–77 mcg/dl, 0.24–1.23 µmol/l (SI units). *Average:* less than 35 mcg/dl; less than 0.56 µmol/l (SI units)

Description.   Zinc protoporphyrin (ZPP) is a screening test to check for lead poisoning and iron deficiency. It can be checked by drawing a blood sample or by use of a hematofluorometer using several drops of blood. With iron deficiency, the ZPP level does not become elevated until after a few weeks. After iron therapy, the ZPP level returns to normal in 2 to $2^{1}/_{2}$ months.

The use of the ZPP test for screening for increased blood lead levels has more than doubled within a year. ZPP is an effective indicator of the total body of lead. After exposure to lead ceases, blood lead becomes more normal in several weeks or months. The Centers for Disease Control (Atlanta, GA) is now recommending that children suspected of lead poisoning be checked using the blood lead test.

Purpose

- To screen for lead poisoning or for iron deficiency

Clinical Problems

Increased level: Lead poisoning, iron deficiency, anemia of chronic disease, sickle cell disease, occupational exposure, accelerated erythropoiesis, acute inflammatory processes

Procedure

- No food or fluid restriction is required.
- Collect 3 to 5 ml of venous blood in a green- or lavender-top tube. Avoid hemolysis. A hematofluorometer with a few drops of blood may be used.

Nursing Implications

- Obtain a history from the client or family concerning the child's ingesting paint containing lead. Older houses may still have lead paint, which might be eaten by a child.
- Obtain a history from the adult client concerning excessive lead exposure due to occupational contact. Other possible contact with lead includes eating or drinking from unglazed pottery, drinking "moonshine" whiskey prepared in lead containers, breathing leaded gasoline fumes.
- Compare the blood lead level with the blood ZPP level.
- Observe for signs and symptoms of lead poisoning, such as lead colic (crampy abdominal pain), constipation, occasional bloody diarrhea, behavioral changes (from lethargy to hyperactivity, aggression, impulsiveness), tremors, and confusion.
- Obtain a history of iron deficiency. Check serum iron level and serum ferritin level. Compare the above levels with the ZPP level.
- Check that blood ZPP levels are repeated after 2 months of iron therapy.

TWO

Considerations for Use
of Diagnostic Tests

Millions of diagnostic tests are performed daily throughout the world. These tests monitor client/patient well-being and assist in the diagnosis of specific conditions.

This introductory chapter to diagnostic tests has a twofold purpose. The first is to disseminate essential information related to all diagnostic tests, and the second is to describe the basic organizational format of the individual tests.

General directions common to most diagnostic tests are normal finding(s), description, purpose(s), clinical problems, procedure, factors affecting diagnostic results, and nursing implications with client teaching. Only facts specific to a given test are given.

Normal Finding(s). Normal size, structure, and function of the organ under examination are stated.

Description. Information about the test is briefly described.

Purpose(s). The purpose(s) is/are given for each diagnostic test.

Clinical Problems. This covers either disease entities or conditions that are associated with abnormal findings or indications for the test.

Procedure.   The procedure usually differs among tests; however, common procedures for most tests are:

1. A signed consent form.
2. Food and fluid restriction.
3. Institutional policies that must be followed.

Factors Affecting Diagnostic Results.   Various factors that could affect test results should be identified. Drugs that affect test results are given in Clinical Problems; therefore, they are not repeated here.

Nursing Implications
1. Be knowledgeable about test.
2. Provide time and be available to answer questions. Be supportive of client and family.
3. Obtain history of allergies to iodine, seafood. Observe for severe allergic reaction to contrast dye.
4. Obtain baseline vital signs. Monitor vital signs as indicated following test.
5. Have client void before test.
6. If sedative is used, instruct client not to drive home.

Client Teaching
7. Explain test procedure to the client or family, or both.
8. Provide teaching related to care of health problem.

List of Diagnostic Tests

DIAGNOSTIC TESTS

AMNIOTIC FLUID ANALYSIS

Normal Findings.   Clear amniotic fluid; no chromosomal or neural tube abnormalities

Description.   Amniotic analysis is useful for detecting chromosomal abnormalities (Down syndrome, trisomy 21), neural tube defects (spina bifida), sex-linked disorders (hemophilia), and for determining fetal maturity. The amniotic fluid is obtained by amniocentesis, performed during the 14th to the 16th weeks of pregnancy, for chromosomal and neural tube defects.

Amnioscopy: Insertion of a fiberoptic, lighted instrument (amnioscope) into the cervical canal to visualize the amniotic fluid. Because of possible infection, the test is rarely performed.

Purposes
- To detect chromosomal abnormalities, neural tube defects, and sex-linked disorders
- To determine fetal maturity

Clinical Problems
Abnormal findings: Chromosomal disorders, neural tube defects (alpha-fetoprotein), hemolytic disease due to Rh incompatibility, X-linked disorders, fetal maturity, fetal stress (meconium), pulmonary maturity of fetus (L/S ratio)

Procedure
- Obtain a signed consent form.
- No food or fluid is restricted.
- Have client void prior to procedure to prevent puncturing the bladder and aspirating urine.
- Cleanse suprapubic area with an antiseptic. A local anesthetic is injected at needle site for the amniocentesis.

- The placenta and fetus are located by ultrasound or manually (fetus only).
- Aspirate 5 to 15 ml of amniotic fluid. Apply dressing to needle insertion site.

Foam stability test: This test determines if surfactant from mature fetal lungs is present in the amniotic fluid. When the test tube of amniotic fluid is shaken, bubbles appear around the surface if adequate amounts of surfactant are present.

Nursing Implications
- Obtain a signed consent form.
- Have the client void before the test.

Client Teaching
- Explain that the test screens only for specific abnormalities.
- Inform the client that normal results do not guarantee a normal infant. The health care provider should tell the woman of potential risks, such as premature labor, spontaneous abortion, infection, and fetal or placental bleeding. Complications are rare.
- Inform the client that the test takes about 30 min.
- Be supportive. Be a good listener.

Post-test
- Encourage the family to seek genetic counseling if chromosomal abnormality has been determined.
- Instruct the client to notify the health care provider immediately of any of the following: bleeding or leaking fluid from the vagina, abdominal pain or cramping, chills and fever, or lack of fetal movement.

ANGIOGRAPHY (ANGIOGRAM)

ARTERIOGRAPHY: CARDIAC (SEE CARDIAC CATHETERIZATION), CEREBRAL ANGIOGRAPHY, PULMONARY ANGIOGRAPHY, AND RENAL ANGIOGRAPHY

Normal Findings.   Normal structure and patency of blood vessels

Description.   The terms angiography (examination of the blood vessels) and arteriography (examination of the arteries) are used interchangeably. A catheter is inserted into the femoral or brachial artery, and a contrast dye is injected to allow visualization of the blood vessels. Angiographies are useful for evaluating patency of blood vessels and for identifying abnormal vascularization resulting from tumors. This test may be indicated when CT or radionuclide scanning suggests vascular abnormalities.

The new contrast medium has a low osmolality; examples include iopamidol, iohexol, and ioxaglate. The older media were hyperosmolar with a high content of iodine.

Cerebral angiography: The injected dye outlines the carotid and vertebral arteries, large blood vessels of the circle of Willis, and small cerebral arterial branches.

Pulmonary angiography: The catheter inserted in the brachial or femoral artery is threaded into the pulmonary artery, and dye is injected for visualizing pulmonary vessels. During the test, the client should be monitored for cardiac dysrhythmias.

Renal angiography: This test permits visualization of the renal vessels and the parenchyma. An aortogram may be performed with renal angiography to detect any vessel abnormality in the aorta and to show the relationship of the renal arteries to the aorta.

Clinical Problems/Purposes

Type of Angiography	*Indications/Purposes*
Cerebral	To detect cerebrovascular aneurysm; cerebral thrombosis; hematomas; tumors from increased vascularization; cerebral plaques or spasm; cerebral fistula
	To evaluate cerebral blood flow; cause of increased intracranial pressure
Pulmonary	To detect pulmonary emboli; tumors; aneurysms; congenital defects; vascular changes associated with emphysema, blebs, and bullae; heart abnormality
	To evaluate pulmonary circulation
Renal	To detect renal artery stenosis; renal thrombus or embolus; space-occupying lesions (that is, tumor, cyst, aneurysm)
	To determine the causative factor of hypertension; cause of renal failure
	To evaluate renal circulation

Procedure
All Angiographies
- Obtain a signed consent form.
- Restrict food and fluids for 8 to 12 h. Anticoagulants (e.g., heparin) are discontinued.
- Record vital signs. Void before test.
- Remove dentures and metallic objects before the test.
- If the client has a history of severe allergic reactions to various substances or drugs, steroids or antihistamines may be given before and after the procedure as a prophylactic measure.
- A sedative or narcotic analgesic, if ordered, is administered 1 h before the test.
- IV fluids may be started before the procedure so that emergency drugs, if needed, can be administered.
- Client is in supine position on an X-ray table. A local anesthetic is administered to the injection/incisional site.
- The test takes 1 to 2 h.

Renal: A laxative or cleansing enema is usually ordered the evening before the test.

Pulmonary: ECG/EKG electrodes are attached to the chest for cardiac monitoring during angiography. Pulmonary pressures are recorded, and blood samples are obtained before the contrast dye is injected.

Factors Affecting Diagnostic Results
- Feces, gas, and barium sulfate can interfere with test results.

Nursing Implications
Pre-test
- Obtain a history of hypersensitivity to iodine, seafood, or contrast dye from other X-ray procedure (e.g., intravenous pyelogram [IVP]).
- Record baseline vital signs.

Client Teaching
- Explain the purpose and procedure of the angiography.
- Inform the client that when the dye is injected there could be a warm, flushed sensation lasting a minute or two. Client must remain still so that the pictures are clear.

- Explain that the test should not cause pain, but there may be moments of discomfort.

Test

- Monitor vital signs.
- Assess for vasovagal reaction (common complication; i.e., decreased pulse rate and blood pressure, cold and clammy). Give IV fluids and atropine IV. This reaction lasts about 15 to 20 min.

Post-test

- Apply pressure on the injection site for 5 to 10 min or longer until bleeding has stopped.
- Monitor vital signs as ordered.
- Enforce bedrest for 12 to 24 h or as ordered. Activities should be restricted for a day.
- Check peripheral pulses in the extremities (i.e., dorsalis pedis, femoral, and radial).
- Check injection site for bleeding.
- Apply cold compresses or an ice pack to the injection site for edema or pain if ordered.
- Monitor ECG tracings, urine output, and IV fluids.
- Inform client that coughing is a common occurrence following a pulmonary angiography.
- Assess for weakness or numbness in an extremity, confusion, or slurred speech following a cerebral angiography. These could be symptoms of transient ischemic attack (TIA).
- Observe for a delayed allergic reaction to the contrast dye (e.g., tachycardia, dyspnea, skin rash, urticaria, decreased BP, and decreased urine output).
- Be supportive of client and family.

ARTHROGRAPHY

Normal Findings
Knee: Normal medial meniscus
Shoulder: Bicipital tendon sheath, normal joint capsule, and intact subscapular bursa

Description.   Arthrography is an X-ray examination of a joint using air or contrast media, or both, in the joint space. It can visualize abnormal joint capsule and tears to the cartilage or ligaments. This procedure is performed when clients complain of persistent knee or shoulder pain or discomfort. It is usually performed on an outpatient basis.

Arthrography is not indicated if the client is having an acute arthritic attack, has a joint infection, or is pregnant. This procedure is usually performed prior to an arthroscopy.

Purposes
- To visualize the structures of the joint capsule
- To detect abnormalities of the cartilage and/or ligaments (tears)

Clinical Problems
Abnormal findings: Osteochondritis dissecans, osteochondral fractures, cartilage and synovial abnormalities, tears of the ligaments, and joint capsule abnormalities. *Shoulder:* adhesive capsulitis, tears of rotator cuff, bicipital tenosynovitis or tears

Procedure
- No food or fluid restriction is required.
- Prepare the knee or shoulder area using aseptic technique.
- Local anesthetic is administered to puncture site.
- A needle is inserted into the joint space (e.g., knee), and synovial fluid is aspirated for synovial fluid analysis.
- Air and/or contrast medium is injected into the joint space, and X-rays are taken.
- The knee may be bandaged.

Nursing Implications
- Obtain a history of type of pain to knee and shoulder, and possible allergies to seafood, iodine, or contrast dye.
- Check vital signs.

Client Teaching
- Explain the procedure to the client (see Procedure).
- Inform the client that changes in body positions may be requested during the procedure. At other times, the client is to remain still. The client will not be asleep.

Post-test
- Apply an Ace bandage to the leg, including the knee, if indicated, to decrease swelling and pain.

Client Teaching
- Instruct the client to rest the joint for a specified time, usually 12 h.
- Inform the client that a crepitant noise may be heard with joint movement; if it persists, the surgeon should be notified.
- Instruct the client to apply an ice bag with a cover to the affected joint to decrease swelling. An analgesic for pain/discomfort may be ordered.

ARTHROSCOPY

Normal Findings.   Normal lining of the synovial membrane; ligaments and tendons intact

Description.   Arthroscopy is an endoscopic examination of the interior aspect of a joint, usually the knee, using a fiber-optic endoscope. Normally, *arthrography* (X-ray examination of a joint using air or contrast media, or both, in the joint space) is performed prior to arthroscopy.

Arthroscopy is used to perform joint surgery and diagnose meniscal, patellar, extrasynovial, and synovial diseases. Frequently, biopsy or surgery is performed during the test procedure. Arthroscopy is contraindicated if a wound or severe skin infection is present.

Purposes
- To diagnose meniscal, patellar, extrasynovial, and synovial diseases
- To perform joint surgery

Clinical Problems

Abnormal findings: Meniscal disease with torn lateral or medial meniscus, patellar disease, chondromalacia, patellar fracture, osteochondritis
dissecans, osteochondromatosis, torn ligaments, Baker's cysts, synovitis,
and rheumatoid and degenerative arthritis

Procedure

- Obtain a signed consent form.
- No food or fluid is restricted for local anesthetic; NPO after midnight with spinal and general anesthesia.
- The arthroscope is inserted into the interior joint for visualization,
  draining fluid from the joint, biopsy, and/or surgery.
- Ace bandage or tourniquet may be applied above the joint to
  decrease blood volume in the leg.

Nursing Implications

- Assess the involved area for possible skin lesion or infection.
- Determine the client's anxiety level, and be available to answer
  questions. Be prepared to repeat information if the level of anxiety
  or fear is determined to be high.

Post-test

- Assess client before, during, and after procedure, including vital
  signs, bleeding, swelling, etc.
- Apply ice to the area as indicated.
- Administer analgesic for pain or discomfort as ordered.

Client Teaching

- Instruct client to avoid excessive use of joint for 2 to 3 days or
  as ordered. Limited walking is usually permitted soon after the
  procedure.

BARIUM ENEMA

LOWER GASTROINTESTINAL (COLON) TEST

Normal Findings.   Normal filling, normal structure of the large colon

Description.   The barium enema is an X-ray examination of the large intestine. Barium sulfate (single contrast) or barium sulfate and air (double contrast) is administered slowly through a rectal tube. The filling process is monitored by fluoroscopy, and then X-rays are taken. The colon must be free of fecal material so that the barium will outline the large intestine to detect any disorders. The double-contrast technique (barium and air) is useful for identifying polyps.

The test can be performed in a hospital, clinic, or at a private health facility.

Purpose
* To detect disorders of the large intestine

Clinical Problems
Abnormal findings: Tumor in the colon; inflammatory disease: ulcerative colitis, granulomatous colitis, diverticulitis; diverticula; fistulas; polyps; intussusception

Procedure.   Abdominal X-rays, ultrasound studies, radionuclide scans, upper gastrointestinal (GI) series, and proctosigmoidoscopy should be done before the barium enema. It is important that the colon is fecal free.

Pre-preparation
* A clear liquid diet for 18 to 24 h before the test (broth, ginger ale, cola, black coffee or tea with sugar only, gelatin, and syrup from canned fruit). Some institutions permit a white chicken sandwich (no butter, lettuce, or mayonnaise) or hard-boiled eggs and gelatin for lunch and dinner; then NPO after dinner.
* Encourage the client to increase water or clear liquid intake 24 h before the test to maintain adequate hydration.
* Prescribe laxatives (castor oil or magnesium citrate), which should be taken the day before the test in the late afternoon or early evening (4 PM to 8 PM).
* A cleansing enema or laxative suppository such as bisacodyl (Dulcolax) may be ordered the evening before the test.

- Saline enemas should be given early in the morning (6 AM) until returns are clear (maximum of three enemas). Some private laboratories have clients use laxative suppositories instead of enemas in the morning.
- Black coffee or tea is permitted 1 h before the test. Some institutions permit dry toast.

Post-preparation

- The client should expel the barium in the bathroom or bedpan immediately after the test.
- Fluid intake should be increased for hydration and to prevent constipation due to retained barium.
- A laxative such as milk of magnesia or magnesium citrate or an enema should be given to get the barium out of the colon. A laxative may need to be repeated on the next day.

Factors Affecting Diagnostic Results

- Inadequate bowel preparation with fecal material remaining in the colon

Nursing Implications

- List the procedure step by step for the client. Most private laboratories have written preparation slips.
- Notify the health care provider if the client has severe abdominal cramps and pain prior to the test. Barium enema should not be performed if the client has severe ulcerative colitis, suspected perforation, or tachycardia.
- Administer a laxative or cleansing enema after the test. Instruct the client to check the color of the stools for 2 to 3 days. Stools may be light in color because of the barium sulfate. Absence of stool should be reported.

Client Teaching

- Emphasize the importance of dietary restrictions and bowel preparation. Adequate preparation is essential, or the test may need to be repeated.

- Explain that he or she will be lying on an X-ray table.
- Inform the client that the test takes approximately 0.5 to 1 h. Tell the client to take deep breaths through the mouth, which helps to decrease tension and promote relaxation.

BIOPSY (BONE MARROW, BREAST, ENDOMETRIUM, KIDNEY, LIVER)

Normal Finding.   Normal cells and tissue from the bone marrow, breast, endometrium of the uterus, kidney, and liver

Description.   Biopsy is the removal and examination of tissue from the body. Usually biopsies are performed to detect malignancy or to identify the presence of a disease process. Biopsies can be obtained by (1) aspiration by applying suction, (2) the brush method, using stiff bristles that scrape fragments of cells and tissue, (3) excision by surgical cutting at tissue site, (4) fine-needle aspiration at tissue site with or without the guidance of ultrasound, (5) insertion of a needle through the skin, and (6) punch biopsy, using a punch-type instrument.

Bone marrow: The bone marrow is composed of red and yellow marrow. The red marrow produces blood cells and the yellow marrow has fat cells and connective tissue. The sternum and iliac crest are the most common sites for bone marrow aspiration.

Breast: Biopsy of the breast is mainly performed to determine if a breast lesion (nodule or mass) is a cyst, benign, or cancerous. The majority of breast lumps are benign. The site of the breast lesion can be identified with the use of a fixed grid on the mammogram.

Endometrium of the uterus: Endometrial biopsy can detect polyps, cancer, inflammatory condition, and defect in ovulation. The biopsy collection using a probe (blind technique) can be performed in the health care provider's office. Complications include perforation of the uterus, excessive bleeding, and aborting an early pregnancy. This procedure should not be performed if there is purulent discharge from the vagina. An endometrial biopsy differs from a D & C (dilation and curettage) in that dilation of the cervix is not needed. D & C requires general anesthesia because the entire endometrium is curettaged. With an endometrial biopsy, the affected tissue in the uterus could be missed with a sample biopsy, while with the D & C the total endometrium is obtained.

Kidney (renal):   A kidney biopsy is usually done with the guidance of ultrasound or fluoroscopy. The biopsy is performed to determine the cause of renal disease, to rule out metastatic malignancy of the kidney, or to determine if rejection of a kidney transplant is occurring. The biopsy can be obtained in three ways: (1) by use of a cystoscope, (2) by excision of the kidney, taking a wedge of issue, and (3) percutaneously, using a needle.

Liver: Liver biopsy is not usually done unless the liver enzymes are greatly increased. It is performed to rule out metastatic malignancy or to detect a cyst or the presence of cirrhosis. Ultrasound is used to guide the biopsy needle to the pathologic site. Prior to a liver biopsy, the following laboratory levels should be checked: prothrombin time (PT), partial thromboplastin time (PTT), and platelet count. The liver is vascular, and if these laboratory results are abnormal, bleeding could occur following the test procedure.

Purposes
- To identify abnormal tissue from various body sites
- To detect the presence of a disease process

Clinical Problems
Indications: Blood disorders, malignancies, cysts, polyps, infectious process, progressive disease entities (cirrhosis, nephrosis, lupus nephritis), ovulative defects, rejection of an organ transplant

Procedure
- A consent form should be signed.
- Baseline vital signs are taken.
- Biopsy site is anesthetized.

Bone Marrow
- A local anesthetic is injected at site (sternum or iliac spine).
- A needle with a stylet is inserted through a skin slit into the bone about 3 mm deep.

- The stylet is removed, and a 10 ml syringe is attached to the needle. Bone marrow is aspirated; part is used for a blood smear, and the remaining amount is placed in a green- or lavender-top tube.

Breast

- Needle aspiration or an excision of breast tissue can be performed.
- The skin is anesthetized; general anesthesia may be used if biopsy tissue is difficult to obtain.
- A mammogram or ultrasound is usually needed to determine the placement of needle or the excision site.
- Tissue obtained from biopsy is placed in formalin and sent immediately to the laboratory. The specimen from a needle aspiration is placed on cytologic slide.

Endometrium of the Uterus

- The client is placed in the lithotomy position.
- A sound (probe) is inserted into the cavity of the uterus to determine its size. This is done as a precaution to prevent perforation of the uterus.
- A suction tube with curette is inserted into the cavity of the uterus, and sample specimens are obtained from the lateral, anterior, and/or posterior uterine wall.
- Specimen(s) is/are placed in formalin solution and sent to the laboratory for histologic testing.

Kidney (Renal).   This test can be performed by use of a cystoscope with the brush method, excision of a wedge of renal tissue, or percutaneously with a special needle.

- The client is placed in the prone position.
- With the percutaneous method, the site is determined with the use of ultrasound or fluoroscopy.
- Anesthetic is given according to the procedure chosen.
- With needle insertion, the client is asked to take a breath and hold it. A small tissue specimen is obtained. Pressure is applied to the site for approximately 20 min to prevent bleeding because the kidney tissue is very vascular.

Liver

- NPO for at least 6 h prior to the test. The liver is less congested without food intake.
- Check that PT, INR, PTT, and platelet count have been done and documented. Abnormal findings should be reported prior to procedure to decrease/avoid excessive bleeding following the biopsy.
- A fine needle is inserted, usually with the guidance of ultrasound.
- The client is asked first to take a deep breath, then to exhale and hold breath. With expiration, the diaphragm is motionless and remains high in the thorax.
- Apply a pressure dressing.
- The tissue specimen is placed in formalin solution, or the specimen is swabbed on a slide and fixed in 95% alcohol.
- Place the client on his or her right side to decrease the chance of hemorrhage.

Factors Affecting Diagnostic Results

- Blind biopsy can result in missing the diseased tissue.
- Improper care of the tissue specimen

Nursing Implications

- Check that the consent form has been signed.
- Check that the prescribed laboratory tests have been done.
- Monitor vital signs as prescribed (i.e., every 15 min for the first hour, every 30 min for the second hour, and then hourly).
- Observe for bleeding and shortness of breath.
- Report absence or decreased bowel sounds following renal or liver biopsy test.

Client Teaching

- Explain the biopsy procedure to the client.
- Instruct the client to report excessive bleeding immediately to the health care provider.
- Instruct the client to report an elevated temperature.
- Instruct the client to take the prescribed pain medication as needed.
- Advise the client to rest for 24 h following the test procedure.

- Instruct the client to avoid heavy lifting for at least 24 h, or longer if indicated (i.e., following liver and renal biopsies).

Kidney
- Increase fluid intake following the biopsy.
- Check bowel sounds for several hours following the test. Abdominal intervention can cause a decrease in bowel sounds (decreased peristalsis).
- Instruct the client to report decreased urination or burning when urinating.

Liver
- Avoid heavy lifting.

BONE DENSITOMETRY

BONE DENSITY (BD), BONE MINERAL DENSITY (BMD), BONE ABSORPTIOMETRY

Normal Finding.   Normal bone densitometry scan is determined according to the client's age, sex, and height.

Normal: 1 standard deviation below peak bone mass level

Osteoporosis: Greater than 2.5 standard deviations below peak bone mass level (WHO standard)

Description.   Bones are made up of minerals and protein. Bone mass peaks in people during their mid-30s. After then, bone is lost at a greater rate than new bone is made. When a woman reaches menopause, bone loss accelerates to about 1% to 3% a year. After age 60, bone loss in women slows, but it does not stop; as she gets older, bone mass loss could be between 35% and 50%. The risk of bone fracture is greater in women than men. Men lose bone also; however, it is at a lower rate than women; 3% to 5% a decade. Usually, men develop osteoporosis about a decade later than women.

A bone density test is done to detect early osteoporosis by determining the density of bone mineral content. Clients who have a loss of bone mineral are readily prone to fractures. The bones that are usually examined are the lumbar spine and the proximal hip (neck of the femur). Another bone site, the heel bone, can be evaluated according to the client's symptoms.

The dual energy X-ray absorptiometry (DEXA) measures bone mineral density and exposes the client to only a minimal amount of radiation. Images from the detector/camera are computer analyzed to determine the bone mineral content. The computer can calculate the size and thickness of the bone.

Purposes
- To evaluate the bone mineral density
- To identify early and progressive osteoporosis

Clinical Problems
Abnormal findings: Loss of bone mineral content, early and progressive osteoporosis

Procedure
- A signed consent form may be required.
- No food or fluid restriction is required.
- Client is to remove all metal objects at the area to be scanned (e.g., keys, coins, zippers, belts).
- The client lies on an imaging table with a radiation source below and the detector above, which measures the bone's radiation absorption.
- The bone density test takes approximately 30 to 60 min.

Factors Affecting Diagnostic Results
- Metallic objects in the bone scanning site
- Previous fractures of the bone may increase the bone density.

Nursing Implications
- Obtain family history of osteoporosis and client's skeletal problems, such as loss of height, fractures, and others.

Client Teaching
- Explain the procedure for bone density test.
- Inform the client that the test should not cause pain and that the radiation is considered minimal.

- Instruct the client to remove all metal objects that would be within the scanning area.
- Tell the client that the test should take approximately 30 to 60 min.

BRONCHOGRAPHY (BRONCHOGRAM)

Normal Finding.   Normal tracheobronchial structure

Description.   Bronchography is an X-ray test to visualize the trachea, bronchi, and the entire bronchial tree after a radiopaque iodine contrast liquid is injected through a catheter into the tracheobronchial space. The bronchi are coated with the contrast dye, and a series of X-rays is then taken. Bronchography may be done in conjunction with bronchoscopy.

Bronchography is contraindicated during pregnancy. This test should not be done if the client is hypersensitive to anesthetics, iodine, or X-ray dyes.

Purpose
- To detect bronchial obstruction, such as foreign bodies, tumors, and the like

Clinical Problems.   Foreign bodies in the bronchial tubes, tumors, cysts, bronchiectasis

Procedure
- Obtain a signed consent form.
- Restrict foods and fluids for 6 to 8 h before the test.
- Oral hygiene should be given the night before the test and in the morning to lessen the number of bacteria introduced into the lung.
- Postural drainage may be performed for 3 days before the test.
- A sedative and atropine are usually given 1 h before the test.
- A topical anesthetic is sprayed into the pharynx and trachea. A catheter is passed through the nose into the trachea, and a local anesthetic and iodized contrast liquid are injected through the catheter.

- The client is usually asked to change body positions so that the contrast dye can reach most areas of the bronchial tree.
- After bronchography, the client may receive nebulization and should perform postural drainage to remove contrast dye. Food and fluids are restricted until the gag (cough) reflex is present.

Factors Affecting Diagnostic Results
- Secretions in the tracheobronchial tree can prevent the contrast dye from coating the bronchial walls.

Nursing Implications
- Obtain a signed consent form.
- Obtain a history of hypersensitivity to anesthetics, iodine, and X-ray dyes.
- Record vital signs.
- Answer client's questions and concerns or refer to other health professionals, if necessary. Reassure the client that the airway will not be blocked. Inform the client that he or she may have a sore throat after the test.

Client Teaching
- Explain the procedure of the test (see Procedure).
- Encourage the client to practice good oral hygiene the night before and the morning of the test. Dentures should be removed before the test.

Post-test
- Assess for signs and symptoms of laryngeal edema (e.g., dyspnea, hoarseness, apprehension).
- Monitor vital signs. The temperature may be slightly elevated for 1 to 2 days after the test.
- Assess for allergic reaction to the anesthetic and iodized contrast dye (i.e., apprehension, flushing, rash, urticaria, dyspnea, tachycardia, and/or hypotension).
- Check the gag reflex before offering fluids and food.
- Check breath signs. Report abnormal findings.
- Have the client perform postural drainage for removal of contrast dye.

- Offer throat lozenges or an ordered medication for sore throat.
- Be supportive of the client and family.

BRONCHOSCOPY

Normal Finding.   Normal structure and lining of the bronchi

Description.   Bronchoscopy is the direct inspection of the larynx, trachea, and bronchi through a standard metal bronchoscope or a flexible fiberoptic bronchoscope called bronchofibroscope (preferred instrument). Through the bronchoscope, a catheter brush or biopsy forceps can be passed to obtain secretions and tissues for cytologic examination. The two main purposes of bronchoscopy are visualization and specimen collection.

Purposes
- To inspect the larynx, trachea, and bronchus for lesions
- To remove foreign bodies and secretions from the tracheobronchial area
- To improve tracheobronchial drainage

Clinical Problems
Abnormal findings: Tracheobronchial lesion (tumor), bleeding site, foreign bodies, mucous plugs

Procedure
- Obtain a signed consent form.
- Restrict food and fluids for 6 h before the bronchoscopy, preferably for 8 to 12 h.
- Dentures, contact lenses, and jewelry should be removed.
- Obtain a history of hypersensitivity to analgesics, anesthetics, and antibiotics.
- Check vital signs and record.
- Administer premedications.

- The client will be lying on a table in the supine or semi-Fowler's position with head hyperextended or will be seated in a chair. The throat will be sprayed with a local anesthetic. The bronchoscope can be inserted through the nose or mouth.
- Specimen containers should be labeled, and specimens should be taken immediately to the laboratory.
- The procedure takes about 1 h.

Nursing Implications
Pre-test
- Obtain vital signs and record.

Client Teaching
- Instruct the client to relax before and during the test. Instruct the client to practice breathing in and out through the nose with the mouth opened; this breathing will be used during the insertion of the bronchoscope.
- Inform the client that there may be hoarseness or sore throat after the test.
- Encourage the client to ask questions, and give client time to express concerns.
- Tell the client the test takes about 1 h.

Post-test
- Recognize the complications that can follow bronchoscopy (i.e., laryngeal edema, bronchospasm, pneumothorax, cardiac dysrhythmias, and bleeding).
- Check blood pressure frequently as prescribed until stable.
- Assess for signs and symptoms of respiratory difficulty (i.e., dyspnea, sneezing, apprehension, and decreased breath sounds).
- Check for hemoptysis. Inform client that blood-tinged mucus is not necessarily abnormal.
- Assess the gag reflex before giving food and liquids.
- Offer lozenges or prescribed medication for mild throat irritation after gag reflex is present.

Client Teaching
- Instruct client not to smoke for 6 to 8 h. Smoking may cause coughing and start bleeding, especially after a biopsy.
- Be supportive of client and family. Answer questions.

CARDIAC CATHETERIZATION*

CARDIAC ANGIOGRAPHY (ANGIOCARDIOGRAPHY), CORONARY ARTERIOGRAPHY

Normal Findings. Patency of coronary arteries; normal heart size, structure, valves; normal heart and pulmonary pressures, normal left ventricular function, wall motion abnormalities

Description. Cardiac catheterization is a procedure in which a long catheter is inserted in femoral vein or artery of the arm or leg. This catheter is threaded to the heart chambers or coronary arteries, or both, with the guidance of fluoroscopy. Contrast dye is injected for visualizing the heart structures. During injection of the dye, cineangiography is used for filming heart activity. The terms *angiocardiography* and *coronary arteriography* are used interchangeably with the term *cardiac catheterization*; however, with coronary arteriography, dye is injected directly into the coronary arteries, and with angiocardiography, dye is injected into the heart, coronary, and/or pulmonary vessels.

The frequency of complications arising from cardiac catheterizations is less than 2%. Complications that can occur, though rare, are myocardial infarction, cardiac dysrhythmias, cardiac tamponade, pulmonary embolism, and CVA and dissection of the coronary arteries. Other rare complications include renal failure, anaphylactic reaction to contrast dye, blood clot at catheter site requiring an anticoagulation drug, or significant inguinal bleeding near insertion site causing retroperitoneal hematomas.

---

*Updated by Dr. Rani Beharry, MD, Christiana Care Cardiology, Newark, Delaware.

With *right cardiac catheterization,* the catheter is inserted into the femoral vein or an antecubital vein and is threaded through the inferior vena cava into the right atrium to the pulmonary artery. Right atrium, right ventricle, and pulmonary artery pressures are measured, and blood samples from the right side of the heart can be obtained. While the dye is being injected, the functions of the tricuspid and pulmonary valves can be observed.

For *left cardiac catheterization,* the catheter is inserted into the brachial or femoral artery and is advanced retrograde through the aorta to the coronary arteries and/or left ventricle. Dye is injected. The patency of the coronary arteries and/or functions of the aortic and mitral valves and the left ventricle can be observed. This procedure is indicated before heart surgery.

Purposes

- To identify coronary artery disease (CAD)
- To determine cardiac valvular disease
- To determine pressure in pulmonary vessels or heart chambers
- To obtain a biopsy of myocardium
- To evaluate artificial valves
- To angioplasty or stent an area of CAD
- To determine left ventricular injection fraction

Clinical Problems

Abnormal findings: *Right-sided cardiac catheterization:* tricuspid stenosis, pulmonary stenosis, pulmonary hypertension, septal defects; *left-sided cardiac catheterization:* coronary artery disease (partial or complete coronary occlusion), mitral stenosis, mitral regurgitation, aortic regurgitation, left ventricular hypertrophy, ventricular aneurysm, septal defect

Procedure

- Obtain a signed consent form. Check that the health care provider has discussed possible risk factors before the consent form is signed.
- No food or fluid is allowed for 6 to 8 h before the test.

- Antihistamines (e.g., Benadryl) and/or steroids may be ordered the evening before and the morning of the test if an allergic reaction is suspected.
- Medications are restricted for 6 to 8 h before the test unless otherwise ordered by the health care provider. Oral anticoagulants are discontinued, or the dosage is reduced to prevent excessive bleeding. Heparin may be ordered to prevent thrombi.
- The weight and height of the client should be recorded. These are used to calculate the amount of dye needed, such as 1 ml/kg of body weight.
- Record baseline VS. Note the volume intensity of pulses. VS should be monitored during the test.
- Premedications may be given 0.5 to 1 h before the cardiac catheterization.
- Client voids before taking premedications (sedative, tranquilizer, analgesic).
- A 5% D_5W infusion is started at a keep-vein-open (KVO) rate for administering emergency drugs, if needed. Occasionally, higher rate IVF NSS or $1/2$ NSS is administered prior to and during catheterization to prevent renal failure from contrast dye.
- The client is positioned on a padded table that tilts. Skin anesthetic is given at the site of catheter insertion. Client lies still during insertion of the catheter and filming.
- ECG leads are applied to the chest to monitor heart activity.
- Vital signs and heart rhythm are monitored during the procedure.
- Coughing and deep breathing are frequently requested. Coughing can decrease nausea and dizziness and possible dysrhythmia.
- The procedure takes 0.5 to 3 h.

Factors Affecting Diagnostic Results
- Insufficient amount of contrast dye could affect results.
- Movement by the client could cause complications and interfere with the filming.
- Premature cessation of catheterization due to complications, for example, anaphylaxis, coronary vasospasm, coronary artery dissection.

Nursing Implications
Pre-test

- Explain to the client that the purpose of the test is to check the coronary arteries for blockage, to check for heart valve defects, to obtain a biopsy of heart tissue, and/or to measure pressures in the pulmonary vessels, and heart chambers. This test is often done before heart surgery to determine if bypass or valvular surgery is necessary.
- Explain the procedure to the client. The cardiologist or cardiac surgeon should explain the purpose, risks, and benefits of the catheterization.
- Obtain a client history of allergic reactions to seafood, iodine, or iodine contrast dye used in other X-ray tests (e.g., pyelography). A skin test may be performed to determine the severity of the allergy. An antihistamine (e.g., diphenhydramine [Benadryl]) and steroids may be given the day before and/or the day of the test as a prophylactic measure.
- Assess the client with renal insufficiency. Premedication with acetylcysteine and/or sodium bicarbonate IV may be administered for renal protection from contrast dye, 24 h before and after the procedure.
- Record baseline VS, and continuously monitor the VS during procedure.
- Check that the catheter insertion site has been prepped (shaved and cleansed with an antiseptic).
- Administer premedication, if prescribed, $^1/_2$ to 1 h before the test.
- Give time for client to express feelings of concern.

Client Teaching

- Inform client that a hot, flushing sensation may be felt for a minute or two when the dye is injected. Explain that clacking noises may be heard as the film advances.
- Inform the client that there may be minimal discomfort at the catheter insertion site and from lying on the back. Tell the client to inform the health care provider of any chest pain or difficulty in breathing during the procedure.

Post-test
- Monitor vital signs every 15 min for the first hour and then every 30 min until stable.
- Watch for cardiac rhythm and rate disturbances.
- Assess patient for complaints of chest heaviness, shortness of breath, and abdominal or groin pains.
- Observe catheter insertion site for bleeding or hematoma. Change dressings as needed.
- Check peripheral pulses below the insertion site.
- Take ECG or check heart monitor.
- Administer analgesics as ordered for discomfort. Give antibiotics if ordered.

Client Teaching
- Instruct the client that he/she is to remain on bed rest for 2 to 4 h. This largely depends on the type of closure device used. The client can turn from side to side, and the bed may be elevated 30 degrees. The leg should be extended if the femoral artery was used. If the brachial artery was used, the head of the bed can be slightly elevated; however, the arm should be immobilized for 3 h. Policy concerning positioning may differ among institutions. Some clients may be discharged the same day, depending on plans for further intervention and complications.
- Encourage fluid intake unless contraindicated (e.g., heart failure).

CERVICOGRAPHY (CERVIGRAM)

Normal Finding.   Normal cervical tissue; no abnormal cells found

Description.   Cervicography is a photographic method to record an image of the cervix. This test may be done in conjunction with a Pap smear, colposcopy, and/or routine gynecologic examination. The Pap smear detects cellular changes, whereas the cervicography is a more sensitive means for detecting cervical cancer. It can identify some cancerous lesions that were missed by the Pap smear.

Purpose
- To detect cervical cancer

Clinical Problems
Abnormal findings: Cancer of the cervix, invasive cervical cancer

Procedure
- A consent form should be signed.
- No food or fluid restriction is required.
- The client is placed in the lithotomy position.
- Acetic acid (5%) is swabbed on the cervical area.
- Pathographs are taken of the cervix.
- Aqueous iodine is then swabbed on the cervix; photos follow.
- An endocervical smear is taken; tissue obtained is applied to a slide(s).

Factors Affecting Diagnostic Results
- Cervical mucus that was not removed from the cervix before applying acetic acid and the photography.

Nursing Implications
- Obtain a signed consent form.
- Obtain a history of any gynecologic health problems (e.g., discharge, abnormal bleeding).

Client Teaching
- Explain the procedure to the client.
- Inform the client that she may experience a brown vaginal discharge following the procedure for a few days. This could be due to the iodine swabbed on the cervix.
- Instruct the client to inform the health care provider if great discomfort or heavy discharge occurs.

CHOLANGIOGRAPHY (IV), PERCUTANEOUS CHOLANGIOGRAPHY, T-TUBE CHOLANGIOGRAPHY

Normal Findings. Patent biliary ducts; no stones or strictures

Description. *IV cholangiography* examines the biliary ducts (hepatic ducts within the liver, the common hepatic duct, the cystic duct, and the common bile duct) by radiographic and tomographic visualization. The contrast substance, an iodine preparation such as iodipamide meglumine (Cholografin), is injected IV, and approximately 15 min later X-rays are taken.

Percutaneous cholangiography is indicated when biliary obstruction is suspected. The contrast substance is directly instilled into the biliary tree. The process is visualized by fluoroscopy, and spot films are taken.

T-tube cholangiography, known as postoperative cholangiography, may be done 7 to 8 h after a cholecystectomy to explore the common bile duct for patency and to see if any gallstones remain. During the operation, a T-shaped tube is placed in the common bile duct to promote drainage. The contrast substance is injected into the T tube.

Clinical Problems/Purposes

Test	*Indications/Purposes*
IV cholangiography	To detect stricture, stones, or tumor in the biliary system
Percutaneous cholangiography	To detect obstruction of the biliary system caused from stones, cancer of the pancreas
T-tube cholangiography	To detect obstruction of the common bile duct from stones or stricture; fistula

Procedure
- Obtain a signed consent form.
- Restrict food and fluids for 8 h before test.

IV Cholangiography
- A laxative may be given the night before the test and a cleansing enema in the morning.

- A contrast agent, iodipamide meglumine (Cholografin) is injected IV while the client is lying on a tilting X-ray table. X-rays are taken every 15 to 30 min until the common bile duct is visualized.

Percutaneous Cholangiography

- A laxative the night before and cleansing enema the morning of the test may be ordered.
- Preoperative medications usually include sedatives/tranquilizers. An antibiotic may be ordered for 24 to 72 h before the test for prophylactic purposes.
- The client is placed on a tilting X-ray table that rotates. The upper right quadrant of the abdomen is cleansed and draped. A skin anesthetic is given.
- The client should exhale and hold breath while a needle is inserted with the guidance of fluoroscopy into the biliary tree. Bile is withdrawn, and the contrast substance is then injected. Spot films are taken.
- A sterile dressing will be applied to the puncture site.

T-tube Cholangiography

- A cleansing enema may be ordered in the morning before the test.
- The client lies on an X-ray table and a contrast agent, such as sodium diatrizoate (Hypaque), is injected into the T tube and an X-ray is taken. Final X-ray is taken 15 min later.

Factors Affecting Diagnostic Results

- Obesity, gas, and fecal material in the intestines can affect the clarity of the X-ray.

Nursing Implications

- List the procedure steps for the client to alleviate anxiety.
- Recognize that obesity, gas, or fecal material in the intestines can affect the clarity of the X-ray.
- Obtain a history of allergies to seafood, iodine, or X-ray dye.
- Permit the client to express concerns. Be supportive.
- Observe for signs and symptoms of allergic reaction to contrast agents (i.e., nausea; vomiting; flushing; rash; urticaria; hypotension; slurred, thick speech; and dyspnea).

- Check the infusion site for signs of phlebitis (i.e., pain, redness, swelling). Apply warm compresses to the infusion site if symptoms are present.
- Monitor vital signs as ordered for percutaneous cholangiography. Instruct the client to remain in bed for several hours following the test.

Client Teaching
- Inform the client having IV cholangiography that the test may take several hours.

CHOLECYSTOGRAPHY (ORAL)

GALLBLADDER RADIOGRAPHY, GALLBLADDER (GB) SERIES

Normal Findings.   Normal size and structure of gallbladder; no gallstones

Description.   Oral cholecystography is an X-ray test used to visualize gallstones. A contrast material (radiopaque dye) is taken orally the night before, and it takes 12 to 14 h for the dye to be concentrated in the gall-bladder. Nonfunctioning liver cells can hamper the excretion of the dye. Immediately after the oral cholecystography test, the client may be given a fat-stimulus meal. Fluoroscopic examination and X-rays are taken to observe the ability of the gallbladder to empty the dye.

When the gallbladder cannot be visualized using an oral contrast substance, the IV cholangiography may be ordered. If GI X-rays are ordered, the gallbladder X-ray should be obtained first because barium could interfere with the test results.

Purposes
- To detect stones or tumor in the gallbladder
- To check for obstruction of the cystic duct

Clinical Problems
Abnormal findings: Cholelithiasis, neoplasms of the gallbladder, chole-cystitis, obstruction of the cystic duct

Procedure

- The client should have a fat-free diet 24 h before the X-ray. Restrict food and fluids except for sips of water 12 h before the test.
- Two hours after the dinner meal, radiopaque tablets are administered according to the directions on the folder. Various commercial contrast agents are available (e.g., iopanoic acid [Telepaque], calcium or sodium ipodate [Oragrafin], iodoalphionic acid [Priodax], and iodipamide meglumine [Cholografin]).
- No laxatives should be taken until after the X-ray tests.
- A high-fat meal may be given in the X-ray department after the fasting X-rays are taken. Post–fatty-meal films will be taken at intervals to determine how fast the gallbladder expels the dye.
- The fasting X-ray test takes 45 min to 1 h, and the post–fatty-meal test takes an hour or two.

Factors Affecting Diagnostic Results

- Diarrhea or vomiting can inhibit absorption of the contrast substance.
- Liver disease.

Nursing Implications

- Obtain a history of allergies to seafood, iodine, or X-ray dye, as many of these agents contain iodine.
- Observe for signs and symptoms of jaundice (i.e., yellow sclera of the eyes, yellow skin, and a serum bilirubin level greater than 3 mg/dl). Test is not done if there is severe liver disease.
- Administer the radiopaque tablets every 5 min with a full glass of water 2 h after the dinner meal. Clients may take the tablets on their own.
- Observe for signs and symptoms of allergic reaction to the radiopaque tablets (i.e., elevated temperature, rash, urticaria, hypotension, thick speech, or dyspnea).
- Report vomiting and diarrhea prior to the test. Tablets may not be absorbed because of hypermotility.

Client Teaching

- Inform the client that the evening meal before the test should be fat free.

- Inform the client that the test does not hurt.
- Inform the client that a second stage of the test may be ordered. It would include a high-fat meal and then more X-rays taken.

CHORIONIC VILLI BIOPSY (CVB)

Normal Finding. Normal fetal cells

Description. Chorionic villi sampling can detect early fetal abnormalities. Fetal cells are obtained by suction from fingerlike projections around the embryonic membrane, which eventually becomes the placenta. The test is performed between the eighth and tenth week of pregnancy. After the tenth week maternal cells begin to grow over the villi.

Advantage of CVB over amniocentesis is that CVB may be performed earlier, and results can be obtained in a few days and not weeks. Disadvantage is that CVB cannot determine neural tube defects and pulmonary maturity.

Purpose
- To detect chromosomal disorders

Clinical Problems
Abnormal findings: Chromosomal disorders; hemoglobinopathies (e.g., sickle cell anemia); lysosomal storage disorders, such as Tay-Sachs disease

Procedure
- Obtain a signed consent form.
- No food or fluid restriction is required.
- Place client in lithotomy position.
- Ultrasound is used to verify the placement of the catheter at the villi. Suction is applied, and tissue is removed from the villi.
- Test takes approximately 30 min.

Factors Affecting Diagnostic Results
- Performing the test 10 weeks after gestation.

Nursing Implications
- Assess for signs of spontaneous abortion resulting from procedure (e.g., cramps, bleeding).
- Be supportive of client and family. Be a good listener.
- Assess for infection resulting from the procedure (e.g., chills, fever).

Client Teaching
- Instruct the client to report if excessive bleeding or severe cramping occurs after the procedure.

COLONOSCOPY*

Normal Finding.   Normal mucosa of the large intestine; absence of pathology

Description.   Colonoscopy, an endoscopic procedure, is an inspection of the large intestine (colon) using a long, flexible fiberscope (colonoscope). The instrument is inserted anally and is advanced through the rectum, the sigmoid colon, and the large intestine to the cecum.

This test is useful for evaluating suspicious lesions in the large colon, such as polyps that could later develop into cancerous tumors, tumor mass, and inflammatory tissue. Biopsy of the tissue or polyp can be obtained. The biopsy forceps passes through the scope to obtain the tissue specimen. Polyps can be removed with the use of an electrocautery snare.

Colonoscopy should not be done on pregnant women near term, after recent abdominal surgery, or in a confused/uncooperative patient. Caution should be taken in performing a colonoscopy following an acute myocardial infarction, in acute diverticulitis, or in severe (active) ulcerative colitis. Rarely colon perforation is caused by the fiberscope. Bleeding may occur after a biopsy or polypectomy.

---

*Updated by Dr. Warren G. Butt, Gastroenterology-Stomach-Colon-Liver, Newark, Delaware.

Screening for polyps for the client over the age of 50 is important. However, if the client has a familial history of colon cancer, a colonoscopy may be recommended before the age of 50. Colon cancer is usually caused by adenomatous polyps, and if the polyps are removed early, cancer of the colon would be unlikely.

Virtual colonography: A virtual colonography is an examination of the colon by CT scanning of the entire large colon. It is currently not as accurate as the traditional colonoscopy, for it is difficult with this procedure to detect small polyps. In a major study, virtual colonoscopy missed 45% of polyps that were 5 mm or smaller. Differentiation of stool from polyps can be difficult.

The client still has to undergo the same "colon prep" before a virtual colonography as the person would with a traditional colonoscopy. Traditional colonoscopy is required to remove a polyp found on a CT scan of the colon. Virtual colonography has advantages over traditional colonoscopy: no sedatives are required, the procedure is less invasive, and additional information outside the colon may also be found, such as incidental renal cell cancer.

Purposes
- To detect the origin of lower intestinal bleeding
- To identify polyps in the large intestine
- To screen for benign or malignant lesions (tumors) in the colon

Clinical Problems
Indications: Intestinal bleeding, periodical screening for polyps or tumors, diverticular disease, benign or malignant lesions, ulcerative colitis

Procedure
- A consent form should be signed.
- Specific laboratory tests may be ordered, such as CBC, INR (if patient has taken Coumadin).
- Withhold medications that interfere with coagulation, such as aspirin, NSAIDs (Advil, Motrin), iron medication, and alcohol, 1 week prior to the test.

- Barium sulfate from other diagnostic studies can decrease visualization; therefore, the colonoscopy should not be attempted within 10 days to 2 weeks of a barium study.
- Avoid using soapsuds enemas. These can irritate intestine.
- Emergency drugs and equipment should be available for hypersensitivity to medications (premedications and anesthetic).
- Specimen containers should be labeled with the client's name, date, and the type of tissue.
- Client should be accompanied by someone who can drive him/her home following the test.
- The procedure takes approximately 15 min to 1 h.
- The day before the procedure, the client may have "clear liquids" only, which includes water, tea, coffee (without milk), strained fruit juices without pulp (apple, white grape, lemonade), plain jello (without added fruits or toppings), clear broths or bouillon (chicken or beef without noodles or solids). Gatorade, carbonated and noncarbonated soft drinks are also allowed. All red fluids should be avoided due to the dye, which can affect the visualization of the test.

Preparation (Use of GoLytely/Colyte Solution)
Day before the Test

- Client should prepare GoLytely or Colyte solution according to instructions and refrigerate solution.
- Client should drink GoLytely/Colyte as instructed, usually 7 PM to 10 PM.

Medication Procedure

- Intravenous fluids with Diprivan (Propofol), midazolam (Versed), or meperidine (Demerol) for conscious sedation is given immediately prior to the test.

Factors Affecting Diagnostic Results

- A soapsuds enema can cause intestinal irritation.
- Barium sulfate from other diagnostic studies can decrease visualization; therefore, the study should not be attempted within 10 days to 2 weeks of a barium study.

- Inadequate bowel preparation with fecal material remaining in the colon will decrease visualization.

Nursing Implications
Pre-test
- The client should follow the pre-test preparation procedure.
- Explain the procedure of the test. The client lies in the Sims position on left lateral position. A lubricated colonoscope is inserted. Air will be insufflated for better visualization. Photos are usually taken of any abnormal tissue or polyps.
- Record baseline vital signs, and if available, pertinent laboratory values.
- Report anxiety and fears to the physician or health professional prior to the test.

Client Teaching
- Instruct the client to bring someone to drive him/her home.
- Instruct the client to breathe deeply and slowly through the mouth during the insertion of the colonoscope.
- Inform the client that the procedure takes approximately 15 min to 1 h.

Post-test
- Monitor vital signs and report abnormal changes.
- Assess for anal bleeding, abdominal distention, severe pain, severe abdominal cramps, and fever; report any of the signs or symptoms immediately.

COLPOSCOPY

Normal Finding.   Normal appearance of the vagina and cervical structures

Description.   Colposcopy is the examination of the vagina and cervix using a binocular instrument (colposcope) that has a magnifying lens and a light. This test can be performed in the gynecologist's office or in the hospital. After a positive Pap smear or a suspicious cervical lesion, colposcopy is indicated for examining the vagina and cervix more thoroughly. A typical epithelium, leukoplakia vulvae, and irregular blood vessels can be identified with this procedure, and photographs and a biopsy specimen can be obtained.

Since the test has become more popular, there has been a decreased need for conization (surgical removal of a cone of tissue from the cervical os). Colposcopy is also useful for monitoring women whose mothers received diethylstilbestrol during pregnancy; these women are prone to develop precancerous and cancerous lesions of the vagina and cervix.

Purpose
- To identify precancerous lesions of the cervix

Clinical Problems
Indications: Vaginal and cervical lesions, abnormal cervical tissue after a positive Pap smear, irregular blood vessels, leukoplakia vulvae, dysplasia and cervical lesions, vaginal and cervical tissue changes for women whose mothers took diethylstilbestrol during pregnancy

Procedure
- A consent form should be signed.
- No food or fluid restriction is required.
- The client's clothes should be removed, and the client should wear a gown and be properly draped.
- The client assumes a lithotomy position (legs in stirrups).
- 3% acetic acid is applied to the vagina and cervix. This produces color changes in the cervical epithelium and helps in detecting abnormal changes.
- A biopsy specimen of suspicious tissues and photographs may be taken.
- A vaginal tampon may be worn after the procedure.
- The test takes approximately 15 to 20 min.

Factors Affecting Diagnostic Results
- Mucus, cervical secretions, creams, and medications can decrease visualization.

Nursing Implications
- Obtain a signed consent form.
- Be present during the test.
- Place the biopsy tissue into a bottle containing a preservative; place the cells, if obtained, on a slide; and spray them with a fixative solution.

Client Teaching
- Inform the client that she should not experience pain but that there may be some discomfort with the insertion of the speculum or when the biopsy is taken.
- Inform the client that the test takes 15 to 20 min.

Post-test Client Teaching
- Inform the client that she may have some bleeding for a few hours because of the biopsy. Tell the client that she can use tampons and that if bleeding becomes heavy and it is not her menstrual period, she should call the gynecologist.
- Instruct the client not to have intercourse for a week, until the biopsy site is healed, or as ordered by the health care provider.
- Inform the client that she should be notified of the results of the test, and tell her to call if she has not heard from the office in a week.

COMPUTED TOMOGRAPHY (CT) SCAN, COMPUTED AXIAL TOMOGRAPHY (CAT)*

CAT SCAN, COMPUTED TRANSAXIAL TOMOGRAPHY (CTT), EMI SCAN

Normal Findings.   Normal tissue; no pathologic findings

Description.   The CT scan, or CAT scan, was developed in England in 1972 and was called the EMI scan. The CT scanner produces a narrow X-ray beam that examines body sections from 360°.

---

*Dr. Stephen Drahovac, Neurologist, Christiana Care, Newark, Delaware.

The CT scanner tubes and detectors rotate around the client who is lying on a table. It produces a series of cross-sectional images in sequence that build up a two-dimensional (2D) picture of the organ and structure. The traditional X-ray takes a flat or frontal picture, which also gives a two-dimensional view. The CT scanner is about 100 times more sensitive than the X-ray machine in separating different soft tissue densities. CT scanning is a costly diagnostic test, although it is popular because it can diagnose at an earlier stage.

The CT scan can be performed with or without iodinated contrast media (dye). It is not an invasive test unless contrast dye is used. The contrast dye causes a greater tissue absorption and is referred to as contrast enhancement. This enhancement enables small abnormalities to be seen.

CT is capable of scanning the head (internal auditory canal, brain, eye orbits, sinuses, head), abdomen (stomach, small and large intestines, liver, spleen, pancreas, bile duct, kidney, and adrenals), pelvis (bladder, reproductive organs, and small and large bowel within pelvis), and chest (lung, heart, mediastinal structure). The CT scan detects most types of body tissue, but NOT nerves. This procedure does not cause pain; however, there may be some discomfort from lying still.

Recent advances in helical (spiral CT) scanning techniques in combination with multirow solid-state detector arrays have allowed greater anatomic coverage with shorter scan times. This allows the imaging without blurring of moving organs such as the heart including such small objects as the coronary arteries. Helical (spiral) CT imaging can take place in 30 seconds and can be performed with one breath held. This new technique is called multislice CT (MSCT).

Head and brain CT: The CT of the brain/head provides two-dimensional views of the brain consisting of cross-sectional images of brain tissue layers. This procedure can differentiate among tumors, aneurysms, cerebral infarction, and intracranial hemorrhage (hematoma). Also this CT scan can detect ventricular displacement or enlargement. Visualization of the pathology can be enhanced with IV iodinated contrast dye.

Chest (thoracic) CT: CT of the chest gives a cross-sectional view of the chest to differentiate among various pathologic conditions, such as tumors, nodules, cysts, abscesses, hematomas, and aortic aneurysms. It can detect pleural effusion and enlarged lymph nodes in the chest area. The use of IV contrast media aids in highlighting blood vessels, thus identifying abnormalities of the vascular structures. CT of the chest can be useful in evaluating the effects of treatment therapy on the tumor and if metastasis has occurred.

The helical or spiral CT imaging can readily detect pulmonary emboli, over 90% of the time.

Abdominal CT: CT of the abdomen is useful for diagnosing tumors, obstructions, cysts, hematomas, abscesses, bleeding perforation, calculi, fibroids, and other pathologic conditions that appear in the liver, biliary tract, pancreas, spleen, GI tract, gallbladder, kidneys, adrenals, uterus and ovaries, and prostate gland. IV contrast dye may be used to enhance visualization. The kidney and urinary flow is easily seen with the use of contrast dye. Oral contrast media may be used for scanning the GI tract. The CT scan is useful for staging tumors and monitoring the effect of treatment therapy on the tumor.

Spine CT: CT scan of the spine gives cross-sectional images that can be reconstructed in the sagittal and coronal plane, or as three-dimensional views on a monitor. It is mainly used to view the bony anatomy. Contrast dye may be injected into the spinal column via lumbar puncture, that is, CT myelography, for clearer visualization of nerve roots and disc herniation. MRI is the preferred study of the spine; however, if MRI is contraindicated or unavailable, then contrast CT would likely be ordered.

Long bones and joints CT: Skeletal CT provides cross-sectional images of the bone. This procedure is useful to detect bone and soft-tissue tumors and bone metastases. Joint abnormalities can be identified with this CT. Contrast dye may be ordered.

Purposes
- To screen for coronary artery disease; head, liver, and renal lesions; tumors; edema; abscess; bone destruction
- To locate foreign objects in soft tissues, such as the eye

Clinical Problems

CT Type	Abnormal Findings
Head	Cerebral lesions: hematomas, tumors, cysts, abscess, infarction, edema, atrophy, hydrocephalus
Internal auditory canal	Acoustic neuroma, cholesteatoma, bone erosion
Eye orbits	Bone destruction, optic nerve tumors, muscle tumor, orbital tumor
Sinus	Bone destruction, sinusitis, polyps, tumors
Neck (soft tissue)	Tumors, abscess, stones in the salivary ducts, enlarged nodes
Abdomen:	
Liver	Hepatic lesions: cysts, abscess, tumors, hematomas, cirrhosis with ascites
Biliary	Obstruction due to calculi
Pancreatic	Acute and chronic pancreatitis; pancreatic lesions: tumor, abscess, pseudocysts
Kidney	Renal lesions: tumors, calculi, cysts, congenital anomalies; perirenal hematomas and abscesses
Adrenal	Adrenal tumors
Chest and thoracic	Chest lesions: tumors, cysts, abscesses; aortic aneurysm; enlarged lymph nodes in mediastinum; pleural effusion
Spine	Tumors, paraspinal cysts, vascular malformation, congenital spinal anomalies (e.g., spina bifida, herniated intervertebral disk)
Bony pelvis, long bones, joints	Bone destruction, fractures, tumors
Guided needle biopsy	For lung or liver masses, adrenal mass, kidney, spine, neck tumors

Procedure
General Preparation for All Scans
- Obtain a signed consent form.
- There is no food or fluid restriction if contrast dye is NOT used.
- For IV contrast injection studies, usually there is NPO 4 h prior to the CT. Diabetics may be given orange juice instead of water; check with the health care provider or CT supervisor. Oral hypoglycemic agents, such as glycophage, are contraindicated for use of iodinated contrast. For PM scheduling, NPO after a liquid breakfast.

- Prescribed medications may be given with a small amount of water prior to the CT scan; check with the health care provider or CT supervisor.
- A mild sedative may be ordered for some clients to alleviate anxiety.
- If contrast media (dye) is ordered and the client is allergic to iodine products, prednisone, diphenhydramine (Benadryl), and ranitidine (Zantac) may be given 1 h prior to CT. With a possible severe allergic reaction, these drugs may be given 6 and 12 h prior to CT.
- IV infusion or heparin lock inserted may be required prior to test.
- CT scanning usually takes 5 to 15 min.

Head CT

- Remove hairpins, clips, and jewelry (earrings) before the test.
- Remove dentures prior to the use of contrast dye.
- A mild sedative or analgesic may be ordered for restless clients or for those who have aches and pains of the neck or back.
- Head is positioned in a cradle, and a wide, rubberized strap is applied snugly around the head to keep it immobilized during test.

Abdominal and Pelvic CT

- Abdominal X-ray (KUB) may be requested before CT scan.
- Laboratory reports of serum creatinine and BUN should be available.
- GI tract must be free from barium. An enema may be ordered.
- For an AM abdominal/pelvic scan, give the oral contrast media (15 oz) between 8 PM and 10 PM the evening before the scan. NPO after 10 PM. One hour prior to the CT, give 1/2 bottle of the oral contrast. One-half hour prior to the CT, give the remaining 1/2 bottle of oral contrast.
- For a PM abdominal/pelvic scan, give 1 bottle (15 oz) of oral contrast media at 7 AM the morning of the scan. NPO after 7 AM. One hour prior to the CT, give 1/2 bottle of the oral contrast. One-half hour prior to the CT, give 1/2 bottle of the oral contrast.
- For pelvic scan, give the oral contrast media (15 oz) between 8 PM and 10 PM the evening before the scan. Additional oral contrast media is usually given the morning of the scan.

Chest CT

- A chest X-ray may be requested before a chest scan.
- IV contrast media is frequently given in left arm.

Spine CT

- NPO is not indicated, as contrast media is usually not ordered.
- Spine X-rays taken prior to scan should be available. When a myelogram has been performed, spine CT should follow myelography.

Neck CT

- IV contrast media is used. Check general preparation for scan for IV contrast injection studies.

Bony Pelvis, Long Bones, and Joints CT

- Nuclear medicine study to locate "hot areas" should be done before the CT scan of the bones and joints.

Factors Affecting Diagnostic Results

- Barium sulfate can obscure visualization of the abdominal organs. Barium studies should be performed 4 days before the CT or after the CT.
- Excessive flatus can cause client discomfort and may cause an inaccurate reading.
- Movement can cause artifacts.
- Metal plates in skull and metal bridges.
- Dental fillings.

Nursing Implications
Pre-test

- Explain the procedure to the client. The CT scanner is circular, with a doughnut-like opening. The client is strapped to a special table, with the scanner revolving around the body area that is to be examined. Clicking noises will be heard from the scanner. The radiologist or specialized technician is stationed in a control room and can observe and communicate with the client at all times through an intercom system. The test is not painful.
- Inform the client that holding breath may be requested several times during an abdominal or thoracic scan.

- Inform the client that the CT of the head takes 5 min without contrast media and 10 min with use of contrast. For body CT, the test takes 5 to 15 min.
- Obtain a history of allergies to seafood, iodine, and contrast dye from other X-ray tests. Contrast enhancement is not always done with CT, especially chest and spinal CT scanning.
- Advise the client that if contrast dye is injected IV, a warm, flushed sensation may be felt in the face or body. A salty, "fishy," or metallic taste, and a sensation of urinating (does not occur) may be experienced. Nausea is not uncommon. These sensations usually last for 1 or 2 min.
- Observe for signs and symptoms of a severe allergic reaction to the dye (i.e., dyspnea, palpitations, tachycardia, hypotension, itching, and urticaria). Emergency drugs should be available.

Post-test
- Observe for delayed allergic reaction to the contrast dye (i.e., skin rash, urticaria, headache, vomiting and/or renal dysfunction). Increased creatinine level can follow IV contrast use. An oral antihistamine may be ordered for mild reactions.
- If contrast dye has been used, instruct the client to increase fluid intake to enhance the excretion of the dye.
- Be supportive of the client and family. The CT scan can be frightening. The major risk involved is an allergic reaction to the dye.

Client Teaching
- Instruct the client to resume his or her usual level of activity and diet, unless otherwise indicated.

CYSTOMETRY, CYSTOMETROGRAM (CMG)

Normal Findings.
Adult: Urine stream: strong and uninterrupted; normal filling pattern and sensation of fullness; bladder capacity: 300–600 ml; residual: 0–30 ml; urge to void: greater than 150 ml; fullness felt: greater than 300 ml
Child: Bladder capacity and urinary flow vary with age.

Description. Cystometry, or cystometrogram (CMG), evaluates the neuromuscular function of the bladder. After the instillation of a measured quantity of fluid, this test measures the efficiency of the detrusor muscle, the intravesical pressure and capacity, and the effect of thermal stimulation. CMG is used for evaluating bladder dysfunction caused by neurologic disorder or disease, such as spinal cord injury, stroke, multiple sclerosis, diabetes mellitus, and by stress incontinence, urinary/stress incontinence, and the effects of drugs the client is taking. Cystometry is contraindicated for a client with a urinary tract infection (UTI).

Urethral pressure profile (UPP) is frequently performed during the cystometry. A special catheter that had been inserted is slowly withdrawn as the urethral pressures are measured. These tests may be conducted in a urologist's office or clinic.

Purposes

- To evaluate the detrusor muscle function and tonicity of the bladder
- To measure the urethral pressures
- To determine the cause of bladder dysfunction

Clinical Problems

Abnormal findings/causes: Stress incontinence; neurogenic bladder from spinal cord injury, stroke, multiple sclerosis, diabetes mellitus, postoperative urinary dysfunction, bladder and prostate obstruction

Procedure

- Obtain a signed consent form.
- No food or fluid restriction is required.
- Have the client urinate into a container attached to a machine that records the force of the urinary flow, amount, and completion time.
- Insert a retention catheter to measure residual urine volume.
- Test for thermal sensation: Instill 30 to 50 ml of room-temperature normal saline solution (NSS) into the bladder. The client should report the sensation that is felt. The NSS is then withdrawn. Instill 30 ml of 30- to 40-degree NSS. Again the client reports his/her sensations, such as a feeling of warmth, flushing, need to void, and/or discomfort. The bladder is then drained.

- Connect the catheter to a cystometer (a tube to monitor bladder pressures). Normal saline solution, sterile water, or gas (carbon dioxide) is *slowly* instilled into the bladder. The cystometer graphically records the data. The client tells when he/she can no longer hold the urine without voiding; the liquid instillation is stopped, and the catheter is removed. The client voids, but does not strain when voiding. Again, the voiding pressure is recorded. If gas is used, the gas is withdrawn and the pressures from the urethral wall are obtained.
- The cholinergic drug bethanechol (Urecholine), an urinary stimulant, may be administered during the cystometric procedure to enhance the bladder tone.
- The test takes approximately 45 min to 1 h.

Factors Affecting Diagnostic Results
- Antihistamines cause relaxation of the bladder muscle and wall, thus, bladder function can be inhibited.

Nursing Implications
- Obtain a history of the client's urinary problem and what drugs the client is taking daily.
- Check vital signs, which may be the baseline VS for the post-test.
- Discuss the procedure with the client.

Client Teaching
- Inform the client that he/she may have a strong urge to urinate during the test and that this is NOT abnormal. Tell the client to let the urologist know what sensations that he/she may have at various times during the test.

Post-test
Client Teaching
- Inform the client that he/she may have bladder spasms after the test. An analgesic is usually prescribed. After 24 h, if the bladder spasms continue, the health care provider should be called.
- Notify the health care provider if blood in the urine occurs 4 to 6 h post-test or after the third voiding.

- Explain to the client who received carbon dioxide gas that it may cause post-test discomfort.
- Instruct the client to report fever, dysuria, or urinary frequency to the health care provider. Urinary tract infection (UTI) may have resulted from this procedure and needs to be reported and treated.
- Encourage the client to increase fluid intake. Measurement of intake and output may be requested.

CYSTOSCOPY, CYSTOGRAPHY (CYSTOGRAM)

CYSTOURETHROSCOPY

Normal Findings.   Normal structure of the urethra, bladder, prostatic urethra, and ureter orifices

Description.   Cystoscopy is the direct visualization of the bladder wall and urethra with the use of a cystoscope. With this procedure, small renal calculi can be removed from the ureter, bladder, or urethra, and a tissue biopsy can be obtained. A *retrograde pyelography,* injection of contrast dye through the catheter into the ureters and renal pelvis, may be performed during the cystoscopy.

Cystography is the instillation of a contrast dye into the bladder via a catheter. This procedure can detect neurogenic bladder, fistulas, tumors, and a rupture in the bladder.

Purposes
- To detect renal calculi and renal tumor
- To remove renal stones
- To determine the cause of hematuria or urinary tract infection (UTI)

Clinical Problems
Abnormal findings: Renal calculi, tumors, prostatic hyperplasia, urethral stricture, hematuria, urinary tract infection

Procedure

- Obtain a signed consent form.
- Provide a full liquid breakfast in the AM if local anesthetic is used. Several glasses of water before the test may be ordered. Restrict food and fluids for 8 h before cystoscopy if general anesthesia is given.
- Record baseline vital signs.
- A narcotic analgesic may be ordered 1 h before cystoscopy. The procedure is done under local or general anesthesia.
- The client is placed in the lithotomy position. A local anesthetic is injected into the urethra. Water may be instilled to enhance better visualization. A urine specimen may be obtained.
- Test procedure takes about 30 min to 1 h.

Nursing Implications

- Obtain history concerning the presence of cystitis or prostatitis, which could result in sepsis following the procedure.
- Check for hypersensitivity to anesthetics.
- Assess urinary patterns—amount, color, odor, specific gravity—and take vital signs.

Client Teaching

- Explain the test procedure.
- Inform the client that there may be some pressure or burning discomfort during or following the test.

Post-test

- Recognize the complications that can occur as the result of a cystoscopy: hemorrhaging, perforation of the bladder, urinary retention, and infection.
- Monitor vital signs. Compare with baseline vital signs.
- Monitor urinary output for 48 h following a cystoscopy.
- Report gross hematuria. Inform the client that blood-tinged urine is not uncommon.
- Observe for signs and symptoms of an infection: fever, chills, tachycardia, burning on urination, pain. Antibiotics may be given before and after the test as a prophylactic measure.

- Apply heat to the lower abdomen to relieve pain and muscle spasm as ordered. A warm sitz bath may be ordered.

Client Teaching
- Advise client to avoid alcoholic beverages for 2 days after the test.
- Inform client that a slight burning sensation when voiding might occur for a day or two.

ECHOCARDIOGRAPHY (ECHOCARDIOGRAM)*

TWO-DIMENSIONAL (2D), SPECTRAL DOPPLER, COLOR FLOW DOPPLER, TRANSESOPHAGEAL, CONTRAST, AND STRESS ECHOCARDIOGRAPHY

Normal Findings.   Normal heart size and structure; normal movements of heart valves and heart chambers

Description.   Echocardiography (echocardiogram) is a noninvasive ultrasound test used to identify abnormal heart size, structure, and function, and valvular disease. A hand-held transducer (probe) moves over the chest area of the heart and other specified surrounding areas. The transducer sends and receives high-frequency sound waves. The sound waves that are reflected (echo) from the heart back to the transducer produce pictures. These pictures appear on a television-like screen and are recorded on videotape and moving graph paper.

There are several types of echocardiographic studies, which include two-dimensional (2D), spectral Doppler, color flow Doppler, transesophageal, contrast, and stress echocardiography. Transesophageal echocardiography (TEE) is gaining popularity for diagnosing and managing a wide range of cardiovascular diseases, such as valvular heart dysfunction and aortic pathology. Stress echocardiography is a valuable tool for assessing myocardial ischemia at half the cost of other cardiac studies.

---

*Updated by Susan L. Chubrik, RN, MSN, CCNRP, Christiana Care Health Services, Newark, Delaware.

Two-dimensional (2D) echocardiography: This test employs 2D echocardiography, which records motion, and provides two-dimensional (cross-sectional) views of the heart structures. It is used to evaluate the size, shape, and movement of the chambers and valves of the heart, and it is useful in detecting valvular disease and in assessing congenital heart disease.

Spectral Doppler echocardiography: Spectral Doppler measures the amount, speed, and dissection of blood passing through the heart valves and heart chambers. A swishing sound is heard as the blood flows throughout the heart. This test can detect turbulent blood flow through the heart valves and may indicate valvular disease. Septal wall defects may also be detected.

Color Doppler echocardiography: The color flow Doppler (red and blue) shows the direction of blood flowing through the heart. It can identify leaking heart valves (regurgitation) or hardened valves (stenosis), function of prosthetic valves, and the presence of shunts (holes) in the heart. The use of the color flow Doppler complements the 2D echocardiogram and the spectral Doppler study.

Transesophageal echocardiography: With transesophageal echocardiography (TEE), a transducer (probe) is attached to an endoscope and is inserted into the esophagus to visualize adjacent cardiac and extracardiac structures with greater acuity than most echocardiography studies, including transthoracic (TTE). TEE can be used in the intensive care unit, emergency department, and operating room, as well as in cardiac testing facilities. This type of echocardiography is useful for diagnosing mitral and aortic valvular pathology; determining the presence of a possible intracardiac thrombus in the left atrium; detecting suspected acute dissection of the aorta and endocarditis; monitoring left ventricular function before, during, or after surgery; and evaluating intracardiac repairs during surgery, guiding pericardiocentesis.

This test is contraindicated if esophageal pathology (e.g., strictures, varices, trauma) exists. Also, TEE should not be performed if undiagnosed active gastrointestinal bleeding is occurring or if the client is uncooperative. A light sedative is frequently given prior to testing. TEE can be performed on an unconscious client. TEE is tolerated well, with approximately 1% of clients being intolerant of the esophageal probe. The rate of complications is less than 0.2%.

Contrast echocardiography: This test assists in determining intracardiac communications and myocardial ischemia and perfusion defects. Microbubbles are injected into the venous circulation for the purpose of recording showers of echoes by 2D tests. The microbubbles pass through the right atrium and ventricle, where they are absorbed in the lung; they do not pass to the left side of the heart. If the microbubbles are detected on the left side of the heart, an intracardiac communication or shunt is present. New contrast agents are used with echocardiography, which may allow visualization of the coronary arteries.

Stress echocardiography: It may be necessary to evaluate the function of the left ventricle under stress. Before starting an exercise, a baseline two-dimensional and Doppler echocardiogram is performed for the evaluation of regional and global left and right ventricular systolic functions, left ventricular diastolic function, and valvular assessment. The client then exercises using a standardized protocol until the predicted maximum heart rate is achieved or until symptoms, electrocardiographic (ECG) or echocardiographic signs of myocardial ischemia, occur. Immediately after exercise, the client returns to a left lateral decubitus position for re-imaging (ideally obtained in less than 1 min). These are compared to those at baseline for any wall motion changes.

The stress modalities used in conjunction with echocardiography include exercise, IV administration of an agent that either increases myocardial oxygen consumption, such as dobutamine or arbutamine, or induces myocardial heterogeneity, such as dipyridamole or adenosine.

Purposes
- To identify abnormal heart size, structure, and function
- To detect cardiac valvular disease and septal wall defects
- To determine the function of prosthetic heart valves
- To detect viable myocardium
- To risk stratification following an acute myocardial infarction (AMI)
- To assess the effects of congenital heart disease
- To monitor left ventricular function before, during, and after surgery
- To evaluate and rule out coronary artery disease (CAD) based primarily on wall motion abnormalities

Clinical Problems

Abnormal findings: Abnormal heart size, structure, and function, heart valvular disease (regurgitation or stenosis of the aortic or mitral valves); congenital heart disease; heart wall damage after a myocardial infarction; cardiomyopathy mural thrombi; pericardial effusion; aortic pathology; and endocarditis

Diagnostic Tests	*Indications to Determine/Detect*
Two-dimensional (2D) echocardiography	Dimension of the left ventricle
	Degree of ventricular dilatation and contractility
	Ventricular hypertrophy
	Function of cardiac valves—stenosis or regurgitation
	Cardiac valvular disease
Spectral Doppler echocardiography	Blood flow through heart chambers and valves
	Septal wall defects
Color Doppler echocardiography	Direction of blood flow through the heart
	Function of cardiac valves—stenosis or regurgitation
	Function of prosthetic valves
	Presence of shunting in the heart
Transesophageal echocardiography	Function of left ventricle before, during, or after surgery
	Cardiac valvular disease
	Presence of intracardiac thrombus in left atrium
	Aortic disease (e.g., dissection of aorta)
	Presence of endocarditis
Contrast echocardiography	Perfusion defects
	Presence of shunting in the heart
Stress echocardiography	Function of left ventricle under stress
	Perfusion defects
	Wall motion abnormalities

Procedure

- Obtain a signed consent form.
- No food or fluid restriction is required.
- No medications should be omitted before the test unless indicated by the institution or health care provider.

- The client undresses from the waist up and wears a hospital gown. The client is positioned on his or her left side or in supine position.
- Vital signs are recorded. Three electrode patches are applied to the chest area to monitor heart rate and changes in cardiac rhythm.
- Water-soluble gel is applied to the skin areas that are to be scanned. The transducer, with slight pressure, moves over different areas of the chest. Some clients may require pictures to be taken under the neck.
- The 2D echo takes about 20 to 30 min, and the 2D echo with Doppler studies take approximately 30 to 45 min.
- The cardiologist interprets the test results and sends report to the client's personal health care provider (HCP). The HCP gives test results to the client.

Transesophageal echocardiography (TEE):
- The client should be NPO for at least 4 h prior to test.
- A light sedative is given prior to the test.
- An IV sedative (e.g., Versed) is given.
- The endoscopic transducer is inserted into the esophagus.
- The test takes 15 to 30 min.
- The client is monitored (Dynamap) during recovery for 1 to 2 h.

Contrast echocardiography:
- An IV line is inserted for injection of contrast media.

Stress echocardiography:
- The client should be NPO for 4 h before the test.
- The client may be placed on a treadmill or receive a pharmacologic agent.
- Images are acquired during rest (pre-test) and then during stress or immediately following stress (post-test).

Factors Affecting Diagnostic Results
- Large body habitus may cause poor image quality.
- Severe respiratory disease may affect test results.

Nursing Implications
- Obtain a history of the client's physical complaints.

- Obtain vital signs and an ECG recording as indicated. These are for baseline readings.
- Check that the consent form has been signed.

Client Teaching

- Explain the procedure to the client (see Procedure).
- Inform the client that he or she will be positioned on his or her back and/or left side during the test procedure.
- Inform the client that a gel will be applied to the skin area and that the transducer (probe) moves over the gel area. The sound waves are transmitted as a picture on videotape and on graph paper.
- Inform the client that he or she will receive test results from either the cardiologist or the health care provider.
- Answer client's questions or refer questions to health care providers.

ELECTROCARDIOGRAPHY (ELECTROCARDIOGRAM—ECG OR EKG), VECTORCARDIOGRAPHY (VECTORCARDIOGRAM—VCG)

Normal Finding. Normal electrocardiogram deflections, P, PR, QRS, QT, S-T, and T

Description. An electrocardiogram (ECG) records the electrical impulses of the heart by means of electrodes and a galvanometer (ECG machine). These electrodes are placed on the legs, arms, and chest. Combinations of two electrodes are called bipolar leads (i.e., lead I is the combination of both arm electrodes, lead II is the combination of right-arm and left-leg electrodes, and lead III is the combination of the left-arm and left-leg electrodes). The unipolar leads are AVF, AVL, and AVR; the A means augmented, V is the voltage, and F is left foot, L is left arm, and R is right arm. There are at least six unipolar chest or precordial leads. A standard ECG consists of 12 leads; six limb leads (I, II, III, AVF, AVL, AVR) and six chest (precordial) leads (V_1, V_2, V_3, V_4, V_5, V_6).

The electrical activity that the ECG records is in the form of waves and complexes: P wave (atrial depolarization); QRS complex (ventricular depolarization); and ST segment, T wave, and U wave (ventricular repolarization). An abnormal ECG indicates a disturbance in the electrical activity of the myocardium. A person could have heart disease and have a normal ECG as long as the cardiac problem did not affect the transmission of electrical impulses.

P wave (atrial contraction or depolarization): The normal time is 0.12 seconds. An enlarged P-wave deflection could indicate atrial enlargement. An absent or altered P wave could suggest that the electrical impulse did not come from the SA node.

PR interval (from the P wave to the onset of the Q wave): The normal time interval is 0.12 to 0.2 seconds. An increased interval could imply a conduction delay in the AV node that could result from rheumatic fever or arteriosclerotic heart disease. A short interval could indicate Wolff–Parkinson–White syndrome.

QRS complex (ventricular contraction or depolarization): The normal time is less than 0.12 seconds. An enlarged Q wave may imply an old myocardial infarction. An enlarged R-wave deflection could indicate ventricular hypertrophy. An increased time duration may indicate a bundle-branch block.

QT interval (ventricular depolarization and repolarization): The normal time interval is 0.36 to 0.44 seconds. A shortened or prolonged QT interval could imply ischemia or electrolyte imbalances.

ST segment (beginning ventricular repolarization): A depressed ST segment indicates myocardial ischemia. An elevated ST segment can indicate acute myocardial infarction (AMI) or pericarditis. A prolonged ST segment may imply hypocalcemia or hypokalemia. A short ST segment may be due to hypercalcemia.

T wave (ventricular repolarization): A flat or inverted T wave can indicate myocardial ischemia, myocardial infarction, or hypokalemia. A tall, peaked T wave, greater than 10 mm in precordial leads, or greater than 5 mm in limb leads, can indicate hyperkalemia.

Vectorcardiogram (VCG): The VCG records electrical impulses from the cardiac cycle, making it similar to the ECG. However, it shows a three-dimensional view (frontal, horizontal, and sagittal planes) of the heart, whereas the ECG shows a two-dimensional view (frontal and horizontal planes). The VCG is considered more sensitive than the ECG for diagnosing a myocardial infarction. It is useful for assessing ventricular hypertrophy in adults and children.

Purposes
- To detect cardiac dysrhythmias
- To identify electrolyte imbalance (e.g., hyperkalemia [peaked T wave])
- To monitor ECG changes during the stress/exercise tests and the recovery phase after a myocardial infarction

Clinical Problems
Abnormal findings: Cardiac dysrhythmias, cardiac hypertrophies, myocardial ischemia, electrolyte imbalances, myocardial infarction, pericarditis

Procedure
- No food, fluid, or medication is restricted.
- Clothing should be removed to the waist, and the female client should wear a gown.
- Nylon stockings should be removed, and trouser legs should be raised.
- The client lies in the supine position.
- The skin surface should be prepared. Excess hair should be shaved from the chest if necessary.
- Electrodes with electropaste or pads are strapped to the four extremities. Chest electrodes are applied. The lead selector is turned to record the 12 standard leads.
- The ECG takes approximately 15 min.

Nursing Implications
- List medications the client is taking and the last time they were taken. The health care provider may want to compare ECG results with prescribed medications.

Client Teaching
- Instruct the client to relax and to breathe normally during the ECG procedure. Tell the client to avoid tightening the muscles, grasping bed rails or other objects, and talking during the ECG tracing.
- Tell the client that the ECG does not cause pain or any discomfort.
- Instruct the client to tell you if he or she is having chest pain during the ECG tracing. Mark the ECG paper at the time the client is having chest pain.
- Allow the client time to ask questions.

ELECTROENCEPHALOGRAPHY, ELECTROENCEPHALOGRAM (EEG)

Normal Finding.   Normal tracing

Description.   The electroencephalogram (EEG) measures the electrical impulses produced by brain cells. Electrodes, applied to the scalp surface at predetermined measured positions, record brain-wave activity on moving paper. EEG tracings can detect patterns characteristic of some diseases (e.g., seizure disorders, neoplasms, strokes, head trauma, infections of the nervous system, and cerebral death). At times, recorded brain waves may be normal when there is pathology.

Purposes
- To detect seizure disorder
- To identify a brain tumor, abscess, intracranial hemorrhage
- To assist in the determination of cerebral death

Clinical Problems
Abnormal tracing: Seizure disorders (e.g., grand mal, petit mal, psychomotor); brain tumor; brain abscesses; head injury; intracranial hemorrhage; encephalitis; cerebral death

Procedure.   The procedure may be performed while the client is (1) awake, (2) drowsy, (3) asleep, (4) undergoing stimuli (rhythmic flashes of bright light), or (5) a combination of any of these.

- Shampoo hair the night before. Instruct the client not to use oil or hair spray on the hair.
- The decision concerning withdrawal or holding of medications before the EEG is made by the health care provider.
- No food or fluid is restricted, with the exception of *no* coffee, tea, cola, and alcohol.
- The EEG tracing is usually obtained with the client lying down; however, the client could be seated in a reclining chair.
- For a sleep recording, keep the client awake 2 to 3 h later the night before the test, and wake the client at 6 AM. A sedative such as chloral hydrate may be ordered.
- The EEG takes approximately 1.5 to 2 h.

Post-Test
- Remove the collodion or paste from the client's head. Acetone may be used to remove the paste.
- Normal activity may be resumed, unless the client was sedated.

Nursing Implications
- Report medications that the client is taking that could change the EEG result.
- Report to the health care provider and EEG laboratory any apprehension, restlessness, or anxiety of client.
- Observe for seizures, and describe the seizure activity.

Client Teaching
- Inform the client that getting an electric shock from the machine does not occur. Also the EEG machine does not determine intelligence and cannot read the mind. Many clients are apprehensive about the test.
- Encourage the client to eat before the test. Hypoglycemia should be prevented because it can affect normal brain activity. Coffee, tea, and any other stimulants should be avoided. Alcohol and tranquilizers are depressants that can affect test results.
- Inform the client that the test does not produce pain.

- Advise the client to be calm and to relax during the test. If rest and stimuli recordings are ordered, inform the client that there will be a brief time when there are flashing lights.
- Instruct the client that normal activity can be resumed following the test.

ELECTROMYOGRAPHY, ELECTROMYOGRAM (EMG)

Normal Findings.   At rest: minimal electrical activity; voluntary muscle contraction: markedly increased electrical activity

Description.   Electromyography (EMG) measures electrical activity of skeletal muscles at rest and during voluntary muscle contraction. A needle electrode is inserted into the skeletal muscle to pick up electrical activity, which can be heard over a loudspeaker, viewed on an oscilloscope, and recorded on graph paper all at the same time. Normally there is no (or minimal) electrical activity at rest; however, in motor disorders, abnormal patterns occur. With voluntary muscle contraction, there is a loud popping sound and increased electrical activity (waves).

The test is useful in diagnosing neuromuscular disorders. EMG can be used to differentiate between myopathy and neuropathy.

Purposes
- To diagnose neuromuscular disorders, such as muscular dystrophy
- To differentiate between myopathy and neuropathy

Clinical Problems
Abnormal findings: Muscular dystrophy; peripheral neuropathy due to diabetes mellitus, alcoholism; myasthenia gravis, myotonia; amyotrophic lateral sclerosis (ALS), anterior poliomyelitis

Procedure
- Obtain a signed consent form.
- No food or fluid is restricted, with the exception of *no* coffee, tea, colas, or other caffeine drinks, and *no* smoking for 3 h before the test.

- Medications such as muscle relaxants, anticholinergics, and cholinergics should be withheld until after the test with the health care provider's approval. If specific medication is needed, the time of the test should be rearranged.
- The client lies on a table or sits in a chair in a room free of noise. Needle electrodes are inserted in selected or affected muscles. If the client experiences marked pain, the needle should be removed and reinserted.
- The procedure takes approximately 1 to 2 h.
- If serum enzyme tests are ordered (e.g., SGOT, CPK, LDH), the specimen should be drawn before the EMG or 5 to 10 days after the test.

Post-test
- If residual pain occurs, analgesics may be given.

Nursing Implications
- Withhold medications that could affect EMG results with permission.
- Draw blood for serum enzymes prior to the test if ordered.
- Administer analgesic if residual pain is present.

Client Teaching
- Inform client that the test will not cause electrocution; however, there may be a slight, temporary discomfort when the needle electrodes are inserted. If pain persists for several minutes, the technician should be told.
- Instruct the client to follow the technician's instructions (i.e., to relax specified muscle(s) and to contract the muscle(s) when requested).

ELECTRONYSTAGMOGRAPHY (ENG)

Normal Findings.   Normal nystagmus, normal vestibular-ocular reflex

Description.   The test, electronystagmography (ENG), records eye movement at rest, with a change in head position, and in response to various stimuli. ENG determines the presence or absence of nystagmus (involuntary rapid eye movement). Nystagmus occurs as the result of vestibular-ocular reflex and is initiated by visual, positional, or caloric stimuli. The degree of nystagmus can be recorded electrically. If nystagmus does not occur, then the test is abnormal and the problem could be due to brain stem, cerebellum, vestibular-cochlear, or auditory nerve pathology. Abnormalities can be caused by ischemia, infection, tumors, or degeneration. The test also helps to differentiate peripheral from central vertigo. It can evaluate the cause of unilateral hearing loss, vertigo, and ringing in the ears. The unilateral hearing loss could be due to middle ear disorder or auditory nerve injury. If nystagmus occurs with stimulation, then the hearing loss is most likely caused by a middle ear problem and not an auditory nerve dysfunction.

Purposes
- To determine the normal response of nystagmus to various stimuli
- To differentiate between peripheral and central vertigo
- To identify that a brain stem, cerebellum, vestibular-cochlear, or auditory nerve pathology may be present because of an absence of nystagmus
- To determine whether the cause of unilateral hearing loss is from a middle ear problem or an auditory nerve injury

Clinical Problems
Abnormal findings: Brain stem lesion, cerebellum lesion, auditory nerve damage, middle ear problem, infection, ischemia to the area, head trauma, tumors, degeneration, unilateral hearing loss, Ménière's disease, congenital disorders

Procedure
- A signed consent form may or may not be needed. Check with the institution.
- Food may be restricted for 6 h before the test to prevent vomiting. Client should not drink caffeine or alcoholic beverages 24 h before the test.
- Test is usually performed in a dark room.

- Place electrodes on the skin at specified positions on both eyes.
- Ear should be free of earwax.
- Various procedures may be used to stimulate nystagmus, such as changing head position, pendulum tracking, changing gaze position, water caloric tests (instilling cold water and then warm water in the ears), optokinetics test (eye motion recorded as client stares straight ahead and then follows a target).
- Avoid CNS stimulants, CNS depressants, sedatives, and antivertigo agents 48 h before the test. A shorter or longer time may be indicated.

Factors Affecting Diagnostic Results
- Drugs: CNS stimulants can increase eye movement, and CNS depressants can decrease eye movement. Taking sedatives and antivertigo agents can affect test results
- A client who will not cooperate during the test
- Poor eyesight, blinking of the eyes
- Electrodes that are not properly applied or that become loose

Caution
- Test is contraindicated for clients with pacemakers.
- The water caloric test should not be performed in the ear canal if the client has a perforated eardrum.

Nursing Implications
- Obtain a history of the client health problems. Report if the client has dizziness prior to the test.
- Record baseline vital signs (VS)
- Note if the client appears cooperative to instructions. Noncooperation can cause false results.
- Ask the client if he/she has a pacemaker or a perforated eardrum. The test is contraindicated if any are present.

Client Teaching
- Inform the client that the room will be dark and electrodes will be placed around the eyes.
- Tell the client that nausea and vomiting may occur during the test. If this feeling occurs, the operator should be informed.

- Explain to the client that several positions and procedures may occur during the test. The client is asked to cooperate.
- Tell the client that bed rest may be ordered following the test if nausea or vertigo is present.
- Inform the client that the test takes 1 h or less.
- Be supportive to the client and answer questions or refer the unknown questions to health professionals.

ENDOSCOPIC RETROGRADE CHOLANGIOPANCREATOGRAPHY (ERCP)*

Normal Findings.   Normal biliary and pancreatic ducts

Description.   Endoscopic retrograde cholangiopancreatography (ERCP) is an endoscopic and X-ray examination of the biliary pancreatic ducts after contrast medium is injected into the duodenal papilla. The purpose of this procedure is to identify the cause of the biliary obstruction, which could be due to stricture, cyst, stones, or tumor. Jaundice is usually present.

ERCP is performed following abdominal ultrasound, CT, liver scanning, or biliary tract X-ray studies to confirm or diagnose hepatobiliary or pancreatic disorder.

Purposes
- To detect biliary stones, stricture, cyst, or tumor
- To identify biliary obstruction, such as stones or stricture
- To confirm biliary or pancreatic disorder

Clinical Problems
Abnormal findings: Biliary stones, stricture, cyst, or tumor; primary cholangitis; pancreatic stones, stricture, cysts or pseudocysts, or tumor; chronic pancreatitis; pancreatic fibrosis; or duodenal papilla tumors

---

*Updated by Dr. Warren G. Butt, Gastroenterology-Stomach-Colon-Liver, Newark, Delaware.

Procedure
- Obtain a signed consent form.
- Restrict food and fluids for 8 h before the test.
- Obtain baseline vital signs. Have the client void.
- Premedicate with mild narcotic or sedative. Atropine may be given prior to or after insertion of the endoscope.
- Local anesthetic is sprayed in the pharynx to decrease the gag reflex prior to the insertion of the fiberoptic endoscope.
- Secretin may be given IV to paralyze the duodenum. Contrast medium is injected after the endoscope is at the duodenal papilla and the catheter is in the pancreatic duct.
- Test takes 0.5 to 1 h.

Factors Affecting Diagnostic Results
- Inability to cannulate biliary and/or pancreatic duct.

Nursing Implications
- Obtain a client history of allergies to seafood, iodine, and contrast dye. Report allergic findings.
- Determine whether anxiety level may interfere with client's ability to absorb information concerning the procedure.
- Monitor the vital signs during the test and compare to baseline vital signs. Rupture within the GI tract caused by endoscope perforation could cause shock.

Client Teaching
- Inform client that the endoscope will not obstruct breathing.
- Explain that there may be a sore throat for a few days after the test.
- Be supportive of the client prior to and during the test procedure.

Post-test
- Monitor vital signs. A rise in temperature might indicate infection.
- Check skin color. Jaundice is an indicator of disease process.
- Check the gag reflex before offering food or drink.
- Check for signs and symptoms of urinary retention caused by atropine.

Client Teaching
- Suggest warm saline gargle and lozenges to decrease throat discomfort, which may persist for a few days after the test.

ENDOSCOPIC ULTRASOUND (EUS)*

Normal Findings.   Normal ultrasonographic views; no irregular borders

Description.   Endoscopic ultrasound (EUS) is an imaging technique that allows fine visualization of structures outside the gastrointestinal tract. An endoscope is attached to an ultrasound transducer providing both a view of the lumen and an ultrasound imaging of deeper structures. EUS is one of the newest diagnostic tests of ultrasonography that improves accuracy by reducing artifacts from anatomic structures and gas.

This technique is mostly utilized for early detection of cancer, staging of cancer, and visualization of the biliary tree. Fine-needle aspiration under EUS guidance allows for pathologic evaluations.

Purposes
- To detect and stage tumors
- To obtain pathology
- To visualize bile duct stones

Clinical Problems
Positive findings: Tumors, staging tumors, lymph node metastasis, bile duct stones

Procedure
- Food and fluids are restricted for 6–8 h before the test.
- Obtain a signed consent form before the procedure.
- Obtain vital signs (VS).
- Anesthesia is given. The scope is then introduced into the mouth or anus.
- Obtain a biopsy when indicated.

---

*Written by Dr. Warren G. Butt, Gastroenterology-Stomach-Colon-Liver, Newark, Delaware.

Factors Affecting Diagnostic Results
- Food in the stomach
- Prior surgery

Nursing Implications
- Obtain a history of prior surgery, especially cholecystectomy.
- Obtain a signed consent form. Discuss the risks of the procedure before client signs.
- Record client's vital signs before, during, and following the procedure.
- Determine the client's anxiety level to see if it may interfere with client's ability to absorb information.
- Remove dentures, glasses, and jewelry.

Client Teaching
- Explain the procedure to the client.
- Inform the client that the test will take approximately 1 h.
- Inform the client that his/her mouth may feel dry and the tongue may feel large or swollen. This will subside.
- Explain to the client that he/she may have a sore throat for a few days after the test. This is due to the endoscope. Suggest warm saline gargle and/or lozenges to decrease throat discomfort.

ESOPHAGEAL STUDIES*

ESOPHAGEAL ACIDITY, ESOPHAGEAL MANOMETRY, ACID PERFUSION (BERNSTEIN TEST)

Normal Finding.   Esophagus secretions of pH 5 to 6

Description.   Esophageal studies are performed mainly to determine pyrosis (heartburn) and dysphagia (difficulty in swallowing). Most esophageal problems result from a reflux of gastric juices into the lower

---

*Updated by Dr. Warren G. Butt, Gastroenterology-Stomach-Colon-Liver, Newark, Delaware.

part of the esophagus because of inadequate closure of the cardio-esophageal (low esophageal) sphincter.

Gastric secretions are highly acidic with a pH of 1.0 to 2.5, whereas the pH in the esophagus is 5.0 to 6.0. Backflow of gastric juices causes esophageal irritation or esophagitis. The three common esophageal studies are esophageal acidity, esophageal manometry, and acid perfusion (Bernstein test).

Esophageal acidity: A pH electrode attached to a catheter is passed into the lower esophagus to measure esophageal acidity. If there is no acid reflux, 0.1 N of HCl is instilled into the stomach. A pH less than 2.0 indicates acid reflux, caused mostly by an incompetent lower esophageal sphincter. The one-time measurement of esophageal acidity has largely been replaced by the 24-h pH monitoring.

24-h pH monitoring: A pH electrode probe is passed through the nostril into the lower esophagus to measure esophageal acidity. The probe is connected to a recording device, which is worn by the client. The client keeps a diary of all symptoms and activities as they occur and marks them by an indicator on the recorder. After 24 h the data is analyzed and interpreted.

Esophageal manometry: This test measures esophageal sphincter pressure and records peristaltic contractions. It detects esophageal motility disorder, such as achalasia (failure to relax GI tract smooth muscles, e.g., lower esophagus when swallowing). In achalasia, the baseline cardio-esophageal sphincter pressure may be as high as 50 mm Hg (baseline cardio-esophageal sphincter pressure is approximately 20 mm Hg), with a relaxation pressure of 24 mm Hg. Food and fluid cannot pass into the stomach until the weight of the contents is increased. With spasms of the esophagus, the sphincter is normal and peristalsis has irregular motility and force.

Acid perfusion (Bernstein test):   This test is useful to distinguish between gastric acid reflux causing "heartburn" or esophagitis, and cardiac involvement (e.g., angina, myocardial infarction). Saline and HCl (0.1 N) are dripped through tubing, one at a time, into the esophagus. If the client complains of symptoms of esophagitis (e.g., epigastric discomfort, heartburn) after 0.5 h of IV HCl drip, the diagnosis is usually acid reflux. Additional GI studies would be needed to confirm the diagnosis.

Purposes

- To distinguish between gastric acid reflux and cardiac involvement
- To diagnose gastric acid reflux
- To determine the cause of heartburn or difficulty in swallowing

Clinical Problems

Esophageal acidity: Incompetent lower esophageal sphincter, chronic reflux esophagitis

Esophageal manometry: Achalasia, spasm of esophagus, esophageal scleroderma

Acid perfusion: Esophagitis, epigastric pain or discomfort

Procedure

- Food and fluids are restricted 8 to 12 h prior to the test. Avoid alcohol intake 24 h prior to the test.
- Place client in high Fowler's position.
- Monitor pulse during test procedure to detect dysrhythmias from catheter insertion.
- Withhold antacids and autonomic nervous system agents for 24 h before the test with health care provider's approval.
- Withhold, proton pump inhibitors 1 week prior to the test.

Esophageal acidity: *One-time measurement*

- A catheter with pH electrode is inserted into the esophagus through the client's mouth.
- The client is asked to stimulate acid reflux by performing Valsalva's maneuver or lifting the legs.
- If there is no acid reflux, 300 ml of HCl 0.1 N is administered over 3 min, and the Valsalva's maneuver or lifting the legs is repeated.

Esophageal acidity: *24-h pH monitoring*

- NPO of solid foods for 8 h prior to the test.
- The catheter with the pH probe is inserted into the esophagus through the client's nostril.
- The probe is taped securely at the nose.
- Secure the recorder to the client's belt or provide a shoulder strap.

- The client records symptoms and activities in a diary and on the recorder over a 24-h period of time.

Esophageal Manometry

- A manometric catheter with a pressure transducer is inserted through the mouth into the esophagus.
- Esophageal sphincter pressure is measured before and after swallowing.
- Peristaltic contractions are recorded.

Acid Perfusion (Bernstein Test)

- A catheter is passed through the nose into the esophagus.
- Saline solution is dripped (6 to 10 ml/min) through the catheter. The client is told to indicate when pain occurs.
- HCl 0.1 N is dripped through the catheter for 0.5 h. The client is told to indicate when pain occurs.
- When pain or discomfort is reported, the HCl line is turned off, and saline solution is started until symptoms have subsided.

Factors Affecting Diagnostic Results

- Antacids, anticholinergics, H_2 antagonists, and proton pump inhibitors may increase the pH, thus reducing acidity and causing false test results.

Nursing Implications

- Explain the test procedure(s) to the client (see Procedure). Note the presence of anxiety and fear. Report findings.
- Monitor pulse and blood pressure during the procedure. Baseline vital signs should be recorded. Report irregularity of pulse rate immediately to the health care provider. Check for signs of respiratory distress during catheter insertion.

Client Teaching

- Instruct the client that food and fluids are restricted for 8 to 12 h before the test. Avoid alcohol for 24 h before the test.
- Instruct the client to sit in high Fowler's position for insertion of the catheter.

Esophageal Acidity
Client Teaching
- Inform the client that a catheter (with electrode) will be swallowed and the pH of the esophagus secretions are recorded.
- Tell the client to perform the Valsalva's maneuver (bear down and hold breath) or to lift legs to stimulate gastric acid reflux as directed by the health care provider.
- Instruct the client to inform the health care provider of any pain or discomfort.

Esophageal Acidity. *24-h pH monitoring*
Client Teaching
- Instruct the client to have a regular diet during the 24 h of recording unless otherwise indicated.
- Inform the client that a catheter with electrode will be inserted through the nostril and that the pH of the esophageal secretions will be recorded for 24 h.
- Instruct the client that a diary will be provided. Symptoms and activities should be noted in the diary at the time they occur.
- Instruct the client not to operate the microwave oven during the 24 h.
- Inform the client that the recorder should not get wet. A sponge bath rather than a shower is suggested.
- Instruct the client to return to the department in 24 h to have the probe removed.

Esophageal Manometry
Client Teaching
- Inform the client that a manometric catheter is to be swallowed. The esophageal pressure and peristaltic contractions are recorded.
- Instruct the client that drinking water may be requested (check with the health care provider first).

Acid Perfusion
Client Teaching
- Inform the client that a catheter is inserted through the nose into the esophagus.

- Tell the client there will be two IV solutions and that only one will be dripping into the catheter at a time.
- Instruct the client to inform the health care provider immediately when pain or discomfort occurs during the procedure.

ESOPHAGOGASTRODUODENOSCOPY, ESOPHAGOGASTROSCOPY

GASTROSCOPY, ESOPHAGOSCOPY, DUODENOSCOPY, ENDOSCOPY

Normal Findings.   Normal mucous membranes of the esophagus, stomach, and duodenum

Description.   Esophagogastroscopy includes gastroscopy and esophagoscopy. If duodenoscopy is included, the term is esophagogastroduodenoscopy. This test is performed under local anesthesia in a gastroscopic room of a hospital or clinic, usually by a gastroenterologist.

A flexible fiberoptic endoscope is used for visualization of the internal structures of the esophagus, stomach, and duodenum. Biopsy forceps or a cytology brush can be inserted through a channel of the endoscope. The major complications are perforation and hemorrhage.

Purposes
- To visualize the internal esophagus, stomach, and duodenum
- To obtain cytologic specimen
- To confirm the presence of gastrointestinal pathology

Clinical Problems
Esophageal: Esophagitis, hiatal hernia, esophageal stenoses, achalasia, esophageal neoplasms (benign or malignant), esophageal varices, Mallory-Weiss tear
Gastric: Gastritis, gastric neoplasm (benign or malignant), gastric ulcer, gastric varices
Duodenal: Duodenitis, diverticula, duodenal ulcer, neoplasm

Procedure
- Obtain a signed consent form.
- Restrict food and fluids for 8 to 12 h before test. Client may take prescribed medications at 6 AM on the day of the test.
- A sedative/tranquilizer, a narcotic analgesic, and/or atropine are given an hour before the test or are titrated IV immediately prior to the procedure and/or during the procedure.
- The client should not drive self home following test because of sedative.
- A local anesthetic may be used.
- Dentures, jewelry, and clothing should be removed from the neck to the waist.
- Record baseline vital signs.
- Test should *not* be performed within 2 days after a GI series.
- The test takes approximately 1 h or less.

Factors Affecting Diagnostic Results
- Barium from a recent GI imaging series can decrease visualization of the mucosa.

Nursing Implications
Client Teaching
- Explain the procedure. Inform the client that the instrument is flexible.
- Have the client void. Take vital signs.
- Explain that some pressure will be felt with the insertion of the endoscope. Fullness in the stomach when air is injected is usually noted.
- Be a good listener. Be supportive.

Post-test
- Keep the client NPO for 2 to 4 h after the test or as ordered. Check the gag reflex before offering food and fluids.
- Monitor vital signs frequently as indicated.
- Give throat lozenges or analgesics for throat discomfort. Inform client that flatus or belching is normal.

- Observe for possible complications, such as perforation in GI tract from the endoscope. These symptoms might include epigastric or abdominal pain, dyspnea, tachycardia, fever, subcutaneous emphysema.

FETAL NONSTRESS TEST (NST), CONTRACTION STRESS TEST (CST)*

Normal Finding.   Negative results

NST: Expressed as a reactive (reassuring) NST; evidenced by acceleration in fetal heart rate (FHR) occurring either spontaneously or in response to fetal movement in utero. The American College of Obstetricians and Gynecologists (ACOG) criteria for a reactive NST is the presence of two or more accelerations of fetal heart rate (FHR) of at least 15 beats per minute (bpm) or more. Above the baseline FHR of 120–160 bpm (each acceleration having a duration of at least 15 seconds) within a 20-min period of monitoring.

Reactive (reassuring) NST implies presence of adequate fetal oxygenation and an intact central and autonomic nervous system.

CST: Expressed as a negative (reassuring) test; evidenced by detecting *NO* late decelerations during a 10-min period when three "effective" quality contractions of 40 seconds or more occur. Additionally, the CST result is expressed as negative if contractions are 3 min apart, of palpable intensity, and of 40- to 60-seconds duration; the fetus shows no late decelerations.

Negative (reassuring) CST implies presence of uteroplacental sufficiency such that the fetus is considered likely to be able to withstand the stressors associated with labor contractions with decreased risk for intrauterine asphyxia.

Description.   The fetal nonstress test (NST) and the contraction stress test (CST) are two diagnostic tests used to help evaluate fetal functioning and well-being in response either to fetal movement (NST) or to spontaneous or induced uterine contraction (CST). The **NST** is inexpensive, is

---

*Jane Purnell Taylor, Associate Professor, Neumann College, Aston, Pennsylvania.

rapidly accomplished, lacks side effects, and is helpful in identifying at-risk fetuses of mothers who exhibit high-risk pregnancy conditions such as diabetes mellitus, intrauterine growth retardation, pregnancy-induced hypertension, decreased fetal movements, and others. Only minimal equipment is required (external transducer for fetal heart rate monitoring). Testing occurs 1 to 2 times per week depending on the reason for doing the testing.

The **CST** is usually employed at 32 to 34 weeks to evaluate high-risk pregnancies, particularly pregnancy conditions that may place the fetus at risk if there is poor placental perfusion, including diabetes, intrauterine growth retardation, and post-term gestation over 42 weeks. In addition, certain fetuses who exhibit a nonreactive NST in the presence of additional data may also have a CST performed. Contraindications to CST testing include presence of a classical uterine incision, presence of placenta previa, multiple gestation, and vaginal bleeding. Equipment required for CSTs includes an external transducer (for FHR monitoring), together with a toco-dynamometer (toco) for monitoring uterine contractions. The NST and CST may be performed in the hospital, office, and clinic settings. The NST may also be conducted in the home care setting with supervision.

Fetal nonstress test (NST): NST is a noninvasive test that monitors FHR with fetal movement. According to the ACOG, the FHR should increase by 15 bpm within a 20-min interval. If there is no fetal movement or increased FHR in 20 min, the mother's abdomen may be rubbed or a loud noise made close to the abdomen to stimulate fetal movement. If after 40 min there is no acceleration of FHR, the NST is nonreactive and a CST may be ordered. With a nonreactive NST after 40 min, fetal distress may be considered; however, the fetus may be in a sleep cycle or the mother may have taken a central nervous system depressant drug. The NST is usually performed at 30 weeks of gestation to allow for sufficient CNS maturation.

Contraction stress test (CST): There are two types of CST: the nipple stimulation test and the oxytocin challenge test (OCT). The nipple stimulation test is a noninvasive test that stimulates the hypothalamus which promotes the release of oxytocin. This can cause uterine contractions. A normal result would be that the FHR does not show late deceleration.

The OCT is somewhat noninvasive but could induce labor in some clients. Oxytocin, a uterine stimulant, is well diluted in IV fluids and thus does not cause continuous contractions. There should be three moderate contractions occurring within 10 min, and the FHR should not show any late deceleration. If there is a late deceleration of FHR with contractions, the test indicates that hypoxia may result during labor due to insufficient placental function. The CST with oxytocin is performed at 32 weeks, preferably 34 weeks of gestation.

Purposes
- To evaluate fetal functioning and well-being
- To evaluate sufficiency of uteroplacental function to support the fetus in labor
- To screen high-risk pregnancies

Clinical Problems
Abnormal findings: Fetal distress, fetal death, placental dysfunction

Procedure
- A signed consent form is required.
- Baseline vital signs are taken for future comparison.
- Position mother in semi-Fowler or lateral position with roll/wedge under right hip to displace uterus slightly to the left.
- Apply transducer (NST) or transducer and toco (CST).
- Monitor maternal blood pressure during the procedure for occurrence of hypotension.

Nonstress Test (NST)
- The client presses the pressure transducer when she feels the body move.
- Monitor for FHR acceleration. There should be 15 bpm (beats per minute) that last for 15 seconds. If the FHR does not increase, rub the mother's abdomen or thump/hit a pan that is close to her abdomen to stimulate fetal movement. If there is no fetal movement in 40 min and no acceleration in FHR, the test indicates a nonreactive fetus.

Contraction Stress Test (CST)
Nipple Stimulation
- The client stimulates one nipple with water-soluble ointment until a contraction occurs. Contraction should occur within 2 min, and if not, nipple stimulation could continue for 15 min.

- If there is no late deceleration in FHR, the test result is considered normal with deceleration of FHR during contraction, and the appropriate health care provider should be notified. It can indicate that the fetus is receiving insufficient blood supply from the placenta.

Oxytocin Challenge Test (OCT)
- Vital signs and FHR are taken at frequent intervals.
- NPO may be suggested in case labor begins.
- Administer oxytocin by IV infusion pump, dosage will be ordered. The oxytocin rate may be slowly increased until the client has a moderate contraction. If a contraction occurs before the oxytocin infusion, withhold the drug.
- A normal test result is a "no late" deceleration of FHR. If late deceleration occurs, it could indicate placental dysfunction that could cause the fetus to receive insufficient oxygen during labor.
- Monitor FHR for 30 to 60 min after oxytocin infusion has been stopped.
- Test takes approximately 1 to 2 h.

Factors Affecting Diagnostic Results
- NST is often nonreactive before 30 to 32 weeks due to central nervous system immaturity.
- NST may be classified as falsely nonreactive because of the occurrence of fetal sleep cycles.
- NST may be more commonly classified as falsely reactive in diabetic clients, post-term pregnancies, and pregnancy-induced hypertension associated with intrauterine growth retardation.
- NST may be falsely nonreactive when smoking has occurred prior to the NST and also in the event of CNS depressant drugs or beta blockers taken by the client.

Nursing Implications
- Obtain a gestation history from the client.
- Determine mother's knowledge level related to high-risk pregnancy condition and purposes of NST/CST testing.
- Attempt to schedule testing times at client's convenience; follow up on missed appointments.

- Monitor blood pressure and other vital signs at stated intervals consistent with agency protocols.
- Incorporate family into discussion and testing process as much as possible and desired.
- Position client correctly to prevent hypotension.
- Remain with the client during testing as often as possible if other supports are lacking.
- Report abnormal changes.

Client Teaching
- Use testing opportunity (NST) to teach importance of observing fetal movements.
- Encourage the client to rest following the test procedure.
- Inform the client to report bleeding, continuous contractions, and lack of fetal movement.

FETOSCOPY*

PERCUTANEOUS UMBILICAL BLOOD SAMPLING (PUBS), CORDOCENTESIS

Normal Findings.   Absence of abnormalities as presented in Clinical Problems, Abnormal Findings

Description
Fetoscopy: Fetoscopy is the direct visualization of the fetus by means of an endoscope inserted through the maternal abdominal wall into the uterine cavity for the purpose of obtaining blood or skin sample or for visualization of external developmental abnormalities. It is rarely used now for blood sampling due to 2% to 5% risk of serious complications. As a result of possible complications, this technique has evolved (particularly in high-risk perinatal center) into the increased use of percutaneous umbilical blood sampling or PUBS, which is known as cordocentesis.

---

*Prepared by Jane Purnell Taylor, MS, RN, Associate Professor, Neumann College, Aston, Pennsylvania.

Cordocentesis or PUBS: It is a technique in which an ultrasound-guided 22- to 26-gauge needle is used to puncture the umbilical cord to obtain fetal blood samples. Reports indicate that many operators find a site about 1 cm from the placenta to be an optimal site for obtaining fetal blood from the umbilical vein. Cordocentesis has been done as early as 12 weeks, but more commonly after 18 weeks until 36 weeks. Early procedures carry a higher risk to the fetus. The amount of blood removed is between 1 and 4 ml; after 20 weeks of gestation, 5 ml may be safely removed. Ultrasound is used to ascertain gestational age of the fetus, position of the fetus, the thickness and location of the placenta, position of tissues to be visualized or sampled, and placement of the needle tip used to obtain the sample. Although fetoscopy is less used today for purposes of fetal blood sampling, the endoscopic technique does allow for direct visualization of aspects of the fetus determined at risk for external abnormalities involving the spine, extremities, face, and genital areas. It may be preferred for skin biopsy sites including the back, thighs, or scalp to aid in the diagnosis of selected skin disorders of genetic origin unable to be otherwise detected. In the event that fetal blood sampling is desired but the umbilical cord is unable to be punctured to obtain fetal blood, a safe alternative for consideration is ultrasound needle-guided *fetal heart puncture.* These procedures, their benefits and risks for fetoscopy, cordocentesis (PUBS), or fetal heart puncture, should be discussed with the client and family.

Purposes

(Overall purpose is to aid in diagnosis, treatment, and monitoring fetal disease)

- To detect inherited blood disorders, including hemophilia A or B, hemoglobinopathies (measurement of hemoglobin concentration to assess fetal anemia), and fetal thrombocytopenia (measurement of fetal platelet count to assess and treat potential risks for perinatal cerebral bleeding)
- To perform rapid fetal karyotyping
- To detect fetal chromosome abnormalities
- To detect fetal infection, including CMV, toxoplasmosis, rubella
- To validate suspected fetal hypoxia or acidosis

- To treat fetal anemia by transfusion
- To assess and treat isoimmunization

Clinical Problems
Abnormal findings: Hemophilia A and B, fetal anemia, fetal thrombocytopenia, chromosome abnormalities, fetal hypoxia, fetal acidosis, fetal infection, isoimmune hemolytic disorders

Procedure (Cordocentesis)
- A consent form should be signed.
- Health care providers should schedule this diagnostic test within ready access to a room suitable for delivery if necessity should arise and decide whether to employ steroid therapy to the mother prior to the procedure.
- A respiratory support (anesthesiologist/anesthetist) should be available should the need arise.
- Monitor vital signs prior to and throughout the test.
- Position the mother to reduce occurrence of supine hypotension; she must remain still during the procedure.
- Ultrasound scanning of the abdomen is performed to visualize chosen area and identify an approach that will protect fetal parts and avoid maternal vessels.
- Local anesthetic is injected into the skin and onto the abdominal and uterine peritoneum.
- Use of prophylactic antibiotics varies by setting; rationale for use generally is to avoid amnionitis (infection to amniotic fluid).
- A paralytic drug, IV pancuronium bromide, may be used to prevent the fetus from moving during the sampling procedure.
- The mother may be given medication to assist her to relax during the procedure; however, it is important that the mother not become sedated to the point that she exhibits deep breathing. Deep breathing could, as a result of the movement created by her diaphragm, interfere with the puncture of the umbilical vein during the procedure.
- Ultrasound is used for confirmation that the needle tip is correctly placed in the umbilical vein (approximately 1 cm from the placental cord insertion site). This allows for removal of the stylet from the

needle and subsequent aspiration of designed quantity of blood into a syringe containing an anticoagulant.

Post-test
- Observe the puncture site (using ultrasound) for bleeding after removal of the needle.
- Employ fetal heart rate (FHR) monitoring for 30 min (minimal) postprocedure, followed by an additional ultrasound 1 h postprocedure to verify no evidence of bleeding/hematoma.

Factors Affecting Diagnostic Results
- Incorrect placement of needle tip resulting in need for additional manipulation; aspiration of sample at wrong time; amniotic fluid contamination of sample (the amniotic fluid has a coagulation effect); or failure to actually obtain a sample
- Amount of sedation received by mother, degree of hyperventilation, and adequacy of placental perfusion (as related to incorrect maternal positioning with resultant supine hypotension) may affect fetal oxygenation levels and outcome of diagnostic studies.
- Placement of sample into incorrect container or container having insufficient or incorrect anticoagulant; loss of portion of the sample; sample contamination; improper labeling of sample

Nursing Implications
- Obtain a history of the client's health problems, familial health disorders, medications, and any pregnancy past or present problems.
- Monitor vital signs. Monitor fetal heart rate (FHR).
- Monitor maternal anxiety level.
- Check medical record to determine if the mother is Rh negative and not sensitized, and if the father is Rh positive or negative or unknown. Plan to administer an IM injection of Rh IgG globulin (RhoGAM) following cordocentesis unless the mother is found to be previously sensitized.
- Discuss the benefits and risks to this procedure with the mother, the physician/health care provider, and the genetic counselor.
- Be available to answer questions and concerns, and if unable, refer the questions to other health professionals.

- Assist mother with proper positioning for the test; assist mother to relax using relaxation exercises and guided imagery.
- Prevent oversedation of the mother for the procedure to reduce chance of occurrence of deep breathing with diaphragm movement that may interfere during the puncture procedure.

Post-test

- Monitor the mother's vital signs and fetal heart rate.

Client Teaching

- Instruct client that she will be ultrasonically monitored for bleeding once the needle is removed.
- Instruct the mother to expect to have fetal monitoring for 30 min or more postprocedure.
- Instruct the mother that if intravascular pancuronium bromide (Pavulon) is used during the procedure, she may not detect the amount of fetal movement she has become accustomed to for a few hours.
- Instruct the Rh negative mother to expect, if not sensitized previously, that she will receive an injection of RhoGAM postprocedure.
- Instruct the client to report any pain or bleeding that might occur.
- Instruct her to rest for at least a day following the procedure and no heavy lifting.
- Encourage her to increase fluid intake.
- Inform her to notify the health care provider with any questions or concerns.

GASTRIC ANALYSIS

Normal Findings.   Fasting: 1.0–5.0 mEq/l/h
Stimulation: 10–25 mEq/l/h
Tubeless: detectable dyes in the urine

Description.   The gastric analysis test examines the acidity of the gastric secretions in the basal state (without stimulation) and the maximal secretory ability with stimulation (e.g., histamine phosphate, betazole hydrochloride [Histalog], pentagastrin). An increased amount of free hydrochloric acid could indicate a peptic ulcer, and an absence of free HCl (achlorhydria) could indicate gastric atrophy, probably caused by a malignancy or pernicious anemia. Gastric contents may be collected for cytologic examination.

Basal gastric analysis: Gastric secretions are aspirated through a nasogastric tube after a period of fasting. Specimens are obtained to evaluate the basal acidity of gastric content, and the gastric stimulation test follows.

Stimulation gastric analysis: The stimulation test is usually a continuation of the basal gastric analysis. A gastric stimulant (e.g., Histalog or pentagastrin) is administered, and gastric contents are aspirated every 15 to 20 min until several samples are obtained.

Tubeless gastric analysis: This test detects the presence or absence of hydrochloric acid (HCl); however, it will NOT indicate the amount of free acid in the stomach. A gastric stimulant (caffeine, Histalog) is given, and an hour later a resin dye (Azuresin, Diagnex Blue) is taken orally by the client. The free HCl releases the dye from the resin base; the dye is absorbed by the GI tract and is excreted in the urine. Absence of the dye in the urine 2 h later is indicative of gastric achlorhydria. This test method saves the client the discomfort of being intubated with a nasogastric tube; however, it does lack accuracy.

There is controversy over the usefulness of gastric acid secretory tests; however, they are still used to document gastric acid hypersecretions (e.g., Zollinger–Ellison syndrome and hypergastrinemia).

Purposes
- To evaluate gastric secretions
- To detect an increase or decrease of free hydrochloric acid

Clinical Problems
Decreased level: Pernicious anemia, gastric malignancy, atrophic gastritis
Elevated level: Peptic ulcer (duodenal), Zollinger–Ellison syndrome

Procedure
Basal and Stimulation
- Restrict food, fluids, and smoking for 8 to 12 h prior to the test.
- Anticholinergics, cholinergics, adrenergic blockers, antacids, steroids, alcohol, and coffee should be restricted for at least 24 h before the test.
- Baseline vital signs should be recorded.
- Loose dentures should be removed.
- A lubricated nasogastric tube is inserted through the nose or mouth.
- A residual gastric specimen and four additional specimens taken 15 min apart should be labeled with the client's name, the time, and specimen number.

Stimulation: Continuation of the basal gastric analysis
- A gastric stimulant is administered (i.e., betazole hydrochloride [Histalog] or histamine phosphate IM; pentagastrin subcutaneously).
- Several gastric specimens are obtained over a period of 1 to 2 h: histamine, four 15-min specimens in 1 h; and Histalog, eight 15-min specimens in 2 h. Specimens should be labeled.
- Vital signs should be monitored.
- The test usually takes 2.5 h for both basal and stimulation tests.

Tubeless Gastric Analysis
- Restrict food and fluids for 8 to 12 h before the test.
- AM urine specimen is discarded.
- Certain drugs are withheld for 48 h before the tests with health care provider's permission (e.g., antacids, electrolyte preparations [potassium], quinidine, quinine, iron, B vitamins).
- Give the client caffeine sodium benzoate 500 mg in a glass of water.
- Collect a urine specimen 1 h later. This is the control urine specimen.
- Give the client the resin dye agent (Azuresin or Diagnex Blue) in a glass of water.
- Collect a urine specimen 2 h later. The urine may be colored blue or blue-green for several days. Absence of color in the urine usually indicates absence of HCl in the stomach.

Factors Affecting Diagnostic Results
- Stress, smoking, and sensory stimulation can increase HCl secretion.

Nursing Implications

- Obtain a history of categories of drugs that can affect test results (e.g., antacids, antispasmodics, adrenergic blockers, cholinergics, and steroids).
- Monitor vital signs. Observe for possible side effects from use of stimulants (e.g., dizziness, flushing, tachycardia, headache, and decreased systolic blood pressure).
- Label the specimens (gastric or urine) with the client's name, date, and time.
- Be supportive of the client.

Client Teaching

- Explain the purpose and procedure of the tube or tubeless gastric analysis test to the client (see Procedure).
- Explain to the client how the nasogastric tube is inserted (through the nose or mouth) and that swallowing during its insertion will be requested.

GASTROINTESTINAL (GI) SERIES, UPPER GI AND SMALL-BOWEL SERIES, BARIUM SWALLOW, HYPOTONIC DUODENOGRAPHY

Normal Findings.   Normal structure of the esophagus, stomach, and small intestine, and normal peristalsis

Description.   Upper GI and small-bowel series are fluoroscopic and X-ray examinations of the esophagus, stomach, and small intestine. Oral barium meal (barium sulfate) or water-soluble contrast agent, meglumine diatrizoate (Gastrografin), is swallowed. By means of fluoroscopy, the barium is observed as it passes through the digestive tract, and spot films are taken. Inflammation, ulcerations, and tumors of the esophagus, stomach, and duodenum can be detected.

If increased peristalsis, a spastic duodenal bulb, or a space-occupying lesion is observed or suspected in the duodenal area during the GI series, a hypotonic duodenography procedure can be performed by giving glucagon, atropine, propantheline (Pro-Banthine), or like drug to slow down the action of the small intestine.

Purposes
- To detect an esophageal, gastric, or duodenal ulcer
- To identify polyps, tumor, or hiatal hernia in the GI tract
- To detect foreign bodies, esophageal varices, or esophageal or small-bowel strictures

Clinical Problems
Abnormal findings: Hiatal hernia; esophageal varices; esophageal or small-bowel strictures; gastric or duodenal ulcer; gastritis or gastroenteritis; gastric polyps; benign or malignant tumor of the esophagus, stomach, or duodenum; diverticula of the stomach and duodenum; pyloric stenosis; malabsorption syndrome; volvulus of the stomach; foreign bodies

Procedure
- Restrict food, fluids, medications, and smoking for 8 to 12 h before the test. A low-residue diet may be ordered for 2 to 3 days before the test.
- Withhold medications 8 h before the test unless otherwise indicated. Narcotics and anticholinergic drugs are withheld for 24 h to avoid intestinal immobility.
- Laxatives may be ordered the evening before the test.
- The client swallows a chalk-flavored (chocolate, strawberry) barium meal or meglumine diatrizoate (Gastrografin) in calculated amounts (16 to 20 oz).
- Spot films are taken during the fluoroscopic examination. The procedure takes approximately 1 to 2 h but could take 4 to 6 h if the test is to include the small-bowel series. A 24-h X-ray film, post-GI series, may be requested.
- A laxative is usually ordered after the completion of the test to rid the GI tract of barium.

Factors Affecting Diagnostic Results
- Excessive air in the stomach and small intestine

Nursing Implications
- Record vital signs. Note in the chart any epigastric pain or discomfort.

Client Teaching
- Inform the client that all of the chalk-flavored liquid must be swallowed. Tell client that the test should not cause pain or any discomfort.

Post-test
- Confirm with the radiology department that the upper GI series or small-bowel studies are completed before giving the late breakfast or late lunch.
- Administer the ordered laxative after the test. Inform the client that the stools should be light in color for the next several days. Barium can cause fecal impaction.

HOLTER MONITORING

AMBULATORY ELECTROCARDIOGRAPHY, DYNAMIC ELECTROCARDIOGRAPHY

Normal Finding.   No abnormal or insignificant ECG findings

Description.   Holter monitoring (ambulatory electrocardiography) evaluates the client's heart rate and rhythm during normal daily activities, rest, and sleep over 24 h (occasionally 48 h). For Holter monitoring, there is a continuous electrocardiogram (ECG) digital recording. The client is given a diary to record symptoms, such as palpitations, chest pain, shortness of breath, syncope, and vertigo, as well as the time of the symptoms. After 24 h the monitor with the tape and diary are returned to the cardiac center, and the tape is scanned or reviewed for abnormal findings, such as cardiac dysrhythmias.

The primary purpose of Holter monitoring is to identify suspected and unsuspected cardiac dysrhythmias which can be correlated between the recorder, event marking of symptoms, and transient symptoms marked in the diary. It is infrequently ordered for clients having Prinzmetal's variant angina, a form of myocardial ischemia, that results from spasms of the coronary arteries. Holter monitoring is more sensitive for identifying the cause of the symptoms than a routine electrocardiogram.

Purpose
- To identify cardiac dysrhythmias related to cardiac symptoms as marked on the monitor and recorded in the diary

Clinical Problems
Indications: Suspected and unsuspected cardiac dysrhythmias (supraventricular and ventricular), correlation of symptoms with the ECG tape, mitral valve prolapse causing dysrhythmia, hypertrophic obstructive cardiomyopathy causing atrial and ventricular dysrhythmias, and pacemaker dysfunction

Procedure
- No food or fluid restriction is required.
- The skin is cleansed, shaved as needed, and electrodes are placed over bony areas for eliminating artifacts that could be caused from skeletal muscle movement and insufficient attachment to the skin due to hair.
- Five to seven electrode patches are placed on the chest area.
- The client is given a diary to record the present activity when symptoms such as palpitations, chest pain, shortness of breath, and others occur.
- The client should not take a bath, shower, or swim until the electrodes are removed.

Post-test
- The client returns the Holter monitor the next day (24 h later) with the diary.
- The tape is scanned (reviewed) by the cardiologist and the diary reviewed. A written report is submitted to the client's health care provider.

Factors Affecting Diagnostic Results
- The client does not record activities correlated with symptoms in the diary.

Nursing Implications
- Check that a consent form has been signed.
- Record the client's history of cardiac disorders and/or symptoms.
- Check that a baseline ECG has been received. A comparison of the baseline ECG with the 24-h ECG monitoring could be requested.

Client Teaching
- Instruct the client that the monitor device will be attached either by a shoulder strap or as a belt.
- Review the procedure for Holter monitoring with the client (see Procedure).
- Emphasize the importance of pushing the event marker button on the monitor when symptoms occur and recording in the diary the time, symptoms, and activity that is present at the time of symptoms.
- Inform the client that the monitor should not get wet. Bathing, showering, and swimming should be avoided. The client should avoid using an electric razor or electric toothbrush during the 24 h of monitoring.
- Instruct the client to return the Holter monitor and diary the next day at approximately the same time the test was started.
- Explain to the client that the cardiologist or health care provider will discuss the findings with him or her.

HYSTEROSALPINGOGRAPHY (HYSTEROSALPINGOGRAM)

Normal Findings.   Normal structure of the uterus and patent fallopian tubes

Description.   Hysterosalpingography is a fluoroscopic and X-ray examination of the uterus and fallopian tubes. A contrast medium, either oil-based Ethiodol or Lipiodol, or water-soluble Salpix, is injected into the cervical canal. It flows through the uterus and into the fallopian tubes and spills into the abdominal area for visualizing the uterus.

The hysterosalpingogram should be done on the seventh to the ninth day after the menstrual cycle. The client should not be pregnant, have bleeding, or have an acute infection.

Ultrasonography is replacing hysterosalpingography, except that the latter test is more effective in determining tubal patency.

Purposes
- To identify uterine fibroids, tumor, or fistula
- To identify fallopian tube occlusion
- To evaluate repeated fetal losses

Clinical Problems
Abnormal findings: Uterine masses (e.g., fibroids, tumor), uterine fistulas, bleeding (e.g., injury), fallopian tube occlusion (e.g., adhesions, stricture), extrauterine pregnancy

Procedure
- Obtain a signed consent form.
- No food or fluid is restricted.
- A mild sedative (e.g., diazepam [Valium]) may be ordered prior to the test.
- A cleansing enema and douche may be ordered prior to the test.
- The client lies on an examining table in the lithotomy position. A speculum is inserted into the vaginal canal, and the contrast medium is injected into the cervix under fluoroscopic control. X-rays are taken throughout the 15- to 30-min procedure.

Nursing Implications
- Obtain a history of hypersensitivity to iodine, seafood, or previous use of contrast dye.
- Ask the client the date of her last menstrual period. If pregnancy is suspected, the procedure should not be done.
- Check for signs and symptoms of infection following the test, such as fever, increased pulse rate, and pain. If the client is at home, instruct her to call the health care provider to report these symptoms.

Client Teaching
- Inform client that some abdominal cramping and some dizziness may be experienced. Explain that it is normal; however, if it is continuous or if severe cramping occurs, the examiner should be notified.

- Encourage the client to ask questions and express concerns. Be a good listener.
- Inform client that there may be some bloody discharge for several days following the test. If it continues after 3 to 4 days, she should notify her health care provider.

HYSTEROSCOPY

Normal Finding.   Normal uterine cavity; normal endometrial uterine tissue

Description.   Hysteroscopy allows visualization of the entire endometrial cavity of the uterus. This test is considered more effective for viewing and obtaining endometrial pathology than the D & C (dilation and curettage) or hysterosalpingography. With D & C, scraping of the endometrial tissue is done without visualization, which may result in failure to obtain the pathologic tissue. With the use of the hysteroscope, a biopsy can be taken and polyp(s) removed.

Hysteroscopy is contraindicated if there is cervical or vaginal infection, pelvic inflammatory disease, or purulent vaginal discharge, or if cervical surgery had been performed previously. Risks of hysteroscopy include perforation of the uterus or infection.

Purposes
- To visualize the uterine cavity
- To obtain a biopsy of the endometrial lining of the uterus
- To remove a uterine polyp

Clinical Problems
Abnormal findings: Hyperplasia of the endometrial tissue in the uterus; endometrial cancer; polyps

Procedure
- Obtain a signed consent form.
- Food and fluids are restricted for 8 h prior to the test.

- The client is placed in the lithotomy position.
- A hysteroscope is placed through the cervical os into the endometrial cavity of the uterus. Carbon dioxide is usually instilled to distend the uterine cavity.
- Biopsy of tissue can be obtained.
- The test takes approximately 30 min.

Nursing Implications
- Obtain a menstrual history. The test should be performed after menstruation and prior to ovulation.

Client Teaching
- Explain the procedure to the client.
- Inform the client that discomfort following the carbon dioxide instillation is possible. Lower abdominal distention (uterus) and bloating can result.

Post-test
- Monitor vital signs.
- Check for excessive bleeding or discharge.

Client Teaching
- Inform the client that cramping or a slight vaginal bleeding may occur following the test for one to two days. Use of a mild analgesic decreases discomfort.
- Instruct the client to report severe discomfort, signs of a fever, heavy vaginal bleeding, or shortness of breath immediately to the health care provider.
- Tell the client that sexual intercourse or douching should be avoided for 2 weeks or as instructed by the health care provider.

INTRAVENOUS PYELOGRAPHY (IVP)

INTRAVENOUS PYELOGRAM, EXCRETORY UROGRAPHY

Normal Findings.   Normal size, structure, and functions of the kidneys, ureters, and bladder

Description.   Intravenous pyelography (IVP) visualizes the entire urinary tract. A radiopaque substance is injected IV, and a series of X-rays is taken at specific times. IVP is useful for locating stones and tumors and for diagnosing kidney diseases.

Purposes
- To identify abnormal size, shape, and functioning of the kidneys
- To detect renal calculi, tumor, cyst

Clinical Problems
Abnormal findings: Renal calculi, tumor, cyst, hydronephrosis, pyelonephritis, renovascular hypertension

Procedure
- Obtain a signed consent form.
- Restrict food and fluids for 8 to 12 h before the test.
- Give client a laxative the night before and a cleansing enema(s) the morning of the test. Check with radiology department for preparation.
- An antihistamine or a steroid may be given prior to the test for those who are hypersensitive to iodine, seafood, and contrast dye.
- Record baseline vital signs.
- The client lies in the supine position on an X-ray table. X-rays are taken 3, 5, 10, 15, and 20 min after the dye is injected.
- Emergency drugs and equipment should be available at all times.
- The test takes approximately 30 to 45 min.
- The client voids at the end of the test, and another X-ray is taken to visualize the residual dye in the bladder.

Nursing Implications
- Obtain a history of known allergies, especially to seafood, iodine preparations, or contrast dye.
- Check the BUN. If BUN levels are greater than 40 mg/dl, notify the health care provider.
- Report to health care provider if client had a recent barium enema or GI series, as these tests can interfere with IVP findings.

Client Teaching

- Inform client that a transient flushing or burning sensation and a salty or metallic taste may occur during or following the IV injection of contrast dye.
- Encourage the client to ask questions and to express any concerns.

Post-test

- Monitor vital signs and urinary output.
- Observe and report possible delayed reactions to the contrast dye (e.g., dyspnea, rashes, flushing, urticaria, tachycardia).
- Check the site where the dye was injected for irritation or hematoma. Apply warm or cold compresses as ordered.

LYMPHANGIOGRAPHY (LYMPHANGIOGRAM)

LYMPHOGRAPHY

Normal Findings.   Normal lymphatic vessels and lymph nodes

Description.   Lymphangiography is an X-ray examination of the lymphatic vessels and lymph nodes. A radiopaque iodine contrast oil substance (e.g., Ethiodol) is injected into the lymphatic vessels of each foot; the dye can also be injected into the hands to visualize axillary and supraclavicular nodes. Fluoroscopy is used with X-ray filming to check on lymphatic filling of the contrast dye and to determine when the infusion of the contrast dye should be stopped. The infusion rate is controlled by a lymphangiographic pump, and approximately 1.5 h are required for the dye to reach the level of the third and fourth lumbar vertebrae.

Other tests, such as ultrasonography, CT, and/or biopsy, may be used to confirm the diagnosis and to stage lymphoma involvement.

Lymphangiography is usually contraindicated if the client is hypersensitive to iodine or has severe chronic lung disease, cardiac disease, or advanced liver or kidney disease. Lipid pneumonia may occur if the contrast dye flows into the thoracic duct and sets up microemboli in the lungs.

Purposes
- To detect metastasis of the lymph nodes
- To identify malignant lymphoma
- To determine the cause of lymphedema
- To assist with the staging of malignant lymphoma

Clinical Problems
Abnormal findings: Malignant lymphoma (e.g., Hodgkin's disease), metastasis to the lymph nodes, lymphedema

Procedure
- Obtain a signed consent form.
- No food or fluid is restricted.
- Antihistamines and a sedative may be ordered prior to the test.
- Contrast dye (blue) is injected intradermally between several toes of each foot, staining the lymphatic vessels of the feet in 15 to 20 min. This is for visualization of the lymphatic vessels.
- A local skin anesthetic is injected, and small incisions are made on the dorsum of each foot.
- The contrast dye is slowly infused with the aid of the infusion pump. The client should remain still during the procedure. X-rays are taken of the lymphatics in the leg, pelvic, abdominal, and chest areas.
- Twenty-four hours later, a second set of films is taken to visualize the lymph nodes. X-ray filming usually takes 30 min. The contrast dye remains in the lymph nodes for 6 months to a year; thus, repeated X-rays can be taken to determine the disease process and the response to treatment.
- The procedure takes 2.5 to 3 h.

Nursing Implications
- Obtain a history of allergies to seafood, iodine preparations, or contrast dye used in another X-ray test.
- Record baseline vital signs.
- Have client void before test.

Client Teaching

- Inform the client that it is a prolonged procedure and that lying still during the test is essential. Give a sedative if one is ordered.
- Inform the client that the blue contrast dye discolors the urine and stool for several days and could cause the skin to have a bluish tinge for 24 to 48 h.
- Tell the client that the test takes about 2.5 to 3 h.

Post-test

- Monitor vital signs as indicated. Observe for dyspnea, pain, and hypotension, which could be due to microemboli from the spillage of the contrast dye.
- Assess the incisional site for signs of an infection (e.g., redness, oozing, and swelling).
- Check for leg edema. Elevate lower extremities as indicated.

MAGNETIC RESONANCE IMAGING (MRI)*

NUCLEAR MAGNETIC RESONANCE (NMR) IMAGING

Normal Findings.   Normal tissue and structure

Description.   Magnetic resonance imaging (MRI) produces cross-sectional images similar to those produced by CT; however, unlike CT, it does not use ionizing radiation and thus is free of the hazards presented by exposure to X-rays. The cost of MRI is approximately one-third more than the cost of CT.

The MRI scanner consists of a magnet encased in a large, doughnut-shaped cylinder. The client lies on a narrow table and is guided into the cylinder until the body part to be imaged is within the magnetic field. The hydrogen nuclei of the cells of the body respond like magnets to the magnetic field and align. When a radio frequency wave is applied, the protons in the nuclei resonate, and when the radio frequency wave is removed, the energy released by the protons as they relax is detected as a radio signal.

---

*Dr. Stephen Grahovac, Neurologist, Christiana Care, Newark, Delaware.

This signal is interpreted by a computer and translated into cross-sectional images.

Since the introduction of MRI in 1983, the quality of images produced by this technique has greatly improved, and the MRI is now the most sensitive technique for defining the structure of internal organs and for detecting edema, infarction, hemorrhage, blood flow, tumors, infections, and plaques on the myelin sheath that cause multiple sclerosis. Many of these conditions would be difficult to distinguish using CT or conventional X-rays. It can differentiate between edema and tumor. MRI excels in diagnosing pathologic problems associated with the central nervous system (CNS), such as tumors, hemorrhage, edema, cerebral infarction, and subdural hematoma. Early after an ischemic stroke, imaging can detect the stroke's location and extent, and can determine the severity of the damage to the brain tissue. MRI can visualize bone, joint, and soft tissue injuries. Bone artifacts do not occur and MRI can identify a tumor adjacent to or within bony structures, such as a pituitary gland tumor.

Pacemakers, wires left in the chest from a previous pacemaker, some aneurysm or some surgical intracranial clips, and certain hearing aids are contraindications to undergoing an MRI procedure. Jewelry, watches, keys, credit cards, hair clips, hearing aids, and mascara must be removed prior to the procedure. Insulin pump should be taken off. Piercing from any part of the body should be removed. When an emergency situation occurs during imaging, the client must be moved from the MRI room so that resuscitation equipment can be used. MRI is difficult to use to study critically ill clients on life-support systems because of the effect of the magnet on the equipment.

MRI and CT can be used for similar tissue studies. MRI involves use of contrast media in certain circumstances, but the IV contrast for MRI is chemically unrelated to the iodinated contrast used in CT and conventional radiography. Presently, the most commonly available contrast for MRI is gadolinium-DTPA. Gadolinium is frequently used to evaluate problems of the brain, base of the skull, and spine. This contrast agent can cross the "leaky" blood–brain barrier. Imaging can occur 5 to 60 min after the start of the gadolinium infusion.

Magnetic resonance of the brain and spine (intracranial IC-MRI): Intracranial MRI gives cross-sectional images of the brain and spine. It can detect neuropathology such as visualizing fluid (edema) within soft tissues. The IC-MRI can identify cerebral thrombosis caused by cerebral vascular accident (stroke), cerebral tumors, abscesses, aneurysms, cerebral hemorrhage, and demyclinated nerve fibers (myelin sheaths) causing multiple sclerosis (MS). It can also detail the abnormalities of the spinal cord and degenerated discs.

Magnetic resonance of the heart and coronary arteries: Cine MRI, or ultrafast MRI, is a fast-moving MRI procedure that can image the heart in a continuous motion. It is useful for perfusion imaging, and it can determine the patency of coronary arteries following coronary grafts. Also it is used to detect the viability of the myocardium and to assess heart chamber volumes. The echo-planar MRI (EPI), like cine MRI, is used for rapid imaging of the heart and coronary arteries.

Magnetic resonance angiography: Magnetic resonance angiography (MRA) is a noninvasive means of displaying vessels by imaging. It maximizes the signals in structures containing blood flow and reconstructs only the structures with flow. It is useful for evaluating vascular lesions. Other structures of lesser interest are subtracted from the image by the computer.

Magnetic resonance spectroscopy: This MRI is a scanner that can evaluate and detect ischemic heart disease and the effects of cancer treatment on tumor. It is especially useful in detecting residual tumors and radiation necrosis. It allows biochemical sampling of the tissue that is being imaged, so that one can distinguish between a demyclinating condition and a neoplasm versus an infection without need for a biopsy. It can also confirm the presence of Alzheimer's dementia, determine the extent of head injury due to trauma and stroke, and identify the cause of coma.

Purpose

- To detect abnormal masses, tissue structures and tears, neurologic and vascular disorders, fluid accumulation

Clinical Problems

Abnormal findings: Tumors, blood clots, cysts, edema, hemorrhage, abscesses, infarctions, aneurysm, plaque formation, demyclinating disease (e.g., multiple sclerosis), dementia, muscular disease, skeletal abnormalities, congenital heart disease, acute renal tubular necrosis (ATN), blood flow abnormalities

Procedure

- Obtain a signed consent form.
- No food or fluid is restricted for adults; NPO for 4 h for children.
- Remove all jewelry, including watches, glasses, hearing aids, hairpins, and any metal objects. Magnetic field can damage watches. Those with pacemakers are not candidates for MRI, and some with metal prosthetics (e.g., hip, knee) may not be candidates for MRI.
- Remove dentures as advised.
- Occupational history is important. Metal in the body, such as shrapnel or flecks of ferrous metal in the eye, may cause critical injury, such as retinal hemorrhage.
- With the closed MRI, the client must lie absolutely still on a narrow table with a cylinder-type scanner around the body area being scanned.
- Contraindications include pregnancy (not recommended in the first trimester of pregnancy). MRI could cause excess heat in the amniotic fluid.
- Sedation may be needed if the client, receiving closed MRI, is extremely claustrophic. A client receiving a sedative should not drive home; therefore, a family member or friend should be available to drive.
- Open MRI may be ordered for clients who are claustrophic, obese, confused, or a child; a family member or friend may be present. A mirror is available to see outside during the procedure. Clients need to remain still during the open MRI. Open MRI uses a lower-field magnet, whereas the closed MRI uses a higher-field magnet; hence lesser quality images are usually produced by open MRI.
- Certain MRI studies require a noniodinated contrast media (gadolinium Magnevist) which may be injected intravenously. Use of MR contrast media may be contraindicated for those with kidney dysfunction; the contrast media is excreted by the kidneys.
- The procedure takes approximately 45 min to 1.5 h.

Blood Flow: Extremities

- The limb to be examined is rested in a cradle-like support. Reference sites to be imaged are marked on the leg or arm, and the extremity is moved into a flow cylinder.
- The procedure takes approximately 15 min for arms and 15 min for legs.

Factors Affecting Diagnostic Results
- Movement during the procedure will distort the imaging.
- Ferrous metal in the body could cause critical injury to the client and distort the image.
- Nonferrous metal may produce artifacts that degrade the images.

Nursing Implications
- Ascertain from the client the presence of a pacemaker, previous pacemaker wire left in the body, any metal prosthetics, or shrapnel left in the body (such as in the eye) which could cause serious tissue injury as the result of the magnetic pull.
- Alert health care provider if client is on an IV pump. MRI can disrupt IV flow.
- Elicit any past problems for claustrophobia. Relaxation technique may need to be tried or a sedative used.
- Assess for body tattoos, especially red in color, for it may get warm during MRI.

Client Teaching
- Explain the procedure. Inform the client that various loud noises (clicking, thumping) from the scanner will be heard. Ear plugs are available. Inform client that the MRI personnel will be in another room but can communicate via an intercom system. With the open MRI, a family member or friend may be in the room with the client while the MRI scanning is taking place. This is also possible with closed MRI.
- Explain that there is no exposure to radiation.
- Instruct the client to remove watches, credit cards, hairpins, jewelry, and makeup. Magnetic field can damage a watch.
- Inform the client that the MRI procedure is painless.
- Inform the client who has metal fillings in teeth that a "tingling sensation" may be felt during imaging.
- Caution clients with cardiac pacemakers not to approach the MRI unit.

MAMMOGRAPHY (MAMMOGRAM)

Normal Findings.   Normal ducts and glandular tissue; no abnormal masses

Description. Mammography is an X-ray of the breast to detect cysts or tumors. Benign cysts are seen on the mammogram as well-outlined, clear lesions that tend to be bilateral, whereas malignant tumors are irregular and poorly defined and tend to be unilateral. A mammogram can detect a breast lesion approximately 2 years before it is palpable.

There have been technical improvements in the equipment, mammographic units, and the recording system used for mammography. The use of radiographic grids has improved the imaging quality of mammograms by decreasing image density. With the use of grids, the visibility of small cancers is increased. Also, the use of magnification mammography has improved the capability to identify cancers; however, the magnification increases the client's radiation dose by prolonging exposure time.

The American Cancer Society and the American College of Radiologists have suggested that women between 35 and 40 years have a mammogram every 2 years and that women over 40 years have an annual mammogram. Radiation received is very low dose.

Purposes
- To screen for breast mass(es)
- To detect breast cyst or tumor

Clinical Problems
Abnormal finding: Breast mass (cyst or tumor)

Procedure
- Food and fluids are not restricted.
- The client removes clothes and jewelry from the neck to the waist and wears a paper or cloth gown that opens in the front. Powder and ointment on the breast should be removed to avoid false-positive result.
- The client is standing, and each breast, one at a time, rests on an X-ray cassette table. As the breast is compressed, the client will be asked to hold her breath while the X-ray is taken. Two X-rays are taken of each breast from different angles.
- The procedure takes about 15 to 30 min.

Nursing Implications

- Ascertain whether the client is pregnant or suspected of being pregnant. Test is contraindicated during pregnancy.
- Ask the client to identify the lump in the breast if one is present.

Client Teaching

- Instruct client not to use ointment, powder, or deodorant on the breast or under the axilla on the day of the mammogram.
- Inform the client not to be alarmed if an additional X-ray is needed.
- Be supportive of the client. Allow the client time to express her fears and concerns.
- Encourage the client to self-examine the breast every month. If premenopausal, breast examination should be done after menstrual period. Demonstrate breast examination if necessary.

MULTIGATED ACQUISITION (MUGA) SCAN

Normal Findings.   Normal heart size, ventricular wall motion, and ejection fractions

Description.   MUGA scan is a rapid, safe method to evaluate the heart size, ventricular wall motion, and ejection fraction. The client's blood is tagged with a radioactive tracer, such as technetium-99m, which permits the heart and its function to be visualized. There is multiple imaging during acquisition (MUGA) scanning. Gated refers to the synchronizing of images with the client's ECG and the computer. MUGA identifies changes occurring with contraction and expansion of the ventricles of the heart. With cardiac disease, there may be reduced ability of the heart to pump blood sufficiently.

Because a radioactive substance is used with the test, the MUGA is a nuclear medicine (scan) procedure. The amount of radiation exposure used is comparable to that of a CT scan. MUGA may be performed with the stress test.

Purposes

- To evaluate the heart's size, ventricular wall motion, and ejection fraction
- To evaluate the effect of an acute myocardial infarction for prognosis
- To evaluate cardiovascular disease
- To detect ventricular aneurysm
- To evaluate pharmaceutical and chemotherapy response

Clinical Problems

Abnormal findings: Congestive heart failure (CHF), valvular disease (regurgitation), ventricular aneurysm, acute myocardial infarction, cardiac ventricular dysfunction

Procedure

- No food or fluid restriction is required.
- A pyrophosphate material which tags to the red blood cells is injected intravenously. A second IV injection of a radioactive tracer is given.
- ECG electrodes are attached and the ECG is monitored.
- Client is in a supine position with a gamma camera over the chest. The radioactive tracer (contains no dye) allows visualization of the heart and its function.

Nursing Implications

- Obtain a history of drugs (e.g., heparin) the client is taking. They may interfere with the test result.
- Monitor vital signs and ECG.

Client Teaching

- Explain the MUGA test procedure (see Procedure).
- Answer client's questions and refer unknown answers to appropriate health professionals.

NUCLEAR SCANS (BONE BRAIN, BRAIN PERFUSION, HEART, KIDNEY, LIVER AND SPLEEN, COLON AND OVARY, GASTROESOPHAGEAL REFLUX, GASTROINTESTINAL BLEEDING, GASTRIC EMPTYING, GALLBLADDER, LUNG, AND THYROID STUDIES)*

RADIONUCLIDE SCANS, RADIOISOTOPE IMAGING

Normal Finding.   Normal; no observed pathology

Description.   Nuclear medicine is the clinical field concerned with the diagnostic and therapeutic uses of radioactive isotopes. A radioactive isotope is an unstable isotope that decays or disintegrates, emitting radiation. Radioisotopes, known as radionuclides, concentrate in certain organs of the body and are distributed more readily in diseased tissues. Scintillation (gamma) camera detectors are used for imaging. Equal or uniform gray distribution is normal, but lighter or brighter areas, referred to as *hot spots,* indicate hyperfunction, and darker areas, *cold spots,* indicate hypofunction. **Note:**   The hot spots can be lighter or darker areas depending on the equipment, display of the images, and the film. Hyperfunction or hot spots, means that more of the tracer is concentrated in the area and can be displayed as light spots on a black screen or as dark spots on a white screen.

There are two types of imaging systems: (1) planar imaging, which projects images acquired from two or three different angles, and (2) single photon emission computed tomography (SPECT), in which the scintillation camera rotates and projects images in an arc of 180° (for cardiac imaging) to 360°, acquiring 32 or more images. The advantage of SPECT over planar imaging is that with SPECT the images are not obscured by overlying organs, tissue, or bone. SPECT uses a conventional Anger camera detector head with a collimator (the part of the camera that absorbs photons) which fits in a rotating gantry. This camera orbits around the

---

*Updated by Cindy Knotts, BS, CNMT, Supervisor Nuclear Medicine, Christiana Care Health Services, Newark, Delaware.

client lying on a special table. Also with SPECT, the images are enhanced with computer processing. The use of a two- or three-headed imaging gamma camera increases the sensitivity and specificity of the SPECT system. With the use of filtering and three-dimensional computer reconstruction of the images, the data analysis can be of great diagnostic value. Nuclear medicine imaging is moving toward a new era with the use of high-speed computers, and new radiopharmaceuticals.

The use of radionuclides as radiopharmaceuticals is considered safe. The radionuclide used in most studies is technetium 99m (Tc-99m), which accounts for 70% of the nuclear imaging procedures. Other radionuclides include, iodine 123 (I-123), thallium (T-201), xenon (Xe-133), indium 111 (In-111)-labeled white blood cells, and gallium (Ga-67) citrate.

Positron emission tomography (PET) is discussed separately in the text.

Clinical Problems

Test	Indications/Purposes
Bone	To detect early bone disease (osteomyelitis); carcinoma metastasis to the bone; bone response to therapeutic regimens (e.g., radiation therapy, chemotherapy)
	To determine unexplained bone pain
	To detect fractures and abnormal healing of fractures; degenerative bone disorders
Brain	To detect an intracranial mass and disorder: tumors, abscess, cancer metastasis to the brain, head trauma (subdural hematoma), cerebrovascular accident (stroke), aneurysm
Brain perfusion study	To diagnose Alzheimer's disease, brain death, AIDS dementia
	To detect frontotemporal dementia (Pick's disease)
	To locate seizure foci
	To determine the location and size of cerebral ischemia
Heart (cardiac) MUGA	To identify cardiac hypertrophy (cardiomegaly)
	To quantify cardiac output (ejection fraction) wall motion
	To detect coronary artery disease (CAD)
	To detect congestive heart failure (CHF) or an aneurysm

(continued)

Test	Indications/Purposes
Kidney	To detect parenchymal renal disease: tumor, cysts, glomerulonephritis, urinary tract obstruction
	To evaluate differential function for renovascular hypertension
	To assess the function of renal transplantation
Liver and spleen	To detect tumors, cysts, or abscesses of the liver and spleen, hepatic metastasis, splenic infarct
	To assess for chronic liver or spleen disease including metastasis, jaundice, cirrhosis, hepatocellular disease, hepatitis, or elevated laboratory results
	To assess liver response to therapeutic regimens (e.g., radiation, chemotherapy)
	To identify hepatomegaly and splenomegaly
	To identify liver position and shape
Lung	To detect pulmonary emboli, tumors, pulmonary diseases with perfusion changes (e.g., emphysema, bronchitis, pneumonia)
	To assess arterial perfusion changes secondary to cardiac disease
Colon and ovary (monoclonal antibodies for cancer)	To detect colon and ovarian cancer cells in the body
Gastrointestinal bleeding study	To detect the localization of gastrointestinal and nongastrointestinal bleeding sites
Gastric emptying study	To diagnose gastric obstruction and the cause of dysmotility
Gastrointestinal reflux	To detect esophageal reflux syndrome
Gallbladder study (CCK hepato-biliary)	To diagnose acute or chronic cholecystitis, cystic or common bile duct obstruction
	To evaluate for biliary dyskinesia
	To evaluate after gallbladder surgery for suspected biliary leakage
	To detect hypercholestasis conditions
Lung	To detect pulmonary emboli; tumors, pulmonary diseases with perfusion changes (e.g., emphysema, bronchitis, pneumonia, COPD)
	To detect right to left cardiac shunt
	To assess arterial perfusion changes secondary to cardiac disease

Test	*Indications/Purposes*
Thyroid	To detect thyroid mass (tumors), diseases of thyroid gland (Graves', Hashimoto's thyroiditis)
	To determine the size, structure, and position of the thyroid gland
	To evaluate and manage thyroid cancer
	To evaluate thyroid function resulting from hyperthyroidism and hypothyroidism

Procedure.   The radionuclide (radioisotope) is administered orally or IV. The interval from the time the radionuclide is given to the time of imaging can differ according to the radionuclide and organ in question. Normally, masses such as tumors absorb more of the radioactive substance than does normal tissue.

For diagnostic purposes, the dose of radionuclide is low (less than 30 mCi) and should have little effect on visitors, other clients, and nursing and medical personnel. There are some food, fluid, and medication restrictions with some procedures. Check with the nuclear medicine staff first.

The procedures for the organ scans are listed according to the radionuclides used, the method of administration, the waiting period after injection, the food and fluid allowed, and other instructions.

Bone

- Radionuclides: technetium (Tc)-99m-labeled phosphate compound (Tc-99m diphosphonate)
- Administration: IV
- Waiting period after injection: 2 to 4 h after injection before imaging
- Food and fluids: no restrictions; for Tc-99m, water is encouraged during the waiting period (six glasses)
- Other instructions: Void before imaging begins. Remove metal objects, jewelry, keys. Scanning occurs 2 to 4 h after IV radionuclicide injection and takes 0.5 to 1 h. A sedative may be ordered if the client has difficulty lying quietly during imaging.

Brain: Radionuclide brain scanning is very effective for identifying metastatic disease, strokes, subdural abscesses, and hematomas.

- Radionuclides: Tc-99m-glucoheptonate, Tc-99m-O$_4$, Tc-99m-DTPA (diethylenetriamine penta-acetic acid), Tl-201 NaCl, Tc-99m-HMPAO (Ceretec), Tc-99m-ECD (Neurolite)
- Administration: IV
- Waiting period after injection: Tc-99m-O$_4$, 1 to 3 h; Tc-99m-DTPA, 45 min to 1 h. With Ceretec or Neurolite, imaging is started immediately. Frequently a few images are taken before the waiting period is over
- Food and fluids: No restrictions
- Other instructions: With Tc-99m-O$_4$, 10 drops of Lugol's solution are given the night before or at least 1 h before the scan, or potassium perchlorate 200 mg to 1 g given 1 to 3 h before brain scan. These agents block the uptake of Tc-99m-O$_4$ in the salivary glands, thyroid, and choroid plexus. Blocking agents are not needed with the other radionuclide. The client should remain still during the imaging (0.5 to 1 h).

Brain perfusion study: Perfusion study to diagnose Alzheimer's disease, locate seizure foci and cerebral ischemia, Parkinson's disease

- Radionuclides: Tc-99m-hexamethylpropyleneamineoxime (Tc-99m-HM-PAO), Tc-99m-ECD (ethyl cysteinate dimer) neurolite
- Administration: IV
- Waiting period after injection: 45 to 60 min after the injection
- Food and fluids: No restriction
- Other instructions: Imaging room should be quiet and lights dimmed. IV line should be inserted before the test. Client lies still 15 min before the Tc-99m-HM-PAO injection. During imaging the client is in supine position with the head in a head holder. The entire brain, including the cerebellum, is imaged.

Heart (cardiac) MUGA: *(For myocardial perfusion imaging studies with stress imaging, see Stress/Exercise Tests.)*

Multigated acquisition (MUGA) scanning is a rapid, safe method to evaluate the heart size, ventricle wall motion, and ejection fraction. The client's blood is tagged with a radioactive tracer, such as technetium-99m, which permits the heart and its function to be visualized. There is multiple imaging during MUGA scanning. MUGA identifies changes occurring with contraction and expansion of the ventricles of the heart. With cardiac disease, the heart's ability to pump blood sufficiently may be reduced. The amount of radiation exposure is comparable to that of a CT scan.

- Radionuclides: Tc-99m-O_4 tagged red blood cells (RBCs)
- Administration: IV
- Waiting period after injection: None
- Food and fluids: None
- Other instructions: The electrocardiogram is monitored. The client is in a supine position with a gamma camera over the chest. The radioactive tracer (containing no dye) allows visualization of the heart and its function.

Heart

- Radionuclides: Tc-99m-pyrophosphate or Tc-99-m-pertechnetate. To confirm if a myocardial infarction (MI) occurred. This test is ordered 2 to 6 days after a suspected myocardial infarction. Tc-99m-labeled RBCs or albumin are used for ejection fraction studies (MUGA)
- Administration: IV
- Waiting period after injection: Tc-99m, 30 min to 1 h
- Food and fluids: NPO may be required from midnight to study
- Other instructions: Client lies quietly for 15 to 30 min during the imaging for a myocardial infarction.

Kidney: For renal blood-flow (renogram) studies and imaging. Two drugs may be used with renal imaging: furosemide (Lasix) for determining renal excretory function, and captopril for identifying renovascular hypertension.

- Radionuclides: Tc-99m-pertechnetate, Tc-99m-glucoheptonate for renal cortical and tubular disorders; Tc-99 diethylenetriamine penta-acetic acid (Tc-99m-DTPA) for evaluating renal function and perfusion disorders; Tc-99m glucoheptonate and I-131 hippuran (for renal perfusion studies); Tc-99m mercaptoacetyltriglycerine (Tc-99m-MAG3) for evaluating renal clearance related to renal insufficiency
- Administration: IV
- Waiting period after injection: Renal perfusion study: Imaging is done immediately after the radiopharmaceutical is given intravenously. Renogram curves are plotted. Renal cortical studies could require delay images up to 24 h.

- Foods and fluids: No restrictions. The client should be well hydrated. Drink 2 to 3 glasses of water 30 min before the scan. Dehydration could lead to false test results.
- Other instructions: Void before the scan. If the client had IVP, the renogram or scan should be delayed 24 h. Lugol's solution, 10 drops, may be ordered if I-131 hippuran is given. Client lies quietly for 30 min to 1 h during imaging.

Liver and spleen: Liver imaging can detect 90% of hepatic metastases and 85% of hepatocellular diseases. It is useful for screening the liver and spleen for lacerations and hematomas following trauma. SPECT improves lesion/mass detection.

- Radionuclides: Tc-99m compounds: Tc-99m-sulfur colloid
- Administration: IV
- Waiting period after injection: Tc-99m-sulfur colloid, 15 min. Spleen scan can be done at the same time.
- Food and fluids: no restrictions. NPO after midnight may be ordered
- Other instructions: Client lies quietly for 30 min to 1 h during the imaging. Client may be asked to turn from side to side and onto abdomen during imaging.

Colon and ovary: The use of radiolabeled monoclonal antibodies: used to identify colon and ovarian cancer cells in areas of the body. The radio-labeled monoclonal antibodies attach to cancer cells. The cancer cells can then be detected with use of a gamma camera.

- Radionuclides: Monoclonal antibodies labeled with 111 Indium (111 In)
- Administration: IV. Infusion takes 5 to 30 min
- Waiting period after injection: 1 to 5 days after radiolabeled mono-clonal antibodies. Usually, two sets of images are taken at different times using the nuclear gamma camera.
- Food and fluids: Light breakfast or lunch
- Other instructions: Regular medications can be taken. Client voids prior to the test. Allergic reaction to the monoclonal antibodies, though uncommon (less than 4%), may occur. Monoclonal antibod-ies are obtained from mice (human cancer cells are injected in the mice to produce antibodies).

Gastroesophageal reflux: Esophageal clearance is determined follow-ing a swallowed radioactive tracer. Numerous esophageal tests, such as endoscopy, barium esophagoscopy, and acid reflux testing may be performed to detect esophageal reflux syndrome. The radionuclide gastroesophageal reflux scan is highly sensitive (99%) for esophageal reflux.

- Radionuclides: Solution containing 150 ml of orange juice, 150 ml of 0.1 N hydrochloric acid, and 300 µCi Tc-99m sulfur colloid (Tc-99m-SC). Child: 250 µCi Tc-99m-SC in 10 ml of sterile water via a feeding tube
- Administration: Orally
- Waiting period: 30 seconds
- Food and fluids: Fasting for at least 4 h prior to the study
- Other instructions: The client is in an upright or supine position. The procedure may require that the client perform a Valsalva maneuver.

Gastrointestinal (GI) bleeding: Upper GI bleeding sites are more difficult to detect than lower GI bleeding sites. Tc-99m-labeled (tagged) RBCs are most effective for detecting active bleeding sites. The radionuclide GI bleeding study is more sensitive than angiography. For a positive test result and accurate identification of the bleeding site, the client must be actively bleeding at the time of imaging.

- Radionuclides: Tc-99m-labeled RBCs
- Administration: Intravenously by bolus injection. For Tc-99m-labeled (tagged) RBCs, withdraw 1 to 3 ml of whole blood into a shielded syringe containing Tc-99m sodium pertechnetate. After processing the blood, Tc-99m-labeled RBCs are injected as a bolus.
- Waiting period after injection: Imaging begins immediately after injection or until the site of bleeding is located. If negative after 2 h, imaging may be repeated when client begins active bleeding or imaging at different time periods during the 24 h after injection.
- Food and fluids: NPO unless otherwise indicated
- Other instructions: Client is in supine position. Imaging is usually over the abdominal and pelvic areas. This test may be done as an emergency study, pre-surgery to locate the site of gastric bleeding, or pre-angiography.

Gastric emptying: Delayed gastric emptying could be due to acute disorders, such as trauma, postoperative ileus, gastroenteritis, or chronic disorders, such as diabetic gastroparesis, peptic ulcers, pyloric stenosis, and Zollinger–Ellison syndrome.

- Radionuclides: 111 In DTPA or Tc-99m-labeled juice and Tc-99m AC-labeled eggs
- Administration: Client ingests scrambled egg sandwich and juice (all radiolabeled). Tc-99m-sulfur colloid–labeled instant oatmeal may be ordered instead of eggs.
- Waiting period after oral meal: Immediately after ingesting the oral meal and continuously for 1 h. A 2-h imaging may also be requested following the oral meal.
- Food and fluids: NPO for 4 h and no smoking prior to the test
- Other instructions: Client is in a mid-Fowler's position for the meal and during imaging. The test should be performed in the morning because during the day the gastric emptying time can vary.

Gallbladder (hepatobiliary scan): Hepatobiliary radioactive scanning is more sensitive for diagnosing acute cholecystitis than other standard gallbladder diagnostic tests. With hepatobiliary scanning, accurate imaging of the biliary tract can be performed even when there is marked hepatic dysfunction and jaundice.

- Radionuclides: Tc-99m disofenin, Tc-99m mebrofenin, or other Tc-IDA derivatives.
- Administration: IV. Cholecystokinin (CCK), a hormone that stimulates the gallbladder (GB) to contract and empty, may be used with normal saline solution as an infusion to promote GB emptying for imaging purposes
- Waiting period after injection: Immediate after CCK and radionuclide infusions
- Food and fluids: NPO for 4 h before the test with use of CCK
- Other instructions: Usually CCK is given pre-radiopharmaceutical injection to stimulate the gallbladder of clients who have not eaten. CCK is short acting (20 to 30 min). Normal value for gallbladder ejection fraction (GBEF%) is greater than 35%. Lower values indicate chronic cholecystitis. Higher values usually indicate hypercholestasis conditions. Nausea and abdominal discomfort may occur for a few minutes after the CCK infusion.

Lung (pulmonary) (V/Q): Lung perfusion and ventilation scannings are sensitive for detecting pulmonary emboli (PE), and obstructive pulmonary disease. Both types of lung scans may be performed to identify the pulmonary disorder.

- Radionuclides: Perfusion study: TC-99m compounds: macroaggregated albumin (Tc-99m-MAA), Tc-99m human albumin microspheres (Tc-99m-HAM). Ventilation study: Xe-133 (more commonly used), Xe-127 (not commonly used), krypton (Kr) 81m, and Tc-99m-DTPA aerosol
- Administration: Intravenously (perfusion) or inhaled (ventilation)
- Waiting period after injection: Tc-99m compounds, 5 min after the injection of the radionuclide
- Food and fluids: No restrictions
- Other instructions: A chest radiograph is usually ordered for comparison with the nuclear medicine study. The ventilation and perfusion lung scan procedure takes 30 min. The camera moves around the client to take multiple images.

Thyroid: Thyroid scintigraphy is effective for determining the functional status of the thyroid nodules and for detecting post-thyroidectomy residual thyroid tissue and metastases. Radioactive iodine is the most frequently used radionuclide because iodine is easily taken up in the thyroid gland. Iodine is a precursor in thyroid hormone synthesis.

- Radionuclides: I-131 sodium iodide, I-123, Tc-99m-pertechnetate
- Administration: I-123, I-131 (orally). I-123 has a short half-life and is the choice radionuclide. Tc-99m-pertechnetate (IV)
- Waiting period after injection: I-123, I-131—2 to 24 h. I-123 is the radionuclide most commonly used because it has a shorter half-life. Tc-99m-pertechnetate, 30 min.
- Food and fluids: No breakfast and NPO for 2 h following oral iodine
- Other instructions: Three days before the scan (imaging), iodine preparations, thyroid hormones, phenothiazines, corticosteroids, aspirin, sodium nitroprusside, cough syrups containing iodides, and multivitamins are usually discontinued with health care provider's permission. Sea foods and iodized salt should be avoided. If the drugs cannot be withheld for 3 days, the drugs should be listed on the nuclear medicine request slip. The client should lie quietly for 30 min during the imaging procedure.

Factors Affecting Diagnostic Results

- Two radionuclides administered in one day may interfere with each other.

• Too short or too long a waiting period after injection of the radio-nuclide could affect test results.

Nursing Implications

• Explain to the client the purpose and procedure for the ordered study. Procedures will differ according to the type of study (see Procedure).
• In some cases, food and fluids are not restricted but check with the nuclear medicine staff about preparations. For the bone scan (Tc-99m), water is encouraged during the waiting period. For the renal scan, the client should be well hydrated before the scheduled scan. Blocking agents, for example, Lugol's solution and potassium perchlorate, are usually ordered before studies that use radioiodine, except for the thyroid scan.
• Check if a consent form is needed. Usually a consent form is not needed unless the radionuclide is greater than 30 mCi.
• Obtain a brief health history in regard to recent exposure to radioiso-topes, allergies that could cause an adverse reaction, being pregnant, breastfeeding, and drugs.
• Adhere to the instructions from the nuclear medicine laboratory con-cerning the client and the procedure. The client should arrive on time.
• Report to the health care provider if the client is extremely appre-hensive.
• Be supportive to the client. Advise the client to ask questions and to communicate concerns.
• List restricted drugs containing iodine that the client is taking on the request slip. This is important if the radionuclide is iodine.

Client Teaching

• Explain that the dose of radiation from radionuclide imaging is usually less than the amount of radiation received from diagnostic X-ray.
• Inform client and family that the injected radionuclide should not affect the family, visitors, other clients, or hospital staff members. The radionuclide is excreted from the body in about 6 to 24 h.
• Explain that the detection equipment will move over a section or sections of the body. No physical discomfort should be felt.

- Inform the client that the scanning may take 30 min to 1 h, depending on the organ being studied.
- Instruct the client to remove jewelry or any metal object.

OCULOVESTIBULAR REFLEX STUDY (OVR STUDY)

CALORIC STUDY

Normal Findings.   Nystagmus with irrigation

Description.   This test is used to evaluate the vestibular area of the eighth cranial nerve. The auditory (ear) canal is stimulated by irrigating the canal with cold water, thus causing nystagmus (involuntary rapid eye movement) away from the ear being irrigated. If hot water is used, nystagmus occurs toward the side of the car being irrigated. If there is no nystagmus, there is likely disease of the eighth cranial nerve or the labyrinth, such as Meniere's syndrome.

This test should not be conducted if the eardrum is perforated. Cold air may be used instead of cold water. The test is contraindicated if the client has Meniere's syndrome. It should not be performed during an acute attack.

Purpose
- To determine the presence of disease in the eighth cranial nerve or the labyrinth

Clinical Problems
Positive findings: Eighth cranial nerve neuritis, Meniere's syndrome, vestibular or cochlear inflammation or tumor, brainstem or cerebellar inflammation or tumor

Procedure
- NPO of solid foods 6–8 h before the test to prevent the urge to vomit.
- Eardrum should be free of wax to ensure that free-flowing of water can occur.

- The external auditory canal is irrigated until nystagmus occurs or the client complains of nausea and/or dizziness, which takes about 15 to 30 seconds. If there is no sign of nystagmus after 3 min, irrigation is stopped.
- If the test is negative, after 5 min, the procedure can be repeated on the other ear.

Factors Affecting Diagnostic Results
- Wax or blockage in the auditory canal
- Presence of nystagmus before the test

Nursing Implications
- Check that there is no blockage in the auditory canal.
- Obtain a history of the client's health problems.

Client Teaching
- Inform the client that he/she may experience nausea and/or dizziness.
- Inform the client that the test takes approximately 15 min.
- Encourage the client to rest for 1 h following the test. This can prevent any reaction, such as nausea or dizziness.

PACEMAKER MONITORING (TRANSTELEPHONIC)*

Normal Findings.   A regular heart rate and rhythm; pacemaker capture verified with magnet placement

Description.   Transmission of a client's heart rate and rhythm over the telephone is now the standard of care for pacemaker follow-up. The ECG is the universally recognized test for detecting abnormal pacemaker function and/or cardiac arrhythmias. The magnet rate provided is for the determination of battery and electronic status and confirms normal pacemaker function as evidenced by capture (the heart's beat in response to the pacemaker's electrical stimulation). Proper sensing (the pacer's ability

---

*Leigh Sibert, RN, MSN, CS, Advanced Practice Nurse, Clinical Nurse Specialist, Cardiology Consultants, Wilmington, Delaware.

to see the client's intrinsic heart rhythm) can also be assessed on the ECG. Telephone monitoring provides maximum safety to the client and is easy to use. The guidelines for follow-up have been largely established by Medicare regulations.

Pacemaker technology has developed rapidly in the last two decades. In general there are two types of pacemakers: dual and single chamber. Aside from the basic function of cardiac electrical stimulation, each pacemaker may have multiple programmable settings. This flexibility determines which chambers (atrium or ventricle) are sensed and a variety of pacemaker responses. Once it has been established that the client has a conduction disorder and warrants permanent pacing, the decision of a single- or dual-chamber device and its programming is based on the following: the client's underlying pathology or conduction disturbance, associated medical problems, exercise capacity, and chronotropic response to exercise.

Single-chamber ventricular pacing (VVI) is usually reserved for clients with chronic atrial fibrillation or flutter. Dual-chamber pacing (DDD) is indicated for clients with sick sinus syndrome or AV conduction disease (i.e., heart block). The Intersociety Commission for Heart Disease (ICHD) codes (i.e., VVI, DDD, etc.) were designed to indicate pacemaker function and whether single or dual chambers are being paced and/or sensed. This code has been widely adopted and is used universally.

A wide variety of transtelephonic pacemaker monitors are available for clients to use. Most equipment has been carefully designed for easy use. The monitor box consists of wristband electrodes; a cradle for the client to place the telephone handset into, and a magnet. This monitor box is powered by a 9-volt battery.

Purposes
- To assess normal pacemaker function
- To evaluate the client's heart rate and rhythm
- To evaluate pacemaker battery status via magnet test

Clinical Problems
- *Failure to pace:* The client could experience symptoms of syncope, presyncope, or lightheadedness.
- *Failure to sense:* The client may experience palpitations or "pacemaker syndrome," which is associated with fatigue, shortness of

breath, dizziness, or hypotension. These symptoms are secondary to a loss of AV synchrony.

- *Atrial or ventricular arrhythmias:* The client may experience palpitations, dizziness, shortness of breath, or even syncope.

Procedure

1. No consent form is necessary.
2. Client may eat and drink without restriction prior to transmission.
3. Client should open monitoring box.
4. The client should dampen the inside of his/her wrists with water prior to putting on the wristband electrodes.
5. Verify that wristband electrodes are on the proper wrists (they are labeled left and right) and that the hard electrode on the band is against the insides of the client's wrists.
6. The client establishes telephone contact with the monitoring nurse or technician. Usually the client is called at a prearranged time by the monitoring clinicians.
7. Instruct the client to turn on the monitoring box via the on/off button.
8. Instruct the client to place his/her telephone handset into the cradle located on the monitoring box. The cradle is labeled so that the receiver must be placed correctly at one end. Instruct the client that once the telephone is placed in the cradle he/she should wait 40 to 45 s before picking the telephone back up.
9. The client should then pick the telephone handset up and verify that the ECG tracing transmitted was acceptable.
10. Instruct the client to place the telephone handset back into the monitor cradle again and then place magnet (included with monitor box) directly over their pacemaker. It is helpful for the client to locate the pacemaker on the chest wall with one hand before applying magnet with the other. Again, the client should wait 40 to 45 seconds with the magnet in place before picking the telephone back up.
11. Verify that the magnet ECG tracing is acceptable.
12. Repeat step 8. The client should then pick the telephone handset back up and verify that the ECG tracing was acceptable. This will then conclude the transmission procedure.
13. The client should place magnet back in monitoring box and turn it off.

Factors Affecting Diagnostic Results

- The telephone is not in good working order.
- The client forgets to wet his/her wrists prior to putting on the wristband electrodes.
- The battery in telephone monitoring box is depleted.
- The client's telephone handset is placed on the monitor box cradle backward.
- Fluorescent lights, televisions, radios, and computers that are turned on in close proximity to the monitor box could cause interference with transmission.
- The client has a condition that causes a lot of uncontrolled shaking or involuntary muscle movements (e.g., Parkinson's disease). This can produce an ECG with a poor baseline, which makes it difficult to assess.

Nursing Implications

- Explain the telephone monitoring box and its components to the client. This equipment is usually given to the client in the hospital prior to discharge or at the first follow-up office visit. Some clients' physicians use a monitoring company, which may mail the telephone box to the client.
- Assess the client's level of understanding on the use of the monitoring box and provide reassurance that transmission is easy and can be reexplained each time the client transmits from home.
- Involve family members or support persons in the teaching of the telephone transmission procedure and equipment, especially if the client suffers from dementia or short-term memory loss.
- Obtain history concerning the presence of symptoms that may be related to pacemaker malfunction and/or may correlate with abnormal findings on the ECG.

Client Teaching
Pre-test

- Answer any questions that the client may have regarding proper transmission.
- Verify that the patient has the monitor box in front of him/her and that wristbands have been applied.
- Remind client of sources of transmission interference.

Post-test

- Instruct client to turn off the monitor box and remove the wrist-bands. The magnet should stay in the monitoring box so that it is not misplaced or lost.
- Inform the client that the transmission will be reviewed by the physician and that if necessary he/she will be contacted via telephone for a follow-up in the physician's office.
- Inform the client of the next scheduled transmission date.
- Remind client not to attempt to telephone transmission without establishing contact with the monitoring clinicians or company.

PAPANICOLAOU SMEAR (PAP SMEAR)*

CYTOLOGY TEST FOR CERVICAL CANCER

Normal Finding.   No abnormal or atypical cells

Description.   The Pap (Papanicolaou) smear became nationally known and was used in the early 1950s for detecting cervical cancer and precancerous tissue. Dr. George Papanicolaou developed the cytology tests in 1928 after spending 18 years in research. Today he is referred to as the father of modern cytology. As a result, the use of the Pap test in the United States as a screening tool for cervical cancer has dramatically increased cure rates.

Because malignant tissue changes usually take many years, yearly examination of exfoliative cervical cells (cells that have sloughed off) allows detection of early, precancerous conditions. It is suggested that women have their first Pap test within 3 years of the onset of sexual intercourse or at age 21. Women younger than 30 should have yearly standard Pap tests, but it is recommended every 2 years if liquid-based collection is

---

*Updated by Ellen K Boyda, RN, MSN, CRNP, Family Nurse Practitioner, PA and Instructor, Widener College, Pennsylvania.

used. Women older than 30 should have a different screening frequency depending on their risk factors:

1. Women with a history of two normal yearly Pap tests in a row can be screened every 2–3 years.
2. Women with a normal Pap test and a human papillomavirus (HPV) test that is negative for high-risk type HPV can be screened every 3 years. Testing more often than every 3 years is not necessary because these women are at low risk for abnormal cervical cell changes.
3. Women with the following risk factors require yearly or more frequent screening:
   - Using birth control pills
   - Having sex with someone who has multiple sexual partners
   - Having three or more sexual partners in a lifetime
   - Starting sexual intercourse before age 18
   - Sexual intercourse with partners who have HPV
   - Cigarette smoking
   - Being infected with Chlamydia
   - Being infected with high-risk type HPV
   - Having an impaired immune system
   - A history of treatment for abnormal cervical cell changes or cervical cancer
   - Infection with HIV (two Pap tests in the first year after diagnosis and yearly after that).
   - Exposure to DES (diethylstilbestrol) in utero (though rare)

The Pap smear (cytology) results are reported by The Bethesda System (TBS). General categories of TBS are as follows:

I. Within normal limits. TBS will also identify if the sample is adequate.
II. Abnormal changes
   A. Benign cellular changes
      1. Differentiates reactive (such as normal cell repair process, radiation and IUD) or inflammatory (such as chlamydia, bacterial vaginosis, trichomoniasis) changes from true dysplastic changes.
      2. Most important features of TBS.
         Management: Repeat smears yearly or as determined by the client's health care provider.

B. Epithelial Abnormalities

1. Atypical squamous cells of undetermined significance (ASCUS): favoring a neoplastic process or a reactive process. **Management:** Repeat smears at closer intervals, recall for colposcopy and/or combine repeat cytology with cervicography or HPV-DNA type.

2. Low-grade squamous intraepithelial lesion (LSIL): shows the earliest abnormal nuclear changes and combines diagnosis of HPV, mild dysplagia, and cervical intraepithelial neoplasia (CIN 1). **Management:** Repeat cytology at close intervals, recall for colposcopy.

3. High-grade squamous intraepithelial lesion (HSIL): includes moderate and severe dysplastic changes, carcinoma in situ (CIS 1), CIN 2, and CIN 3. **Management:** Recall for colposcopy.

4. Squamous cell carcinoma: changes consistent with invasive cancer. **Management:** Recall for colposcopy.

5. Glandular cell abnormalities

   a. Atypical cells of undetermined significance, atypical endocervical cells, or endometrial cells. **Management:** In young women, check for endocervicitis, repeat smear, refer to colposcopy; in older women; refer for colposcopy with endocervical sample.

   b. Adenocarcinoma **Management:** Refer for colposcopy.

For suggestive or positive Pap smears, colposcopy and/or a cervical biopsy is frequently ordered to confirm the test results. Atypical cells can occur following cervicitis and after excessive or prolonged use of hormones.

Purposes

- To detect precancerous and cancerous cells of the cervix
- To assess the effects of sex hormonal replacement
- To identify viral, fungal, and parasitic conditions
- To evaluate the response to chemotherapy or radiation therapy to the cervix

Clinical Problems

Positive findings: Precancerous and cancerous cells of the cervix; cervicitis; viral, fungal, and parasitic conditions

Procedure

- Food and fluids are not restricted.
- The client should not douche, insert vaginal medications, or have sexual intercourse for at least 24 h (preferably 48 h) before the test. The test should be done between menstrual periods.
- The client is generally asked to remove all clothes, because the breasts are examined before the Pap smear is taken. A paper or cloth gown is worn.
- Instruct the client to lie on the examining table in the lithotomy position (heels in the stirrups).
- A speculum is inserted into the vagina. The speculum may be lubricated with warm running water.
- A curved spatula (Pap stick) or spatula/brush combination is used to scrape the cervix. The obtained specimen is transferred onto a slide and sprayed with a commercial fixation spray or the whole stick is immersed in a container of liquid-based fixative. Label the slide or container with the client's name and date.
- The Pap smear procedure takes approximately 10 min.

Factors Affecting Diagnostic Results

- Allowing cells to dry on the slide before using the fixative solution or spray.
- Douching, use of vaginal suppositories, or sexual intercourse within 24 h before the test.
- Menstruation can interfere with the test results.
- Drugs (e.g., digitalis preparations, tetracycline, female hormones) could change the cellular structure.
- Lubricating jelly on the speculum can interfere with the test results.
- Inadequate specimen.

Nursing Implications

- Explain the procedure to the client. Emphasize to the client that she should not douche, insert vaginal suppositories, or have sexual intercourse for at least 24 h before the Pap smear. Douching could wash away the cervical cells.

- Obtain a client history regarding menstruation and any menstrual problems (i.e., the date of the first day of the last menstrual period, bleeding flow, vaginal discharge, itching, whether she is taking hormones or oral contraceptive, or previous abnormal Pap test).
- Answer the client's questions, and refer questions you cannot answer to other health professionals. Try to alleviate the client's anxiety, if at all possible. Be a good listener.
- Label the slide or container with the client's name and date. The laboratory slip should include the client's age and the specimen site(s).

Client Teaching

- Inform the client that a manual examination of the vagina, lower abdomen, and breast will precede the Pap smear.
- Explain to the client that the frequency of the test depends on her risk factors and is determined by her health care provider. See section on Risk Factors under Description. Usually women over 30 years should have a Pap smear once a year.
- Inform the client that test results should be back in 7 to 10 days. Physicians and health care providers differ in the way they report test results; some send cards to the client stating that the Pap smear is normal, while others send cards only if the test is abnormal.

PERICARDIAL FLUID ANALYSIS

PERICARDIOCENTESIS

Normal Findings.   Appearance: Clear, pale yellow, straw color

Abnormal Findings

Bacteria present
Red and white blood cells
Blood streaks
Milky appearance

Description. The pericardial membrane surrounds the heart and contains a small amount of serous fluid, which is produced and absorbed at the same rate. When there is an excess of fluid in the pericardium, a pericardiocentesis is usually ordered. The procedure involves the insertion of a needle through the intercostal space into the lower part of the pericardium. Echocardiography helps to locate the site for the needle insertion. Excess fluid is aspirated; the fluid is evaluated to determine the cause of the problem.

This procedure is contraindicated if the client is taking an anticoagulant, has a bleeding disorder, or has thrombocytopenia. Potential complications might occur such as air embolism, coronary artery or myocardial laceration, dysrhythmias, excess bleeding, pleural infection, pneumothorax, and ventricular fibrillation.

Purposes
- To identify the cause of pericardial fluid excess
- To determine the presence of a bacterial infection

Clinical Problems
Abnormal findings: Pericarditis, bacterial infection, metastatic cancer, congestive heart failure, cardiac trauma, cardiac surgery, heart transplant rejection, acute rheumatic fever, and tuberculosis

Procedure
- Obtain a signed consent form.
- Restrict fluids and food for 6 to 8 h
- Start an IV line for possible IV medications.
- Start an EKG; echocardiography may be used to guide the insertion of the needle.
- Insert pericardial fluid in a red- or lavender-top tube (according to the policy).

Factors Affecting Diagnostic Results
- Blood from the insertion of the needle into the heart chamber.

Nursing Implications

- Obtain a history of cardiac problems.
- Record the medications the client is taking.
- Take baseline vital signs (VS). Record on chart.
- Check that consent form has been signed.
- Note any signs or symptoms of chest pain, dizziness, shortness of breath (SOB) during the procedure.

Client Teaching

- Have the client void before the test.
- Monitor VS. Record VS on chart.
- Monitor EKG during and after the procedure.
- Inform the client that the procedure should take 30 to 45 min.
- Explain the importance of remaining still during the procedure.
- Explain to the client that a local anesthetic will be administered prior to the insertion of the needle.
- Answer client and/or family's question(s) before and after the test or refer questions to appropriate health professionals.

PERITONEAL FLUID ANALYSIS

PARACENTESIS, PERITONEAL TAP

Normal Findings

Appearance: Clear, pale yellow, light yellow
Red blood cells: None to less than 100,000 mm^3
Protein: Less than 4.0 g/dl
Glucose: Same as serum glucose
Amylase: Same as serum amylase
Alkaline phosphatase: Same as serum alkaline phosphatase
Bacteria: None

Description.   The peritoneal cavity contains two layers of serous membranes (the peritoneum) that line the walls of the abdominal and pelvic cavities. The fluid between these two layers of membrane is called the serous fluid; excess fluid is known as the ascites fluid. Normally there is small amount of fluid present; the fluid production and absorption are about the same. The procedure to remove excessive amounts of fluid is called paracentesis. A needle or catheter is inserted into the peritoneal cavity to remove the ascites fluid for therapeutic purpose (relief of client's symptoms) and/or for diagnostic purpose (cause of the effusion of fluid).

The client with cirrhosis of the liver may develop ascetic fluid, which causes shortness of breath (SOB), also called shortness of air (SOA), and abdominal distention. Removal of the fluid can help alleviate these symptoms. Excessive amount of fluid removal may cause fluid reoccurrence in the peritoneal cavity. For diagnostic purposes, the fluid that has been removed is analyzed to determine the cause of the peritoneal effusion. It also could be caused by infectious or neoplastic conditions. Bloody fluid could be the cause of the needle penetrating a blood vessel, which may be referred to as a traumatic tap.

Purposes
- To remove peritoneal fluid for therapeutic purposes
- To remove peritoneal fluid for diagnostic purposes

Clinical Problems
Abnormal Findings: Cirrhosis of the liver, heart failure (HF), portal hypertension, nephrotic syndrome, hypoproteinemia, metastatic cancer, peritonitis, pancreatitis, trauma, gastrointestinal diseases

Procedure
- Obtain a signed consent form.
- There is no food or fluid restriction.
- Have client void prior to the procedure to prevent an accidental bladder tap.
- Have client in a high-Fowler's position.
- Use strict sterile technique to clean skin, during needle insertion, and for collection of fluid.
- A scalpel may be needed to allow needle or catheter insertion.
- Send the specimen(s) immediately to the laboratory.
- Usually 2 (2,000 ml) of fluid is removed at one time. Excessive amount of fluid removal could cause hypovolemia.
- Antibiotic therapy may be ordered following the procedure.

Factors Affecting Diagnostic Results
- Bloody fluid as the result of a traumatic tap

Nursing Implications
- Obtain baseline vital signs (VS); continue monitoring VS.
- Measure abdominal girth.
- Record client's weight before and after the procedure.
- Have client urinate before the procedure.
- Obtain the necessary equipment. Keep a sterile field.
- Observe the client for signs and symptoms of hypovolemia (excess fluid loss). Watch for signs of hypotension and rapid pulse.
- Check dressing for blood or leaking of ascitic fluid after the procedure.

Client Teaching
- Inform the client that a local anesthetic will be used to eliminate the pain during the needle insertion. The client may feel some pressure during the insertion of the needle.
- Instruct the client to report any excessive abdominal pain.
- Inform the client that the procedure usually takes 30 to 45 min.
- Be supportive to the client. Answer questions and refer unknown questions to appropriate health professionals.

POSITRON EMISSION TOMOGRAPHY (PET)*

Normal Findings. Normal brain, lung, heart, and gastrointestinal activities and blood flow

Description. Positron emission tomography (PET), a relatively noninvasive test, measures the body's abnormal molecular cell activity. PET is used to study the brain, heart, lungs, and abdominal organs, and for oncologic

---

*Updated by Susan L. Chudzik, CRNP, Christiana Care Health Services, Newark, Delaware.

purposes. For brain studies, PET assesses normal brain function; regional cerebral blood flow and volume; glucose, protein, and oxygen metabolism; blood–brain barrier function, neuroreceptor–neurotransmitter systems; and the pathophysiology of neurologic and psychiatric disorders. For heart studies, PET assesses cardiac perfusion or blood flow; glucose and oxygen metabolism; and receptor functions. PET perfusion imaging provides information concerning the severity of coronary artery disease (CAD). In oncology, PET has recently been approved for lung and breast nodules and colorectal imaging.

The client receives a substance tagged with a radionuclide by gas or injectable form (e.g., radioactive glucose, rubidium-82, oxygen-15, nitrogen-13). Fluorodeoxyglucose (FDG) is the most common radioisotope used in PET. Tomographic slices from cross sections of tissue are detected and visually displayed by computer. PET is most effective in determining blood flow (brain, heart). Radiation from PET is a quarter of that received by CT.

Purposes
- To detect a decreased blood flow or perfusion with coronary artery disease
- To determine the size of infarct and myocardial viability
- To detect transient ischemia
- To detect decreased oxygen utilization and decreased blood flow with brain disorders such as cerebral vascular accident (CVA)
- To detect viable myocardium
- To differentiate between types of dementia (e.g., Alzheimer's disease and other dementias, such as parkinsonism)
- To identify stages of cranial tumors
- To identify lung and breast nodules
- To identify colorectal metastasis

Clinical Problems
Abnormal findings: Hypoperfusion to brain and heart, stroke, epilepsy, migraine, Parkinson's disease, dementia, Alzheimer's disease, AMI for first 72 h

Procedure
- Obtain a signed consent form.
- Start two IVs, one for radioactive substance and the second to draw blood gas samples. A blindfold may be used to keep the client from being distracted, since alertness is necessary.
- No coffee, alcohol, or tobacco is allowed for 24 h before the test.
- Check glucose levels.
- Empty bladder 1 to 2 h before the test.
- No sedatives are given, since client needs to follow instructions.
- Test takes 1 to 1.5 h.

Nursing Implications
- Explain procedure (see Procedure).
- Obtain a signed consent form.
- Monitor vital signs.

Client Teaching
Pre-test
- Inform the client that instructions given during test should be followed.
- Assess IV site.
- Listen to the client's concerns.

Post-test
- Encourage fluid post-test to get rid of radioactive substance.
- Avoid postural hypotension by slowly moving the client to upright position.

PULMONARY FUNCTION TESTS*

PULMONARY DIAGNOSTIC TESTS

Normal Findings.   Normal values according to patient's age, sex, and height; greater than 80% of the predicted value. 95% confidence levels are also being used; these confidence ranges give a normal and a low or

---

*David C. Sestill, CRTT, RPFT, Technical and Research Coordinator, Pulmonary Function Laboratory, Temple University Hospital, Philadelphia, Pennsylvania.

minimal normal value. This is done to account for physiologic differences in body types

Description. Pulmonary function tests (PFTs) are useful in differentiating between obstructive and restrictive lung diseases and in quantifying the degree (mild, moderate, or severe) of obstructive or restrictive lung disorders. Other purposes of PFTs include establishing baseline test results for comparison with future tests; evaluating pulmonary status before surgery; determining pulmonary disability for insurance; tracking the progress of lung disease; assessing the response to therapy; pulmonary evaluation; determining pulmonary status before rehabilitation and post rehabilitation to document outcomes.

In pulmonary physiology testing, the lungs are monitored by many complex devices and tests. The most basic device is the spirometer; it is used to measure flows, volumes, and capacities.

A number of pulmonary tests are conducted, because no single measurement can evaluate pulmonary performance. The most frequently performed PFTs are the slow vital capacity tests; lung volume tests; forced vital capacity, flow-volume loop, and diffusion-study tests; bronchodilator response studies; exercise studies; and nutritional studies.

Pulmonary Rehabilitation. Many pulmonary laboratories incorporate pulmonary rehabilitation into their outpatient programs because it is important for clients with pulmonary diseases to keep active. Activities and exercises prescribed in the pulmonary rehabilitation program have been demonstrated to reduce the amount of oxygen required for muscle use. Other benefits gained from exercise for clients with pulmonary disease include a decrease in the sedentary lifestyle that can lead to depression, decrease in dyspnea, increase in activities of daily living, lesser dependence on significant others to assist in basic care; a decrease in complications and increase in the recovery time for clients having transplant and lung reduction surgery (pre- and post-operatively); and improvement in respiratory status for clients with interstitial fibrosis, cystic fibrosis, asthma, emphysema, primary pulmonary hypertension, or alpha-l-antitrypsin deficiency.

Pulmonary rehabilitation incorporates a multidisciplinary approach. Specialists in the program include the dietitian; exercise physiologist; nurse; occupational, physical, and respiratory therapists; and social worker.

Purposes

- To assess pulmonary/respiratory function
- To detect the occurrence of pulmonary dysfunction
- To differentiate between obstructive and restrictive lung diseases
- To evaluate the response to drug therapy (i.e., some cardiac drugs, and chemotherapy may induce hyperactivity or fibrosis where response to bronchodilator therapy and steroids may increase function)
- To be informed of program(s) for improving respiratory status for clients with pulmonary dysfunction or for clients prior to or following lung surgery

Pulmonary Function Tests

1. Slow Vital Capacity (SVC) Tests
   - *Tidal volume (TV, V):* The amount of air inhaled and exhaled during rest or quiet respiration or normal breathing.
   - *Inspiratory capacity (IC):* The maximal inspired amount of air from end-expiratory tidal volume in normal breathing.
   - *Expiratory reserve volume (ERV):* The maximal amount of air that can be exhaled from end-expiratory tidal volume in normal breathing.
   - *Inspiratory reserve volume (IRV):* The maximal amount of air that can be inspired from end-inspiratory tidal volume in normal breathing.
   - *Vital capacity (VC):* The maximal amount of air exhaled after a maximal inhalation.

$$VC = ERV + IC$$

Note: These pulmonary measurements are done slowly, without force. Individuals with obstructive lung disease will be able to expire more volume with this test than during the forced vital capacity maneuver that may lead to early airway closure.

2. Lung Volume Studies
   - *Lung volume tests using indicator gas:* Helium dilution and nitrogen washout are special studies that use the data generated in the slow vital capacity test to obtain the lung volumes. Tracer gases such as 10% helium or 100% oxygen is required. Using one of the gases, the person breathes in and out as the tracer gas is equilibrated

in the lung; the functional residual capacity (FRC) is calculated from the changes. This method will tend to underestimate persons with advanced obstructive lung disease. This underestimation is a result of the trapped air in the lung which does communicate with the airways.

- *Lung volumes by plethysmography method:* Lung volumes can be obtained by total body plethysmography. Body plethysmography uses a device that resembles an air-tight telephone booth in which the subject sits. This method is a more accurate means to measure total volume of the lungs than the tracer gas method. Volumes measured in the box will be larger than those measured by the indicator gas method. The body plethysmography is able to measure trapped air that does not communicate with the airways.
- *Lung volume measurements:* See Figure 2–1.
- *Residual volume (RV):* The amount of air that remains in the lungs after maximal expiration.

$$RV = FRC - ERV$$

- *Functional residual capacity (FRC):* The amount of air left in the lungs after tidal or normal expiration.

$$FRC = ERV + RV$$

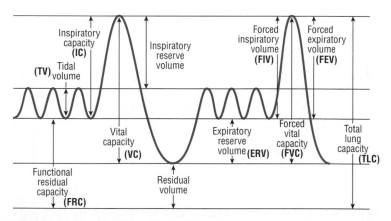

FIGURE 2–1. Graphic of lung volume and capacity.

In obstructive disorders, FRC is increased because of hyperinflation and/or air trapping in the lungs. This value may normalize in clients with asthma post exacerbation but will not for clients with COPD. In classical restrictive disorders, FRC, TLC, and RV are all reduced.

- *Total lung capacity (TLC):* The total amount of air that is in the lungs at maximal inspiration.

$$TLC = VC + RV \text{ or } TLC = FRC + IC$$

3. Lung Volumes and Capacity. See Figure 2–1
- *Forced vital capacity (FVC):* The maximal amount of air that can be forced out of the lungs as hard, as fast, and as long as possible before a forceful inspiration. In obstructive lung disease, the FVC is decreased; in restrictive lung disease, the FVC is normal or decreased.

$$FVC = IC + ERV$$

- *Forced inspiratory volume (FIV):* The greatest amount of air inhaled after a maximal expiration.
- *Forced expiratory volume timed (FEV_T):* This value reflects the air flow through the bronchial tubes from the greatest to the smallest. It is reported as a time-based value as in 0.5 seconds FEV_5, 1 second FEV_1, 2 seconds FEV_2, and 3 seconds FEV_3. See Figure 2–2.

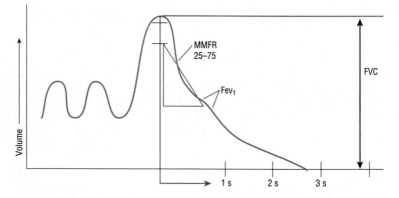

FIGURE 2–2. Graphic of forced expiratory volume timed (Courtesy of David C. Sestifi, CRTT, RPFT).

The American Thoracic Society (ATS) has suggested reporting the FEV_6 which is the amount of air expired in 6 seconds. This reflects the minimum exhalation time suggested for a forced vital capacity maneuver. The parameter of choice for evaluation of asthmatics and other obstructive lung disease and to evaluate the response to bronchodilator therapy is still FEV_1. An improvement of greater than 15% after bronchodilator therapy is considered significant and indicates the presence of reversible airway obstruction, such as bronchospasm.

4. Flow-Volume Loop (FVL)

   Another method to visualize FVC measurement is by graphing flow versus volume, as seen in Figure 2–3. Abnormal FVLs in Figure 2–4 indicate types of pulmonary problems. This test yields the same basic information as the FVC test but in addition provides the following useful visual information, such as small-airway disease and upper-airway obstruction. Its usefulness in screening people with some

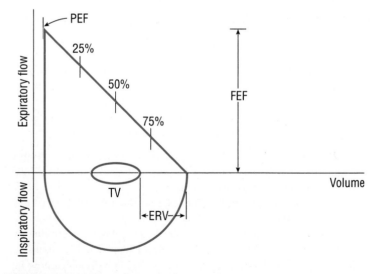

FIGURE 2–3. Flow-volume loop (FVL) and forced expiratory flow (FEF) (Courtesy of David C. Sestifi, CRTT, RPFT).

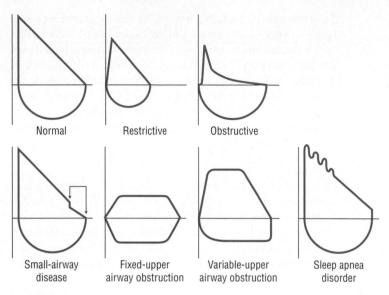

Normal	Restrictive	Obstructive
Small-airway disease	Fixed-upper airway obstruction	Variable-upper airway obstruction	Sleep apnea disorder

FIGURE 2–4. Abnormal flow-volume loops (FVLs) (Courtesy of David C. Sestifi, CRTT, RPFT).

types of sleep disorder problems has been recently documented. It is used as a non-invasive tool to evaluate clients who may have some type of upper-airway obstruction from thermal injury, polyps on the vocal cords, vocal cord paralysis, edema of the epiglottis, scar tissue from old tracheotomy site, and floppy trachea.

- *Peak expiratory flow (PEF):* The highest flow rate achieved at the beginning of the FVC; reported in liters per second. *Note:* Peak flow meters measure in liters per minute.
- *Peak inspiratory flow (PIF):* The highest flow rate achieved at the beginning of the forced inspiratory capacity.
- *Forced expiratory flow (FEF):* Figure 2–3 demonstrates the rate of flow at selected points on the flow-volume loop. The FEF looks at flow at the 25%, 50%, and 75% of the FVC and evaluates flow in various size airways. It can evaluate the effectiveness of bronchodilator therapy. FEF 25% reflects flow through large airways;

FEF 50% reflects flow through medium airways; and FEF 75% reflects flow through small airways. Decreased FEF 75% is indicative of small-airway disease.

5. Impulse Oscillometry Spirometry (IOS) / Forced Oscillatory Technique (FOT)

IOS also known as FOT is a noninvasive test that employs sound waves to measure the resistance, impedance, and reactance of the airways. This testing modality has been gaining popularity with the commercial availability of equipment (1997). The device generates a sound signal that is superimposed on the normal tidal breathing of the subject. Du Boise et al. first described this technique in 1956 as a noninvasive method to measure resistance to breathing. As a historical note the total body plethysmograph was also developed at the same time.

The computer creates small impulses of air at random frequencies between 3 and 40 Hz and oscillates a base speaker. The reflected returning signals from the airways are analyzed using the fast Fourier transformation equation. The FOT device is compared to the plethysmography method of airway resistance measurement (see Figure 2–5). Total body plethysmography makes a single measurement of the total respiratory system resistance. In contrast, FOT is a spectral analysis, which

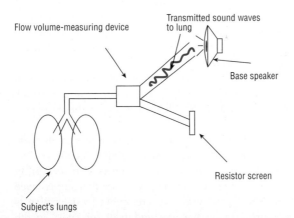

Flow volume-measuring device

Transmitted sound waves to lung

Base speaker

Resistor screen

Subject's lungs

FIGURE 2–5. Forced oscillometry device (Courtesy of David C. Sestili, CRTT, RPFT).

reflects the resistances of the central and peripheral airways. The measurements for these airways are in two well-published values—R20 that reflect the resistance in the large airways and R5 that reflect the resistance in the peripheral airways.

The test requires the client to perform normal tidal breathing only for a minimum of 30 seconds. The client is required to hold his/her cheeks, or an operator will hold them, while breathing through a filter mouthpiece, and a nose clip is used. What is unique about this testing method is that complicated breathing maneuvers are not required like spirometry. An added advantage for clients with obstructed disease is that FOT will not alter the tone of their airway that can lead to air trapping and thus to increased hyperinflation of the lungs.

The IOS/FOT method has demonstrated great potential in its ability to test very young children and adults who may have difficulty in performing spirometry or more complicated testing. IOS/FOT has shown great promises of being more sensitive than spirometry testing. Asthmatics may have normal spirometry yet have higher airway resistances than normal subjects. FOT can also be used to determine bronchodilator reversibility, evaluate airway hyperreactivity as part of a bronchial challenge study with exercise; cold air; hypertonic saline, methacholine, or other drugs.

A downside of this method is the small number of population used to develop the predicted normalcy at this time. The more practical approach would be to use the client as his/her own control by serial testing change. Unfortunately, most laboratories use a predicted group that is decided on by more of a preference or by what came with their device than by a universal standard that not everyone agrees on. The power in monitoring a trend of the pulmonary data is that one is able to see a change in the clients' data after establishing a mean to follow over a period of time.

The author (David Sestili) is currently evaluating and monitoring lung and heart/lung transplant clients for organ rejection, stenosis of the anastomosis, and central airway collapse. The team is also measuring pathological samples recovered during biopsy from the surveillance bronchoscopies in these subjects. What we are trying to determine is whether we can measure airway diameter and wall thickness in the peripheral airways less than 5 mm and correlate the actual measurements.

Preparation for the Test

The client preparation for testing requires him/her not to use inhaled bronchodilators medication unless so directed by the ordering practitioner and not to perform any exercising prior to the testing. Also, he/she must refrain from caffeine, smoking, and large changes in temperature. Instructions to the client should include that the test does not hurt; it will require them to perform relaxed normal tidal breathing only for a minimum of 30 seconds. The IOS unit makes a light popping sound like popcorn. During testing the client will be required to hold his/her cheeks, or an operator can hold them. The client will be breathing through a filter mouthpiece and a nose dip will be used. Total test time will be between 30 and 45 min.

6. Exhaled Nitric Oxide (eNO)

In the lungs, inflammatory processes can lead to increased production of nitric oxide gas in the bronchial tree. Nitric oxide (NO) is released by the leukocytes in the bronchial wall in response to inflammation. Normal lung nitric oxide levels are less than 12 parts per billion (ppb). Abnormal levels of exhaled nitric oxide (eNO) have been published as greater than 30 ppb in clients with diseases such as asthma and interstitial disease. In moderate to severe chronic obstructive pulmonary disease (COPD) patients, eNO may be downregulated from normal levels and may be much lower than 12 ppm. This is thought to be the result of the destruction of airways and the alveolar capillary bed.

In the sinus cavity, normal nasal NO levels are greater than 200 ppb. Nitric oxide is also elevated in the stomach. In geographical locations where air pollution is high, such as in cities, atmospheric NO levels have been recorded at greater than 300 ppb. Studies have been published demonstrating that the inspired atmospheric NO levels do not affect the expired NO. Nevertheless it is recommended that atmospheric or inspired NO levels be monitored and recorded in the client data report. Some laboratories use NO scrubbers on the inspired side of the valve.

The most popular method of measuring eNO is via the chemiluminescent technique. There are two methods of collecting the NO sample. The first method is the off-line method in which the sample is collected in a special Mylar bag and is measured off-line at a later time. The second method is the on-line method. NO is measured in real time as the client exhales through the valve. The same type of valve configuration is used to collect the samples in both the methods.

The client is instructed to take a deep breath in through a one-way valve. On the exhalation side is a restrictor to help maintain a predetermined exhalation rate at a constant pressure. The patient is instructed to exhale at a target pressure, and flows are displayed on a monitor for more than 6 seconds. No nose clip is used as the backpressure generated by the client as he/she exhales is used to close the velum of the nose. This prevents contamination of the exhaled nitric oxide in the sinus cavity by mixing with the exhaled lung gas. The client must be able to follow commands and be able to exhale for more than 6 seconds.

For more detailed information on the methods and uses, the American Thoracic Society has published recommendations for the collection of exhaled nitric oxide in adults and children, and these are available at www.thoracic.org.

Exhaled nitric oxide is useful in monitoring subjects with asthma, allergic reactions, interstitial fibrosis, and cystic fibrosis, just to name a few. By monitoring exhaled nitric oxide in asthmatic subject compliance to prescribed therapy can be monitored and adjusted.

Preparation of the Client for Exhaled Nitric Oxide

Preparation for the exhaled nitric oxide is extensive and should be documented via a client questionnaire or a checklist.

The client must be able to follow commands and be able to exhale for more than 6 seconds.

The subject must abstain from some foods and drinks that may alter the exhaled nitric oxide values. They must refrain from alcohol (including mouthwash), water, salads, and foods with nitrates, for example, luncheon meat, pickled products, bacon, ham, and hot dogs. Refrain from smoking and medications that block nitric oxide production, to name a few. The subject is also required not to exercise and to limit his/her exposure to cold air or sudden changes in temperature as this may also affect the eNO levels.

7. Diffusion Capacity Test

Diffusion tests can be done using a number of techniques. The most commonly used is the single breath test. This requires the client to inspire from RV to TLC. The gas inhaled is mixture of helium 10%, carbon, monoxide 0.3%, oxygen 21%, and the balance is nitrogen. The client holds his/her breath for 10 seconds prior to expiration. After the first 750 ml is discarded to wash out dead-space gas, an alveolar sample is collected in a bag and analyzed for helium and carbon monoxide concentration. Results of this reflect the state of the alveolar capillary barrier.

Decreased diffusing capacity occurs in such disease states as interstitial fibrosis, pulmonary edema, and emphysema. It will also decrease in persons with abnormal hemoglobin, such as occurs in anemias including methemoglobin and increased carboxyhemoglobin in smokers. Cardiac output can affect this result. Increased DLCO values can be caused by pulmonary hemorrhage.

8. Bronchial Provocation Studies

Inhalation of pharmacological and antigenic substances is used to test the sensitivity or hyperactivity of the airways. Types of challenge would include; methacholine, histamine, ASA, cold air, hypertonic saline, antigens, and others. Serial spirometry tests are performed to document the amount or degree of reactivity (a drop in FEV_1 greater than 20% of baseline spirometry). A baseline test followed by a challenge substance is given first, followed by a bronchodilator to assure reversal. Indications for these tests are: (1) normal spirometry test, (2) a history of symptoms such as wheezing, or coughing without a cause, and (3) symptoms related to exposure to industrial substances.

Methacholine chloride is usually the testing drug of choice because it causes bronchoconstriction rapidly. The client inhales progressively larger doses of the drug until all levels are administered without change in FEV_1 or a drop of 20% of baseline FEV_1 is reached. The drug is then reversed by administration of a bronchodilator.

9. Exercise Studies

Pulmonary function studies are done at a resting or static state. Exercise studies evaluate the patient during an active or dynamic state. These tests are performed by having the subject walk on a treadmill or pedal an ergometer to a set protocol to stimulate activity at progressive workloads. During this test, the heart rate and rhythm is monitored by a 12-lead electrocardiogram (ECG). The client will also be breathing through a mouthpiece during the test to measure ventilation, expired carbon dioxide

(VCO$_2$) and oxygen consumption (VO$_2$). Blood gases may be drawn at rest and at peak exercise. Pulse oximetry may also be monitored, as well as blood pressure. These tests are used to determine the amount of disability and to evaluate persons with exertion dyspnea. This information can have an exercise prescription for activities for fitness programs, pulmonary, and cardiac rehabilitation.

Types of exercise testing can be designed to simulate activity-related problems, of which *exercise induced bronchospasm (EIB)* is an example. A common complaint of clients active in sport activities is bronchospasm. Several theories suggestive of the cause include allergy-triggered airway, production of nitric oxide by the airway hyper-reactivity in association with physical activity and mouth breathing required when the participant increases activity. When the individual breathes rapidly in and out through the mouth, the nose, which warms and filters air, is by-passed. This dry air causes chilling of the airway, leading to instability of the airways and can lead to bronchoconstriction in some persons.

10. Pulse Oximetry (POX). This is a noninvasive procedure to measure the oxygen saturation (SaO$_2$) of the blood. The device measures the SaO$_2$ by passing two wavelengths of infrared light through an extremity such as a finger. The device (sensor probe) measures the saturation of oxyhemoglobin in the pulsatile fraction of blood. This method is an excellent noninvasive trending device; when values vary, a blood gas analysis of the partial pressure of oxygen (PO$_2$) and/or CO-oximetry to measure oxyhemoglobin (%HbO$_2$) and SaO$_2$ should be done to validate the results. A note of caution: Blood gas analyses normally do not measure SaO$_2$; they are calculated. Check with your blood gas laboratory for this information.

Pulse oximetry is a very useful test but it has some drawbacks. It should be trusted after direct comparison to CO-oximetry is done. Abnormal hemoglobin levels (i.e., carboxyhemoglobinemia, methemoglobinemia, and sulfhemoglobinemia) could fool the device. These abnormal levels are detected at the same infrared wavelengths as O$_2$ and may falsely be interpreted by the oximeter to be oxygen. Impeded blood flow to an area will also affect the pulse oximetry. Correlation with the client's true pulse will assist in correcting this problem. Light sources may also affect the results; thus the area should be guarded against external light sources.

11. Nutritional Studies. *Indirect calorimetry* is the measurement of oxygen consumption (VO_2) to derive energy expenditure (EE) and carbon dioxide production (VCO_2) allowing us to derive respiratory quotient (RQ). Respiratory quotient obtained from the calorimetry yields the type and amount of substrate used in metabolism (carbohydrate, protein, fats). It is calculated as:

$$RQ = VO_2/VCO_2$$

This noninvasive test gives useful information as to the resting energy expenditure (REE), the amount of calories needed for minimal existence expressed in kilocalories per 24 h. What it measures is the output side of the nutrition question since we know and measure the input side. The RQ will indicate the type of fuel substrates being metabolized. For example, an RQ of 1.0 indicates carbohydrates; an RQ of 0.80 indicates mixed carbohydrates, fats, and protein; an RQ 0.75 indicates lipids metabolism; and an RQ of 0.65 could be seen in an individual in ketosis. If 24 h urine urea nitrogen is known, nonprotein R can be calculated along with the actual amount of carbohydrates, fats, and protein metabolized in grams and percent of EE.

12. Body Plethysmography (Body Box). Body plethysmography is a method to measure the exact amount of air in the thorax. This is accomplished by having the subject sit inside an airtight box and breathe through a flow-measuring device. A panting maneuver is employed, and a shutter is closed to measure pressure at the mouth, and a second pressure measures the changes of the box. By measuring the mouth and box pressure, the measurements can be applied to Boyle's Law. The thoracic gas volume (TGV), which correlates to functional residual capacity (FRC), can be measured. The compliance of the lungs can be measured but it requires the subject to swallow an esophageal balloon. This device can also measure airway resistances of the lung. Advantages are that the body box measures all air in the thorax that causes volumes to be larger in box studies than by other methods. Disadvantages to the body box test are that some clients have claustrophobia, and persons with perforated eardrums will tend to have readings much higher than normal which could be misleading. Obese clients may not be able to be tested due to weight limitations of the equipment. This test requires total client cooperation and ability to follow commands.

Clinical Problems

Obstructive diseases: Emphysema, chronic bronchitis, bronchiectasis, bronchospasm, bronchial secretions, airway inflammation caused by bacterial or viral infections, asthma

Restrictive diseases: Pulmonary fibrosis, pneumonia, lung tumors, kyphoscoliosis, neuromuscular diseases, chest trauma, obesity, scleroderma, pulmonary edema, surgical removal of lung tissue, high abdominal incisions

Procedure.   For most pulmonary testing the following are good guidelines. It is always wise to contact the laboratory for specific restrictions, as they vary.

- Eating a heavy meal before the test should be discouraged.
- Smoking should be avoided 4 to 6 h before the test.
- The client should wear nonrestrictive clothing.
- Record the client's age, height, and weight, which may be used to predict the normal range.
- Bronchodilator therapy is normally restricted prior to the test, because it is usually administered in the pulmonary function laboratory to evaluate response to the drug.
- Usually sedatives and narcotics are not given. Other medications are given prior to the test unless otherwise indicated by the health care provider.
- Postpone procedure if the client has an active cold, is running a fever, or is under the influence of alcohol.
- Dentures may be left in during testing.
- A nose clip is applied and the client is instructed to breathe in and out through their mouth while attached to a mouthpiece.
- Practice sessions on fast-and-deep breathing. Normally the test is repeated until two efforts are reproducible and the best tracing is used. Check with your laboratory to find out the length of time the client may be in the laboratory as it may take anywhere from 1 to 4 h for testing according to the tests ordered.
- The test or tests may be repeated after using a bronchodilator.

Bronchial Provocation Studies.   The routine test is methacholine. Make sure to contact the pulmonary laboratory to check for restrictions and the type of test used at your facility.

- Informed consent is needed for this test.
- It is recommended that the client has a pre- and post-bronchodilator test done before being referred for this test. History of severe reactions, hives, anaphylaxis, and so on, may be contradictive for this test.
- There are many restrictions associated with this test and the laboratory should be contacted. Some include: no exercise, smoking, or caffeine (coffee, cola, or chocolate) consumption for a minimum of 6 h before testing. Any bronchodilator or antihistamine therapy (PO or inhaled) should be discontinued; some may need to be withheld up to 72 h prior to testing.
- Avoid methacholine challenge testing for women who are pregnant and breastfeeding or who are trying to become pregnant. Its safety has not been documented. Other testing such as cold air challenge may be employed.

Nutritional Studies

- The client should be NPO for 12 h prior to and until completion of the test.
- Physical activity must be restricted before the test.
- Nutritional studies are usually performed 0.5 h after awakening, if possible.
- The client's exhalation is analyzed for oxygen consumption (VO_2) and carbon dioxide production (VCO_2). Clients on ventilators, receiving continuous hyperalimentation, and/or tube feeding can be tested as long as there are no changes in the diet or ventilator settings until the test is completed.
- Clients with a leaking endotracheal tube, tracheotomy tube, or chest tubes cannot be tested as the gas leaking will alter the results. Clients weaning on various ventilator modalities may also have variations in their metabolic rate. Clients on dialysis of any type cannot be tested because of CO_2 removal and variation in metabolic status. Check with your laboratory for restrictions.

Exercise Studies.   Exercise induced bronchospasm (EIB) stress testing is a form of bronchoprovocation testing that can be performed by one of the two methods.

In the first method:

- The client refrains from pulmonary medications, caffeine, exposure to cold air, and physical exercise as in the methacholine procedure prior to testing.
- A 12-lead ECG is applied.
- A baseline spirometer test is done, which acts as the control.
- The client exercises on a treadmill or a bicycle ergometer until the target heart rate of 85% of maximum is met or the client has symptoms limiting the exercise.
- Exercise is terminated and serial spirometry is performed immediately postexercise and at 1, 3, and 5 min and then every 5 min for a period up to 45 min postexercise. A drop of greater than 10% to 15% of the FEV_1 indicates a positive response.

In the second method:

The procedures of the first method arc followed with the following additions:

- The client inhales cold ($-20°C$), dry air, which is generated by a chilling device driven by compressed air prior to and during the exercise test.
- Spirometry is performed as above; see the first method.

Factors Affecting Diagnostic Results
- Use of bronchodilator 4 h before the pulmonary function test may produce falsely improved pulmonary results. Other medications used may also cause other changes. Check with the physician to see what is being diagnosed and the pulmonary laboratory regarding the medication list.
- Activity/exercise may cause bronchodilation.
- Sedatives and narcotics given before the test could decrease test results.
- Lack of cooperation by the client due to not understanding the specific test procedure or malingering may affect results.

Nursing Implications
- List on the request slip oral/inhaled bronchodilators and steroids the client is taking. Record client's age, height, and weight.
- Record vital signs.

- Assess for signs and symptoms of respiratory distress (i.e., breathlessness, dyspnea, tachycardia, severe apprehension, and gray or cyanotic color). Notify the physician and the laboratory. If the client is too ill or a recent exacerbation has occurred, pulmonary testing may yield little useful information. These tests require total client effort, cooperation, and the ability to follow instructions. The majority of this type of testing is performed on an out-patient bases.
- Be supportive of the client, and answer client's questions if you can or contact the laboratory for more information. Many laboratories will come and access clients prior to testing. Clients with recent mental status changes, uncontrolled blood pressure, acute MI or stroke may not do well with these procedures.

Client Teaching

- Instruct the client to eat a light breakfast, except in nutritional studies; to take medications, except for bronchodilators, sedatives, narcotics, and others as stated by health care provider orders; and to avoid smoking for 4 to 6 h before test. For any questions, contact the pulmonary laboratory.
- Explain to the client that the test should not be performed if he/she has an active cold, is running a fever, or has a communicable disease such as active TB, unless approved by the health care provider and the pulmonary laboratory chief.
- Practice breathing patterns for pulmonary function tests with the client (i.e., normal breathing, rapid breathing, and forced deep inspiration and forced deep expiration).

RADIOACTIVE IODINE (RAI) UPTAKE TEST

I-131 UPTAKE TEST, RADIOIODINE THYROID UPTAKE TEST

Normal Findings.   Adult: 1%–13% (thyroid gland); 6 h: 2%–25% (thyroid gland); 24 h: 15%–45% (thyroid gland)

Description.   The radioactive iodine uptake test is used to determine the metabolic activity of the thyroid gland by measuring the absorption of

I-131 or I-123 in the thyroid. The uptake test is one of the tests used in diagnosing hypothyroidism and hyperthyroidism. It tends to be more accurate for diagnosing hyperthyroidism than for diagnosing hypothyroidism. It is also useful for differentiating between hyperthyroidism (Graves' disease) and an overactive toxic adenoma.

A calculated dose of I-131 or I-123, in liquid or capsule form, is given orally. The client's thyroid is scanned at three different times. The tracer dose has a small amount of radioactivity and is considered harmless. The client's urine may be checked for radioactive iodine excretion.

Purposes
- To determine the metabolic activity of the thyroid gland
- To diagnose hypothyroidism and hyperthyroidism
- To differentiate between hyperthyroidism and an overactive toxic adenoma

Clinical Problems
Decreased level: Hypothyroidism (myxedema)
Drugs that may decrease RAI uptake: Lugol's solution, vitamins, expectorants (SSKI), antithyroid agents, cortisone preparation, ACTH, aspirin, antihistamines, phenylbutazone (Butazolidin), anticoagulants, thiopental sodium (Pentothal)
Foods that may cause false negatives: Seafood, cabbage, iodized salt
Increased level: Hyperthyroidism (Graves' disease), thyroiditis, cirrhosis of the liver
Drugs that may increase RAI uptake: Barbiturates, estrogens, lithium carbonate, phenothiazines

Procedure
- Restrict food and fluids for 8 h prior to the test. The client can eat an hour after the radioiodine capsule or liquid has been taken.
- The amount of radioactivity in the thyroid gland may be measured three times (after 2, 6, and 24 h).

- The client should return to the nuclear medicine laboratory at specified times to measure the I-131 uptake level with the scintillation counter.

Factors Affecting Diagnostic Results

- Severe diarrhea, intestinal malabsorption, and X-ray contrast media studies may cause a decreased I-131 uptake level, even in normal thyroid glands.
- Renal failure could cause an increased iodine uptake.

Nursing Implications

- Ask client for any known allergic reaction to iodine.
- Write down the times for returning to the nuclear medicine laboratory. Emphasize the importance of being on time for each determination.
- List on the request slip the X-ray studies and drugs the client has received in the last week, which could affect test results.
- Draw blood for T_3 and/or T_4 tests, if ordered, before the client takes the radioiodine capsule or liquid.
- Observe for signs and symptoms of hyperthyroidism (i.e., nervousness, tachycardia, excessive hyperactivity, exophthalmos, mood swings, and weight loss).

Client Teaching

- Inform client that eating an hour after the radioiodine capsule or liquid has been taken is usually permitted unless otherwise indicated by the nuclear medicine laboratory.
- Inform the client that the test should not be painful and that the amount of radiation received should be harmless.
- Inform client that the radioactive substance should not harm family members, visitors, or other clients, since the dosage is low and gives off very little radiation. Women who are pregnant should not be given this test.

SCHILLING TEST (URINE)

CO-57-TAGGED VITAMIN B$_{12}$ (COBALT-57-TAGGED CYANOCOBALAMIN)

Normal Finding
Adult: Greater than 7% excretion of radioactive vitamin B$_{12}$ within 24 h. Usual range is 10%–40% of vitamin B$_{12}$ excretion. Pernicious anemia: excretion of vitamin B$_{12}$ is less than 3%. Intestinal malabsorption: excretion is 3%–5%

Description.
The Schilling test is primarily ordered to diagnose pernicious anemia, a macrocytic anemia. The test determines whether the client lacks the intrinsic factor in the gastric mucosa that is necessary for the absorption of vitamin B$_{12}$ from food. With impaired absorption due to the lack of intrinsic factor or from intestinal malabsorption, little to no vitamin B$_{12}$ is absorbed and therefore less is excreted in the urine.

A vitamin B$_{12}$ deficiency affects the bone marrow, the gastrointestinal tract, and neurologic system. The bone marrow becomes hyperplastic, having many bizarre red blood cell forms. The gastrointestinal mucosa atrophies, and there is a decrease in hydrochloric acid. Classic symptoms of pernicious anemia include a beefy, red tongue; indigestion; abdominal pain; diarrhea; and tingling and numbness of the hands and feet.

The test consists of collecting a 24-h urine specimen after the client has taken a radioactive capsule of vitamin B$_{12}$ administered by a technician from the nuclear medicine laboratory and an injection of intramuscular vitamin B$_{12}$ given by the nurse. The intramuscular vitamin B$_{12}$ will saturate the liver and the protein-binding sites, thus permitting the absorption of the capsule cobalt-tagged vitamin B$_{12}$ by the small intestines and its excretion in the urine. There are various types of radioactive cobalt (Co-57, Co-56, Co-60), but Co-57 is preferred because of its shorter half-life and its low-energy gamma radiation.

Purposes
- To determine whether there is a vitamin B$_{12}$ deficiency
- To detect pernicious anemia and intestinal malabsorption syndrome

Clinical Problems

Decreased level: Pernicious anemia, intestinal malabsorption syndrome, liver diseases, hypothyroidism (myxedema), pancreatic insufficiency, sprue

Procedure

- Obtain a signed consent form.
- Restrict food and fluids for 8 to 12 h before the test. Food and fluids are permitted after the IM vitamin B_{12} dose.
- Avoid ingestion of B vitamins for 3 days prior to the test and no laxatives for 1 day prior to test.
- A sample of urine (25–50 ml) should be collected before cobalt-tagged vitamin B_{12} is given to determine if there are radionuclide contaminants. A recent radionuclide scan within 7 days prior to the test could affect test result.
- The radioactive Co-57-tagged vitamin B_{12} capsule(s) or liquid is/are administered orally by a technician from nuclear medicine.
- Vitamin B_{12} (usually 1 mg) is given IM by the nurse 1 to 2 h after the radioactive dose.
- Collect urine in a large container for 24 h, according to the institution's procedure. No preservative is needed in the urine container. Check laboratory's policy.
- Label the urine container with the client's name, date, time, and room.
- Rubber gloves should be worn to handle the 24-h urine specimen.

Nursing Implications

- Assess for signs and symptoms of pernicious anemia, such as beefy, red tongue; indigestion; abdominal pain; diarrhea; and tingling and numbness of the hands and feet.
- Assess urine output; low urine output affects test results.
- Do not administer laxatives the night before the test, as they could decrease absorption rate.
- Observe the client for at least 1 h after the administration of the radionuclide for possible anaphylactic reaction.
- Release the breakfast tray after the nonradioactive vitamin B_{12} is given.

- Label the urine container and laboratory slip with the exact dates and times of collection. Tell client and family not to throw away the urine.

Client Teaching

- Discuss the test procedure with the client (see Procedure).
- Explain to the client that the radioactive substance should not be harmful to family members, visitors, or self unless the person is pregnant.
- Instruct the client that foods high in vitamin B_{12} are mostly animal products, such as milk, eggs, meat, and liver. Vitamin B_{12} is low in vegetables. Refer the client to the dietitian as needed.

SEX CHROMATIN MASS, BUCCAL SMEAR, BARR BODY ANALYSIS

Normal Finding.   Barr body in 25% to 50% of the female buccal mucosal cells

Description.   The sex chromatin test is a screening method to detect the presence or absence of Barr chromatin body (an inactivated X chromosome in a mass lying at the periphery of the cell nucleus) in the buccal mucosal cells. Buccal smears are used to check for Barr body when chromosomal abnormalities are suspected (e.g., Turner's syndrome [absent or less than 20% Barr body in females] and Klinefelter's syndrome [presence of Barr body in males]). This test is also indicated if amenorrhea or abnormal sexual development is present.

Abnormal findings should be followed up by chromosome analysis (karyotype). The sex chromatin test should not be used for sex determinations.

Purposes

- To detect Barr chromatin body
- To check for the presence of Turner's syndrome or Klinefelter's syndrome

Clinical Problems

Abnormal findings: Turner's syndrome (female); absence of Barr body, amenorrhea, sterility, underdeveloped breasts; Klinefelter's syndrome (male); presence of Barr body, small penis and testes, sparse facial hair, gynecomastia, sterility.

Procedure

- There is no food or fluid restriction.
- The client should rinse his or her mouth well.
- Wooden or metal spatula is used to scrape the buccal mucosa twice; the first scraping is discarded, and the second is spread over a glass slide. The slide should be sprayed with a fixative solution and sent to the laboratory for identifying a Barr body in the cells. The specimen should be labeled with the client's name, sex, and age, as well as the date and the specimen site.
- Check that the specimen is not saliva. The smear is stained and examined under a microscope.
- The procedure usually takes 10 to 20 min.

Factors Affecting Diagnostic Results

- If the specimen is saliva and not cells, the test result could be inaccurate.
- Failure to use a preservative spray on the buccal smear specimen will cause cell deterioration.

Nursing Implications

- Record in the chart any abnormal sexual characteristics or problems (e.g., amenorrhea, gynecomastia) and note them on the request slip.
- Be supportive of the client and his or her family. Be a good listener. Answer questions or refer them to the appropriate health professionals.

Client Teaching

- Explain to the client and/or parents that the purpose of the test is to determine the cause of abnormal sexual development. Inform them that this is a screening test and that other tests, such as chromosome analysis, may be indicated.

- Explain the procedure to the client and parents. Inform the client that the cells from inside the mouth (buccal smear) are used because they are easy to obtain. Tell them that the test has a high percentage of accuracy. The procedure usually takes 10 to 20 min; however, the results from the test may take several weeks.
- Inform the client that there should be a minimal amount of discomfort. Light pressure will be applied when scraping the mucosa.

SIGMOIDOSCOPY*

Normal Finding. Normal mucosa and structure of the rectum and sigmoid colon

Description. Sigmoidoscopy is an examination of the anus, rectum, and sigmoid colon using a flexible sigmoidoscope to visualize the descending colon. This test is usually performed for screening for colon polyps and can be performed in a physician's office, clinic, or hospital. It may be part of an annual physical examination. Sigmoidoscopy may be requested when the client does not want a colonoscopy. With this procedure the rectum and distal sigmoid colon can be visualized, and specimens can be obtained by a biopsy forceps or a snare.

Purposes
- To examine the anus, rectum, and sigmoid colon
- To detect blood, polyps, or tumor in the sigmoid colon
- To obtain a culture of tissue or secretion for cytologic study

Clinical Problems
Abnormal findings: Hemorrhoids; rectal and sigmoid colon polyps; fistulas, fissures; rectal abscesses, benign or malignant neoplasms; ulcerative or granulomatous colitis; infection and/or inflammation of the rectosigmoid area

---

*Updated by Dr. Warren G. Butt, Gastroenterology-Stomach-Colon-Liver, Newark, Delaware.

Procedure
- A consent form should be signed.
- The client should follow the pre-test preparation given by the physician or health care provider. The client is usually allowed a light dinner the night before the test and then NPO afterwards. Usually heavy meals, vegetables, and fruits are prohibited within 24 h of the test.
- No barium studies should be performed within 3 days of the test.
- Fleet enema(s), which is (are) hypertonic salt enema(s), is (are) given the morning of the test. If enemas are contraindicated, then a rectal suppository, such as bisacodyl (Dulcolax), may be prescribed. Fecal material must be evacuated before the examination. Preparation with GoLytely could be used. Oral cathartics are seldom used, because they may increase fecal flow from the small intestine during the test.
- The client should assume a Sims (side-lying) position.
- A lubricated, flexible endoscope is inserted into the rectum. The client should be instructed to breathe deeply and slowly. Air may be injected into the bowel to improve visualization.
- Specimens can be obtained during the procedure.
- The procedure takes approximately 15 to 30 min.

Factors Affecting Diagnostic Results
- Barium can decrease the visualization, so barium studies should be performed a week before the test or afterward.
- Fecal material in the lower colon can decrease visualization.

Nursing Implications
- Explain the purpose of the sigmoidoscopy to the client. The test could be a part of the routine physical examination for preventive health care, or the cause of the symptoms, such as bright blood or mucus in stools, constipation, bowel changes.
- Explain the procedure to the client, such as the pre-test preparation.
- Check the chart to determine whether the client has had a barium study. If so, when, and notify the physician.
- Obtain the client's history in regard to health problems and being pregnant. Caution should be taken with some health problems such as ulcerative colitis.

- Record baseline vital signs before the test and following the test.
- Allow the client time to ask questions and express concerns. Refer questions you cannot answer to a physician or to the appropriate health professional.

Client Teaching

- Inform the client that the procedure may cause some discomfort but should not cause severe pain. Encourage the client to breathe deeply and slowly and to relax during the test. Explain that there may be some gas pains if a small amount of air is injected during the procedure for better visualization.

Post-test

- Monitor vital signs as indicated.
- Observe for signs and symptoms of bowel perforation, such as pain, abdominal distention, and rectal bleeding. These problems rarely occur. Report all symptoms immediately to the physician or health professional.
- Be supportive of the client and his or her family.

Client Teaching

- Encourage the client to rest for several hours or as indicated after the test if possible. This procedure may be done in a physician's office, clinic, or hospital. If the test is done on an outpatient basis, the client should rest for 1 h before leaving.

SINUS ENDOSCOPY

Normal Finding.   Normal sinuses; no infection or structural abnormalities noted

Description.   Sinus endoscopy examines the anterior ethmoids and the middle meatal sinus areas. The primary purposes are to correct structural abnormalities and alleviate an infectious process. Sinus endoscopy is frequently prescribed for clients with chronic sinusitis who are nonresponsive to antibiotic therapy.

Purpose
- To diagnose the presence of a chronic sinus infection or structural abnormality

Clinical Problems.   Acute or chronic sinusitis, cysts, sinus erosion, structural abnormality

Procedure
- Obtain a signed consent form.
- Restrict food and fluids after midnight or 12 h prior to the procedure.
- Remove dentures, jewelry, and hairpins if present.
- Intravenous fluids are usually started prior to the procedure.
- Eye pads may be used to protect the eyes from injury during the procedure.
- The nostrils are sprayed with topical anesthetic. The procedure may be performed in the health care provider's office or in an outpatient department.
- CT scan may be needed during the procedure to visualize the sinus area.
- Nasal packing may be inserted into the nostril(s) post-procedure.

Factors Affecting Diagnostic Results
- Severe nasal septal defect.

Nursing Implications
- Obtain a history of the sinus problem(s) from the client.
- Check that the consent form is signed.
- Monitor vital signs.

Client Teaching
- Explain the procedure for sinus endoscopy (see Procedure). Answer questions that the client may have or if unknown, refer questions to appropriate health professionals.

Post-test
- Continue monitoring client's vital signs until stabilized.
- Check for excessive bleeding or discharge.

Client Teaching

- Instruct client to call health care provider if excessive bleeding or discharge occurs and for elevated body temperature.
- Instruct the client to take prescribed drugs (antibiotic and pain medication). Discuss post-test care as indicated by the health care provider.

SKIN TESTS (TUBERCULIN, BLASTOMYCOSIS, COCCIDIOIDOMYCOSIS, HISTOPLASMOSIS, TRICHINOSIS, AND TOXOPLASMOSIS)

Normal Finding. Negative results

Description. Skin testing is useful for determining present or past exposure to an infectious organism: bacterial (tuberculosis); mycotic (blastomycosis, coccidioidomycosis, histoplasmosis); or parasitic (trichinosis and toxoplasmosis). The types of skin tests include scratch, patch, multipuncture, and intradermal. With intradermal, the antigen of the organism is injected under the skin, and if the test is positive in 24 to 72 h, the injection site becomes red, hard, and edematous.

Bacterial organism and disease: Tuberculosis: The tuberculin skin test indicates whether a person has been infected by the tubercle bacilli.

Testing Methods

- *Mantoux Test:* Purified protein derivative tuberculin (PPD) is injected intradermally. PPD has several strengths, but the intermediate strength is usually used unless the client is known to be hypersensitive to skin tests. The client should not receive PPD if there was a previous positive test. The test is read in 48 to 72 h.
- *Tine Test or Mono-Vacc Test:* These are multipuncture tests that use tines impregnated with PPD. Method is for mass screening. The tine test is read in 48 to 72 h, and the Mono-Vacc Test is read in 48 to 96 h.
- *Vollmer's Patch Test:* This test "patch" resembles a Band-Aid; however, the center piece is impregnated with concentrated old

tuberculin (OT). The patch is removed in 48 h, and the test result is read.

Mycotic Organisms and Diseases

- *Blastomycosis:* The organism *Blastomyces dermatitidis* causes blastomycosis. The antigen blastomycin is injected intradermally, and if an erythematous area greater than 5 mm in diameter occurs, the test is positive. The skin test should be read in 48 h. Positive sputum and tissue specimens will confirm the blastomycin skin test.
- *Coccidioidomycosis:* The organism *Coccidioides immitis* causes the fungal disease coccidioidomycosis. The antigen, coccidioidin, is injected intradermally, and the skin test is read in 24 to 72 h.
- *Histoplasmosis:* The organism *Histoplasma capsulatum* causes histoplasmosis. On chest X-ray the lung infection resembles tuberculosis. The histoplasmin test is not always reliable. The antigen is injected intradermally, and the skin test is read in 24 to 48 h. To confirm the skin test result, sputum and tissue specimens should be obtained.

Parasites

- *Trichinosis:* The parasitic organism *Trichinella spiralis* causes trichinosis. Symptoms of nausea, diarrhea, pain, colic, fever, and swelling of the muscles occur approximately 2 weeks after ingesting the organism. The antigen is injected intradermally, and the test is read in 15 to 20 min. A positive test is a blanched wheal with an erythematous area surrounding it.
- *Toxoplasmosis:* The organism *Toxoplasma gondii* causes toxoplasmosis. This organism is found in the eye ground and brain tissue of man. The antigen, toxoplasmin, is injected intradermally, and the test result is read in 24 to 48 h. A positive test is an erythematous area over 10 mm in diameter.

Purposes

- To determine the present or past exposure to an infectious organism
- To determine if the client has been infected by the tubercle bacilli using the TB skin test

Clinical Problems

Antigen Skin Test	Organism	Disease
Tuberculin	Tubercle bacilli	Tuberculosis
Blastomycin	*Blastomyces dermatitidis*	Blastomycosis
Coccidioidin	*Coccidioides immitis*	Coccidioidomycosis
Histoplasmin	*Histoplasma capsulatum*	Histoplasmosis
Trichinella	*Trichinella spiralis*	Trichinosis
Toxoplasmin	*Toxoplasma gondii*	Toxoplasmosis

Procedure

- No food or fluid is restricted.
- Cleanse the inner aspect of the forearm with alcohol and let it dry.
- Inject intradermally 0.1 ml of the antigen into the inner aspect of forearm.
- Indicate injection site for reading of test result.

Nursing Implications

- Obtain a client history about hypersensitivity to skin tests. Ask the client if the skin test was performed before and if so, the result. The skin test should only be repeated if it was negative.
- Report if the client has taken steroids or immunosuppressant drugs in the last 4 to 6 weeks, since false test results could occur.

Client Teaching

- Inform the client that a pinprick will be felt. A small amount of solution is injected under the skin.
- Inform the client that the result of the skin test must be read during the stated time.
- Ask the client about contact with a bacterial, fungal, or parasitic organism.
- Tell the client that a positive skin test does not always indicate active infectious disease. However, the positive test does indicate that the organism is present in the body in either an active or a dormant state.

SLEEP STUDIES

POLYSOMNOGRAPHY (PSG)

Normal Findings.   Normal sleep pattern with normal ECG, EEG, EMG, O$_2$ saturation

Description.   Sleep studies, primarily called polysomnography (PSG), determine the cause of sleep disorders, including daytime sleepiness, obstructive sleep apnea (OSA) or sleep disordered breathing, insomnia, nocturnal awakening, and snoring problems. OSA occurs when there is no ventilation for 10 seconds. It may be attributed to oxygen desaturation, cardiac dysrhythmia, or sleep interruption. Also PSG is indicated for persons having difficulty staying awake during the day or who fall asleep at inappropriate times.

Testing for sleep disorders is performed in a sleep laboratory at night over an 8-h period of time. The client is monitored during the night by electrocardiogram (ECG or EKG), pulse oximetry to determine heart rate and oxygen saturation, electroencephalogram (EEG), electrooculogram (EOG), electromyogram (EMG), airflow monitoring, and snoring sensor. All these testing devices may not be indicated.

Purpose
- To determine the cause of the sleep disorder

Clinical Problems
Abnormal findings: Obstructive sleep apnea (OSA), insomnia, nocturnal awakening, and snoring

Procedure
- A consent form should be signed.
- Keep a sleep log for 1 to 2 weeks prior to the PSG test.
- Avoid caffeine products, alcohol, sedatives, and naps 1 to 2 days before testing.

- Omit prescribed medications until the sleep studies are completed, if indicated.
- Sleep studies are scheduled in the sleep laboratory at night usually 10 or 11 PM until 6 or 7 AM (8-h period of time).
- Attach electrodes for ECG, EEG, EMG.
- Attach the pulse oximetry.
- Place a commode by the bedside. Electrode leads may inhibit bathroom use.
- Lights are turned off.
- In the AM, have the client evaluate his/her sleep experience.

Factors Affecting Diagnostic Results
- Defective electrodes or those that become loose or fall off
- Inability to sleep
- Drugs such as sedatives, caffeine taken prior to the test

Nursing Implications
- Obtain a history from the client in regard to medications, past stroke, head injury, headaches, seizures.
- Review the sleep log that the client has given.
- Check vital signs. Note if there is respiratory distress.

Client Teaching
- Explain to the client that electrodes will be attached to the head, chest, and legs.
    ECG: selected leads attached
    EEG: 2 sets of electrodes to the scalp
    EOG: 1 electrode to canthus eye
    EMG: electrodes attached to the leg muscles
    Pulse oximeter: attached to the finger to determine heart rate and oxygen saturation.
- Answer client's questions or refer the questions to other health professionals.

STRESS/EXERCISE TESTS (TREADMILL EXERCISE ELECTROCARDIOLOGY, EXERCISE MYOCARDIAL PERFUSION IMAGING TEST [THALLIUM/TECHNETIUM STRESS TEST], NUCLEAR PERSANTINE [DIPYRIDAMOLE] STRESS TEST, NUCLEAR DOBUTAMINE STRESS TEST)*

Normal Findings.   Normal ECG with little or no ST-segment depression or arrhythmia with exercise; normal myocardial perfusion

Description.   Stress testing is based on the theory that clients with coronary artery disease will have marked ST-segment depression when exercising. Depression of the ST-segment and depression or inversion of the T wave indicate myocardial ischemia. ST-segment depression usually occurs before the onset of pain and remains present for some time after the pain has subsided. Mild segment depression after exercise can occur without coronary artery disease (CAD).

Treadmill and bicycle exercise electrocardiology: This type of stress test is frequently prescribed to determine the presence of CAD. The bicycle ergometer test may be used; however, the treadmill seems to be the choice. The body muscles do not seem to tire with the treadmill method as much as leg muscles with the bicycle ergometer. For clients who cannot walk (e.g., hemiplegics, amputees), an arm ergometer can be used. With the treadmill stress test, the work rate is changed every 3 min for 15 min by increasing the speed slightly and the degree of incline (grade) by 3% each time (3%, 6%, 9%, etc.). The clients will exercise until they are fatigued, develop symptoms, or reach their maximum predicted heart rate (MPHR).

Exercise thallium perfusion test: The radioisotope thallium-201, which accumulates in the myocardial cells, is used during the stress test to deter-

---

*Updated by Susan L. Chudzik, CRNP, Christiana Care Health Services, Newark, Delaware.

mine myocardial perfusion during exercise. With severe narrowing of the coronary arteries, there is less thallium accumulation in the heart muscle. If a coronary vessel is completely occluded, no uptake of thallium will occur at the myocardial area that the vessel supplies.

Clients with coronary artery disease (CAD) may have normal thallium perfusion scans at rest; however, during exercise, when the heart demands more oxygen, myocardial perfusion can decrease. In the resting state, blood flows through a coronary artery with stenosis, and it remains normal until the stenosis exceeds 85%. The client returns 2 to 3 h later for a second scan of the heart at rest. Frequently second scans are done to differentiate between an ischemic area and an infarcted or scarred area of the myocardium.

Uses for the stress/exercise test or the exercise myocardial perfusion test include screening for CAD, evaluating myocardial perfusion, evaluating the work capacity of cardiac clients, developing a cardiac rehabilitation program, and preoperative assessment for noncardiac surgery.

Exercise technetium perfusion test: This is a useful stress test for detecting myocardial ischemia using technetium 99m-laced (Tc-99m) compounds, such as Tc-99m-sestamibi (Cardiolite). The technetium compounds are used for perfusion scanning because they are trapped in the myocardium and do not cause redistribution of the compound. Technetium compounds provide more clinical information by allowing the assessment of perfusion, wall motion, and ejection fraction in one test procedure. Other technetium agents approved by the U.S. Food and Drug Administration (FDA) are Tc-99m-teboroxime and Tc-99m-tetrofosmin.

Cardiolite imaging is perhaps the most useful noninvasive test for diagnosing and following CAD at the present time. Positive stress Cardiolite scanning usually indicates CAD; however, a more markedly abnormal scan is more likely to indicate serious CAD. It is important to correlate the scan findings with the ECG, the exercise stress test, and the client's symptoms. The use of gated single positron emission (SPECT) (gated refers to the synchronizing of images with the computer and the client's heart rhythm) greatly improves the sensitivity and specificity of the Cardiolite scan.

Nuclear Persantine (dipyridamole) stress test: This is an alternative stress test usually ordered when the client is not physically able to exercise or to walk on a treadmill. Persantine is administered intravenously to dilate the coronary arteries and increase blood flow to the myocardium.

Arteries that have become narrowed because of coronary artery disease (CAD) cannot expand.

Thallium-201, Cardiolite, or other Tc-based compounds, administered intravenously, detect decreased blood flow to the heart muscle (myocardium). The isotope is administered 3 min after the 4-min IV Persantine infusion. The client must avoid foods, beverages, and medications containing xanthines (caffeine and theophyllines) 24 h prior to the test, and theophylline preparations 36 h prior to the test.

Nuclear Persantine stress testing is contraindicated for clients who have severe bronchospastic lung disease, such as asthma or advanced atrioventricular heart block. Other unfavorable conditions in which this test is not indicated include acute myocardial infarction (AMI) within 48 h of the test, severe aortic or mitral stenosis, resting systolic blood pressure less than 90 mm Hg, and allergy to dipyridamole.

Nuclear dobutamine stress test: Dobutamine is an adrenergic (sympathomimetic) drug that increases myocardial contractility, heart rate, and systolic blood pressure, which increases the myocardial oxygen consumption and thus increases coronary blood flow. If the client has heart block or asthma and takes a theophylline preparation daily, this test may be ordered instead of the nuclear Persantine (dipyridamole) stress test. Dobutamine is an alternative stressor test.

Contraindications for nuclear dobutamine test include clients having acute myocardial infarction (AMI) within 10 days, acute myocarditis or pericarditis, unstable angina pectoris (prolonged episodes, episodes at rest), ventricular and atrial antidysrhythmias, severe aortic or mitral stenosis, hyperthyroidism, and acutely severe infections. Propranolol (Inderal) should be available for any possible adverse reaction to the dobutamine infusion.

Purposes

- To screen for coronary artery disease (CAD)
- To evaluate myocardial perfusion
- To differentiate between an ischemic area and an infarcted or scar area of the myocardium
- To develop a cardiac rehabilitation program
- To evaluate cardiac status for work capability
- To evaluate drug efficiency

Clinical Problems

Abnormal finding: Positive: greater than 2 mm ST depression, coronary artery disease, myocardial hypoperfusion

Procedure

- Obtain a signed consent form.
- NPO for 2 to 3 h before the test. Avoid alcohol, caffeine-containing drinks, and smoking for 2 to 3 h before the test. Most medications should be taken.
- Comfortable clothes should be worn (e.g., shorts or slacks, sneakers with socks, and *no* bedroom slippers).
- The chest is shaved as needed, and the skin is cleansed with alcohol.
- Electrodes are applied to the chest according to the lead selections.
- Baseline ECG, pulse rate, and blood pressure are taken and then monitored throughout the test.
- The test is stopped if the client becomes dyspneic, suffers severe fatigue, complains of chest pain, has a rapid increase in pulse rates or blood pressure, or both, or develops life-threatening arrhythmias (i.e., ventricular tachycardia, premature ventricular contractions [PVCs] over 10 PVC in 1 min).
- The test takes approximately 30 min, which includes up to 10 to 15 min of exercising.

Treadmill stress test: Usually, there are five stages: first the speed is 2 mph at a 3% incline for 3 min. In the second stage the speed is 3.3 mph at a 6% incline for another 3 min. The speed usually does not go beyond 3.3 mph. With each stage the incline is increased 3% and the time is increased by 3 min, unless fatigue or adverse reactions occur.

Bicycle ergometer test: The client is instructed to pedal the bike against an increased amount of resistance. A shower or hot bath should *not* be taken for 2 h after testing.

Exercise thallium perfusion test: An IV line is inserted. Exercise time for the stress test is determined. The client obtains the maximal exercise level, and thallium is injected intravenously 1 min before the test ends. The client continues to exercise for 1 more min. A scan taken by a nuclear camera (scintillator) visualizes thallium perfusion of the myocardium. Client returns in 3 or more h for a second scan.

Exercise technetium perfusion test: With the Cardiolite stress test, the client receives two injections intravenously, one at rest and one at stress. The client should be NPO for 2 to 3 h prior to the test. Any medications that may affect the blood pressure or heart rate should be discontinued 24 to 36 h prior to the test unless the test is used to evaluate the efficacy of cardiac medication. The total time for the test is 3 h, a shorter time than thallium imaging.

Nuclear Persantine (dipyridamole) stress test: The client remains NPO after midnight except for water. A diabetic client should check with the health care provider concerning diet. Caffeine-containing drugs, food, and beverages such as colas must be avoided 24 h prior to the test. Decaffeinated beverages should also be avoided. Certain drugs (e.g., theophylline preparations) should be stopped 36 h before the test.

The client is in a supine position during the test. The client receives a total of 0.56 mg/kg/dose of IV Persantine (dipyridamole) over a period of 4 min. Three minutes after the Persantine infusion, the isotope (thallium, Cardiolite, or other Tc-based compound) is injected intravenously. Aminophylline should be available to reverse any adverse reaction to Persantine. Imaging procedure begins 15 to 30 min after the isotope infusion. Heart rate, blood pressure, and ECG will be monitored before and during the test.

The test is terminated if any of the following occur: ventricular tachycardia, second degree heart block, severe ST-segment depression, severe hypotension (less than 90 mm Hg), or severe wheezing. The asthmatic client may use the beta-agonist inhaler if necessary during the procedure.

Nuclear dobutamine stress test: The client remains NPO after midnight except for water. Beta blockers, calcium channel blockers, and ACE inhibitors should be discontinued for 36 h prior to the test. Nitrates should not be taken 6 h before the test. Dobutamine is administered IV using an infusion pump. The dobutamine is mixed in 1 L of normal saline solution, and the dose and infusion rate are increased until the client's heart rate reaches approximately 85% of his or her maximum predicted heart rate. If the heart rate is less than 110 beats per minute, IV atropine sulfate may be given. The isotope is injected when the maximum heart rate is achieved.

The test is terminated if any of the following occur: atrial or ventricular tachycardia, atrial flutter or fibrillation, severe ST-segment depression, progressive anginal pain, severe hypotension (less than 90 mm Hg systolic), and severe hypertension (greater than 220 mm Hg systolic or greater than 120 mm Hg diastolic). Nitroglycerin may be given for angina pain. Propranolol (Inderal) should be available for adverse reaction to dobutamine. Imaging procedure occurs 15 min after the completion of the dobutamine infusion.

Factors Affecting Diagnostic Results
- Certain drugs (e.g., digitalis preparations) can cause a false-positive test result.
- Leaning on support rails of the treadmill or the handlebars of the bicycle.

Nuclear Persantine (Dipyridamole) Stress Test
- Taking theophylline preparations within 24 h of the test.
- Ingesting caffeine products (beverages, chocolates) 6 h before the test.
- Ingesting decaffeinated beverages 4 h before the test.

Nuclear Dobutamine Stress Test
- Taking beta blockers, calcium channel blockers, ACE inhibitors, 24 h before the test.
- Taking nitrates 4 h before the test.
- Ingesting a full meal 4 h before the test.

Nursing Implications
- Recognize when the stress/exercise test is contraindicated (i.e., with recent myocardial infarction; severe, unstable angina; uncontrolled cardiac dysrhythmias; congestive heart failure; or recent pulmonary embolism).
- Check that the consent form has been signed.
- Recognize whether a treadmill stress test or pharmacological stress test is appropriate.
- Review medications that may interfere with test, for example, beta blockers to decrease heart rate.

Client Teaching
Treadmill Stress Test
- Explain the procedure to the client in regard to NPO 2 to 3 h prior to test; not smoking; continuing with medications; the clothing and shoes that should be worn; shaving and cleansing the chest area;

electrode application; continuous monitoring of the ECG, pulse rate, and BP; and not leaning on the rails of the treadmill or the handlebars of the bike.

- Instruct the client to inform the cardiologist or technician if he or she experiences chest pain, difficulty in breathing, or severe fatigue. The risk of having a myocardial infarction during the stress test is less than 0.2%.

- Inform the client that after 10 to 15 min of testing or when the heart rate is at a desired or an elevated rate, the test is stopped. It will be terminated immediately if there are any severe ECG changes (e.g., multiple PVCs, ventricular tachycardia).

- Allow the client to ask questions. Refer questions you cannot answer to other appropriate health professionals (i.e., a cardiologist, a specialized technician, or a nurse in the stress test laboratory).

- Instruct the client to continue the walking exercise at the completion of the test for 2 to 3 min to prevent dizziness. The treadmill speed will be decreased. Tell the client that he or she may be perspiring and may be "out of breath." Profuse diaphoresis, cold and clammy skin, severe dyspnea, and severe tachycardia are not normal, and the test will be terminated.

- Inform the client that an ECG and vital signs are taken after the stress test (recovery stage) until returning to baseline.

- Encourage the client to participate in a cardiac/exercise rehabilitation program as advised by the health care provider/cardiologist. Tell the client of the health advantages—constant heart monitoring, improved collateral circulation, increased oxygen supply to the heart, and dilating coronary resistance vessels.

- Discourage the client over 35 years of age from doing strenuous exercises without having a stress/exercise test or a cardiac evaluation.

- Inform the client that he or she can resume activity as indicated.

- Explain to the client that a written report is submitted to the client's personal physician from the cardiologist. The client should check with the health care provider for the test results.

Exercise Thallium Perfusion Test
- Explain the procedure for the test (see Procedure). Explain that the difference between the routine stress test and the exercise thallium

perfusion test is an injection of thallium 201 during the routine stress test followed by scans and/or X-rays. Nursing implications are the same for both tests.

- Instruct the client to return for additional pictures in 2 to 4 h as indicated by the technician or cardiologist.

Exercise Technetium Perfusion Test
- Explain the procedure (see Procedure).
- The client should lie quietly for approximately 30 min during the imaging.
- Inform the client that the test should last no more than 3 h.
- Instruct the client taking medications that affect the blood pressure or heart rate to check with the health care provider as for discontinuing the medications for 24 to 48 h prior to testing.

Nuclear Persantine (Dipyridamole) Stress Test
- Explain the procedure for the test to the client (see Procedure). The client should be NPO after midnight except for water.
- Instruct the client to avoid food, beverages, and drugs that contain caffeine. Beverages and foods rich in caffeine include colas (Coke and Pepsi), Dr. Pepper, Mountain Dew, Tab, chocolate (syrup and candy), tea, and coffee. Decaffeinated coffee and tea should also be avoided. Drugs containing caffeine include Anacin, Excedrin, NoDoz, Wigraine, Darvon compound, cafergot, fiorinal. Theophylline preparations should be avoided 36 h before the test; the client should check with the health care provider in case it is not possible to discontinue the theophylline drug for that period of time.
- Explain to the client that first Persantine will be given intravenously and then an isotope. The client is positioned under a camera with his or her left arm over the head. The camera will be moving very close to the chest for taking pictures (imaging). The imaging takes approximately 20 to 30 min.
- Instruct the client to return for additional pictures in 2 to 4 h as indicated by the technician or cardiologist.
- Explain to the client that a written report is submitted to the client's personal health care provider from the cardiologist.

Nuclear Dobutamine Stress Test

- Explain the procedure for the test to the client (see Procedure). The client should be NPO after midnight except for water.
- Instruct the client to discontinue drugs that are beta blockers, calcium channel blockers, or ACE inhibitors for 36 h prior to the test with the health care provider's approval. Give the client the date and time for stopping the drug. Nitrates should not be taken 6 h before the test unless necessary (check with the health care provider).
- Warn clients of side effects that may occur, such as chest pain, palpitations, headache, paresthesia, nausea, tremor, ventricular arrhythmias, ST-segment depression, and hypotension, which resolve with the discontinuation of the infusion.

THORACOSCOPY

Normal Findings.   Free of pleural and lung disease

Description.   With thoracoscopy, an endoscope (thoracoscope) tube is inserted into the thoracic cavity to visualize the pleural space, thoracic wall, pericardium, and the mediastinum. This test is replacing the thoracotomy procedure. Biopsies and fluid can be obtained with this procedure; also fluid can be drained. Wedge resection to remove blebs or disease tissue and laser procedure may be performed during this test.

Purposes

- To obtain biopsy specimens
- To assess tumor growth, pleural effusion, pleural and pulmonary infections, emphysema
- To perform laser procedure to the thoracic area

Clinical Problems

Abnormal findings: Pleural or lung tumors, metastatic cancer in the lungs and/or pleura, emphysema, empyema, inflammatory process in the thoracic cavity

Procedure

- A signed consent form is required.
- Nothing by mouth (NPO) for 8 to 12 h prior to the test.
- *Pre-test requirements:* Pulmonary function tests, chest X-ray, ECG (EKG), selected laboratory tests. These tests should be completed before the thoracoscopy.
- IV line is inserted for IV medications.
- Client is anesthetized and an endobronchial tube is inserted.
- The lung on the operative side is collapsed.
- The thoracoscope is inserted through a trocar to view the thoracic cavity.
- Following the thoracoscopic procedure, the lung is reexpanded and a chest tube is placed in the thoracic cavity with a water-sealed drainage tube attached (closed drainage system).
- A thoracoscopy takes approximately 1 h.

Factors Affecting Diagnostic Results

- Previous thoracic surgery can inhibit the test procedure.

Nursing Implications

- Obtain a history of the client's health problems and drugs that are taken daily.
- Obtain vital signs.
- Check that the client has completed the pre-test orders. Report any abnormal findings.

Client Teaching

- Explain the procedure to the client and refer unknown questions to other health professionals.
- Inform the client that pain medication will be available if the client has discomfort following the procedure.
- Inform the client that he/she will have a chest tube with a drainage system after the test. The chest tube is to ensure that any fluid left in the chest will be removed.

Post-test

- Monitor vital signs as indicated.
- Check patency of the drainage tube frequently or as ordered.

- Assess respiratory status.
- Report frank bleeding that appears in the drainage tube.
- Administer analgesics for pain as ordered and as needed.
- A chest X-ray will be ordered to determine whether the lung has expanded. Chest tube remains in the thoracic cavity until the lungs have expanded.

ULTRASONOGRAPHY (ABDOMINAL AORTA, BRAIN, BREAST, CAROTID, DOPPLER — ARTERIES AND VEINS, EYE AND EYE ORBIT, GALLBLADDER, HEART, KIDNEY, LIVER, PANCREAS, PELVIS [UTERUS, OVARIES, PREGNANT UTERUS], PROSTATE, SCROTUM, SPLEEN, THORACIC, AND THYROID)*

ULTRASOUND, ECHOGRAPHY (ECHOGRAM), SONOGRAM

Normal Finding. A normal pattern image of the organ or Doppler spectral analysis

Description. Ultrasonography (ultrasound or sonogram) is a diagnostic procedure used to visualize body tissue structure or wave-form analysis of Doppler studies. An ultrasound probe called a transducer is held over the skin surface or in a body cavity to produce an ultrasound beam to the tissues. The reflected sound waves or echoes from the tissues can be transformed by a computer into either scans, graphs, or audible sounds (Doppler).

Ultrasound can detect tissue abnormalities (e.g., masses, cysts, edema, stones). It cannot be used to determine bone abnormalities or for air-filled organs. In obese persons it is difficult for sound waves to pass through fat layers.

---

*Updated by Dr. Sharon W. Gould, Director; Radiology Residency Program, Christiana Care Health Services, Newark, Delaware.

Diagnostic ultrasound examinations are relatively inexpensive and cause no known harm to the clients. Most ultrasound studies (e.g., gallstones) do not need other modalities for confirmation; however, CT, MRI, or radionuclide scanning may be used to confirm certain ultrasound results.

Abdominal aorta: The area for abdominal scanning includes the xyphoid process to the umbilicus. Ultrasound can detect aortic aneurysms with 98% accuracy and can determine whether they are fusiform, saccular or dissecting types.

Arteries and veins (Doppler): Doppler ultrasonography evaluates the blood flow in arteries and veins anywhere in the body. The Doppler transducer can detect decreased blood flow caused by partial arterial occlusion or by deep-vein thrombosis. It can be used in fetal monitoring during labor and delivery. A Doppler instrument is available to nurses for monitoring blood flow for those who have altered circulation. Low-frequency waves usually indicate low-velocity blood flow. This procedure may also be used to evaluate the patency of a graft.

Brain: Brain echoencephalography is ultrasound of the brain. If the third ventricle, which is normally midline, is shifted to one side, then pathologic findings, such as intracranial lesion or intracranial hemorrhage, may be suspected. It is most useful to evaluate hydrocephalus and intracranial hemorrhage in newborns.

Breast: Ultrasound of the breast is helpful for (1) diagnosing breast lesions in women who have dense breasts, (2) differentiating between cystic and solid lesions, (3) follow-up of fibrocystic breast disease, and (4) evaluating women with silicone breast implants for breast lesions. The breast ultrasound may be suggested for pregnant women as well as any woman with a palpable breast mass. X-ray mammography remains the *screening* examination of choice, as ultrasound cannot detect microcalcification. Still, ultrasound serves as a valuable adjunctive tool.

Carotid artery with Doppler: Blood flow in the carotid artery can be measured by using Doppler technique to determine carotid stenosis. During a carotid sonogram, vertebral arteries can be visualized by this Doppler technique to determine antegrade or retrograde blood flow through these vessels.

Eye and eye orbit: Ultrasound of the eye and eye orbital area may be used to (1) determine abnormal tissue of the eye (vitreous adhesions, retinal detachment) when opacities within the eye are present, and (2) detect orbital lesions. With this test, orbital lesions can be distinguished from orbital inflammation.

Gallbladder and bile ducts: Ultrasonography can evaluate the size, structure, and position of the gallbladder and can determine the presence of gallstones.

Heart: Echocardiography is ultrasound of the heart. It can determine the size, shape, and position of the heart and the movement of heart valves and chambers. The methods commonly used are the M-mode and the two-dimensional. The M-mode records the motion of the intracardiac structures, such as valves, and the two-dimensional records a cross-sectional view of cardiac structures (see Echocardiography for detailed data).

Intravascular ultrasonography: An ultrasound transducer mounted on a catheter is used to obtain pathologic changes to the arterial wall and to evaluate vascular procedures such as angioplasty placement. This test is usually performed in large medical centers.

Kidneys (Renal): Ultrasound is a reliable test to identify and to differentiate renal cyst and tumor. The cyst is echo free, and the tumor and renal calculi record multiple echoes. This test is highly recommended when the client is hypersensitive to iodinated contrast dye used in X-ray tests (e.g., IVP).

Liver (Hepatic): The liver was one of the first organs examined by ultrasound. It is useful for distinguishing between a cyst or tumor and for determining the size, structure, and position of the liver. It is very helpful in differentiating obstructive from nonobstructive jaundice.

Pelvis: *Uterus:* Ultrasonography may be used to distinguish between cystic, solid, and complex masses as well as to localize free fluid and inflammatory processes. *Ovaries:* The dimensions of the ovaries, as well as ovarian cysts and solid lesions, can be identified by pelvic sonography. Pelvic ultrasonography is a valuable tool but should not replace a gynecologic examination. *Pregnancy:* In pregnancy the amniotic fluid enhances reflection of sound waves from the placenta and fetus, thus revealing their size, shape, and position. Echoes from the pregnancy may be seen after as few as 4 weeks of amenorrhea. For visualization of pelvic structures, a full bladder is indicated in the nongravid and first-trimester pregnancy.

The uterus is sometimes evaluated with a transvaginal transducer with the bladder empty.

Pancreas: The pancreas is a more difficult organ to examine and may require distending the stomach with water to create an acoustic window. Ultrasonography does not measure pancreatic function, but it can determine overall size of the gland and detect pancreatic abnormalities, such as pancreatic tumors, pseudocysts, and pancreatitis. This test is useful for clients who are too thin for adequate CT scanning.

Prostate (transrectal): Ultrasound of the prostate gland is used to (1) evaluate palpable prostate nodules and seminal vesicles, (2) determine if urinary problems may be related perhaps to benign prostatic hypertrophy (BPH), (3) detect early small prostate tumor, and (4) identify tumor location for biopsy and/or radiation purposes. A rectal examination and the laboratory test, prostate-specific antigen (PSA), should be included for diagnosing prostatic lesions.

Scrotum/testes: Ultrasound of the scrotum sac contents is helpful in diagnosing abscess, cyst, hydrocele, spermatocele, varicocele, testicular tumors, torsion, and chronic scrotal swelling.

Spleen: Ultrasonography can be used for determining the size, structure, and position of the spleen. This procedure can identify splenic masses. In some cases it is a useful tool for evaluating the need for splenectomy, follow-up of pathologies such as hematoma or abscess.

Thoracic: Ultrasound is useful in identifying lesions, but it is not diagnostic on air-filled cavities such as the lungs unless a lesion is present adherent to the chest wall. It may be used to identify pleural fluid, malposition of the diaphragm, and the presence of an abscess. Ultrasound of the thoracic area may be used in combination with X-ray and thoracic scans.

Thyroid: Ultrasonography of the thyroid is 85% accurate in determining the size and structure of the thyroid gland. It can differentiate between a cyst and tumor and can determine the depth and dimension of thyroid nodules.

Purposes

- To evaluate the size, structure, and position of body organs
- To evaluate the blood flow in arteries and veins
- To detect cysts, tumors, and calculi

Clinical Problems

Organ	*Abnormal Findings*
Abdominal aorta	Aortic aneurysms, aortic stenosis
Arteries and veins (Doppler)	Arterial occlusion (partial or complete), deep-vein thrombosis, chronic venous insufficiency, arterial trauma
Brain	Intracranial hemorrhage, lesions (tumors, abscess), hydrocephalus
Breast	Cysts, tumors (benign or malignant), metastasis to the lymph nodes and muscle tissue
Carotid artery	Carotid plaque, thrombus, degree of stenosis
Eye and eye orbit	Vitreous opacities, detached retina, foreign bodies, orbital lesion, orbital inflammation, meningioma, glioma, neurofibroma, cyst, keratoprosthesis
Gallbladder	Acute cholecystitis, cholelithiasis, biliary obstruction
Heart (Cardiac)	Cardiomegaly, mitral stenosis, aortic stenosis and insufficiency, pericardial effusion, congenital heart disease, left ventricular hypertrophy, ischemic heart disease, septal defects
Kidney (Renal)	Renal cysts and tumors, hydronephrosis, perirenal abscess, acute pyelonephritis, acute glomerulonephritis
Liver (Hepatic)	Hepatic cysts, abscesses, tumor; hepatic metastasis; hepatocellular disease, congenital abnormalities
Pancreas	Pancreatic tumors, pseudocysts, acute pancreatitis
Pelvis	
Uterus	Uterine tumor, fibroids; hydatiform mole, endometrial changes
Ovaries	Ovarian cysts or tumor
Pregnancy	Fetal age, fetal death, placenta previa, abruptio placenta; hydrocephalus; breech fetal presentation
Prostate	Cancer of the prostate gland, benign prostatic hypertrophy (BPH), prostatitis
Scrotum	Hydrocele, spermatocele, varicocele, testicular tumors, torsion, acute/chronic epididymitis, cyst, abscess, chronic scrotal swelling
Spleen	Splenomegaly; splenic cysts, abscesses, tumor, congenital anomalies
Thoracic	Pleural fluid, abscess formation, malposition of the diaphragm
Thyroid	Thyroid tumors (benign or malignant), thyroid goiters or cysts

Procedure

- Obtain a signed consent form, if necessary.
- Restrict food and fluids for 4 to 8 h before test for abdominal aorta, gallbladder, liver, spleen, and pancreas ultrasound studies.

- The client should eat a fat-free meal the night prior to the test for abdominal, gallbladder, liver, pancreas, and kidney sonograms.
- Premedications are seldom given unless the client is extremely apprehensive or has nausea and vomiting.
- Conductive gel is applied to the skin surface at the site to be examined. The transducer is hand held and moved smoothly back and forth across the oiled or gel-skin surface.
- The client's position may vary from supine to oblique, prone, semi-recumbent, and erect.
- The average time for a procedure is 30 min.
- The client should not smoke or chew gum prior to the examination to prevent swallowing air.

Brain

- Remove jewelry and hairpins from neck and head.

Breast

- Hand-held, real-time contact scanning over palpable mass is the most widely used method for breast imaging.
- An automated system utilizing full-breast water immersion and a reproducible, systematic survey is less widely used due to higher cost, space requirements, and lack of real-time capability.
- No lotion or powder should be applied under the arm or breast area the day of the test.

Doppler

- Blood pressure will be taken at certain limb sites.

Eye and Eye Orbit

- Anesthetize the eye and eye area.
- With contact method, the probe touches the corneal surface.

Heart and Liver

- Ask the client to breathe slowly and to hold breath after deep inspiration.

Obstetrics (First Trimester), Pelvic and Renal

- The client should drink 24 ounces of water 1 h prior to the examination, or three to four 8-ounce glasses of clear liquid 90 min prior to the test. The client should not void until the test is completed. Second- and third-trimester clients need not drink large amounts of water *unless* bleeding has occurred, in which case the above procedure is followed.

Prostate
- Administer an enema 1 h prior to the test.
- The client should drink two 8-ounce glasses of clear fluid 1 h prior to the test.
- The client should *not* void 1 h prior to the test.
- The client lies on his left side.
- Rectal examination is usually performed before the transducer is inserted into the rectum. Lubricate the rectal probe and insert it into the rectum. The test takes approximately 30 min.

Scrotum
- The penis is strapped back to the abdominal area or covered with a towel.
- Gel is applied and the transducer is passed over the scrotum.

Factors Affecting Diagnostic Results
- Residual barium sulfate in the GI tract from previous X-ray studies will interfere with ultrasound results. Ultrasonography should be performed before barium studies.
- Air and gas (bowel) will not transmit the ultrasound beam.
- Excess fecal material in the colon and rectum (prostate).

Nursing Implications
- Obtain a signed consent form if needed.
- NPO for 6 h prior to all abdominal studies (e.g., gallbladder, aorta).
- Confirm that the client has not had any other tests that may interfere with test results (e.g., upper GI series).

Client Teaching
- Explain the procedure to the client (see Description and Procedure).
- Inform the client that this is a painless procedure, that there is no exposure to radiation, and that the ultrasound test is considered to be safe and fast.
- Instruct the client to remain still during the procedure. Inform him or her that the test usually takes 30 min or less, except for a few

ultrasound tests (e.g., arterial, venous, and carotid ultrasonography), which could take 1 h.

- Encourage the client to ask questions and to express any concerns. Refer questions you cannot answer to the ultrasonographer or the health care provider.
- Be supportive of the client and the family.

Eye

- Avoid rubbing the eyes until the anesthetic effect has worn off in order to avoid corneal abrasion.
- Inform the client that blurred vision may be present for a short time until the anesthetic has worn off.

Abdominal Studies

- Inform the client that she/he should be NPO for 6 h prior to all abdominal studies.
- Confirm that the client has not had other tests that may interfere with the ultrasonography, such as upper GI series.

VENOGRAPHY (LOWER LIMB)

PHLEBOGRAPHY

Normal Finding.   Normal, patent, deep leg veins

Description.   Lower-limb venography is a fluoroscopic or X-ray examination of the deep leg veins after injection of a contrast dye. This test is useful for identifying venous obstruction caused by a deep-vein thrombosis (DVT). This procedure is frequently done after Doppler ultrasonography to confirm a positive or questionable DVT. *Radionuclide venography* using I-125 fibrinogen IV with scintillation scanning may be done for clients who are too ill for venography or are hypersensitive to contrast dye. It may take 6 to 72 h for the isotope to collect at the thrombus site, and so the scanner could be used to check the leg daily for 3 days. This type should not be used for screening purposes.

Purposes
- To detect deep-vein thrombosis (DVT)
- To identify congenital venous abnormalities
- To select a vein for arterial bypass grafting

Clinical Problems
Abnormal findings: Deep-vein thrombosis, congenital venous abnormalities

Procedure
- Obtain a signed consent form.
- Restrict food and fluids for 4 h before the test; some permit clear liquids before the test.
- Anticoagulants may be temporarily discontinued.
- The client lies on a tilted radiographic table at a 40- to 60-degree angle. A tourniquet is applied above the ankle, a vein is located in the dorsum of the client's foot, a small amount of normal saline is administered IV into the vein, and then the contrast dye is injected slowly over a period of 2 to 4 min.
- Fluoroscopy may be used to monitor the flow of the contrast dye, and spot films are taken.
- Normal saline is used after the procedure to flush the contrast dye from the veins.
- A sedative may be indicated prior to the test for clients who are extremely apprehensive and for those who have a low threshold of pain.
- The test takes 30 min to 1 h.

Factors Affecting Diagnostic Results
- Weight on the leg being tested can cause a decrease in the flow of the contrast dye.

Nursing Implications
- Obtain a history of allergies to iodine, iodine substance, and seafood. Antihistamines or steroids may be given for 2 to 3 days before the test.
- Record baseline vital signs. Have client void before test.

Client Teaching

- Inform the client that a slight burning sensation may be felt when the dye is injected. Instruct the client not to move the leg being tested during the injection of the dye or during X-ray filming.

Post-test

- Monitor vital signs as indicated.
- Check the pulse in the dorsalis pedis, popliteal, and femoral arteries for volume intensity and rate.
- Observe for signs and symptoms of latent allergic reaction to the contrast dye (i.e., dyspnea, skin rash, urticaria, and tachycardia).
- Observe the injection site for bleeding, hematoma, and signs and symptoms of infection (i.e., redness, edema, and pain).
- Elevate the affected leg as ordered.
- Be supportive of the client.

VENTILATION SCAN (V/Q)*

PULMONARY VENTILATION SCAN

Normal Finding.   Normal lung tissue with normal gas distribution in both lungs

Description.   The ventilation scan is a nuclear scan of the lungs. The client inhales a mixture of air, oxygen, and radioactive gas (xenon [Xe-127 or Xe-133] or krypton-81m [Kr-81m]). A single-breath scan is taken first. Then three phases of scanning follow: (1) the wash-in phase single inspiration which is the build-up of gas distribution in the lungs; (2) the equilibrium phase in which radioactive gas reaches a steady state; and (3) the wash-out phase in which room air is breathed to remove radioactive gas from the lungs.

The pulmonary ventilation scan is usually performed with the *pulmonary perfusion scan* to differentiate between a ventilatory problem

---

*Updated by Cindy Knotts, BS, CNMT, Supervisor, nuclear medicine, Christiana Care Health Services, Newark, Delaware.

and vascular abnormalities in the lung. The pulmonary perfusion scan indirectly evaluates problems related to blood flow to the lungs (e.g., pulmonary embolism). The radioactive substance used is technetium and images are taken by a gamma camera. A ventilation scan can reveal decreased ventilation (uptake of radioactive gas) caused by chronic obstructive pulmonary disease (COPD), atelectasis, and pneumonia; the pulmonary perfusion scan is normal. However, pulmonary embolus can cause an abnormal perfusion scan and a normal ventilation scan.

Purposes
- To differentiate between a ventilatory problem and vascular abnormalities in the lung.
- To evaluate low blood oxygen saturation.
- To evaluate and stage persons with COPD, lung cancer and bronchial obstruction.

Clinical Problems. Parenchymal lung disease (COPD), vascular abnormalities (pulmonary emboli), tuberculosis, sarcoidosis, lung cancer, hypoventilation due to excess smoking or COPD

Procedure
- No food or fluid restriction is required.
- Remove all metal objects (jewelry) from around the neck and chest.
- The client inhales radioactive gas. The client will be asked to take a deep breath and to hold it for a short time (single breath) while the scanner takes an image of the lung. Other images will be recorded during three phases of the test: wash-in, equilibrium, and wash-out.

Factors Affecting Diagnostic Results
- Metal objects could cause inaccurate recorded images.

Nursing Implications
- Record and report any respiratory distress the client is having. Check breath sounds.
- Report if the client is having chest pain, especially if pulmonary embolism is suspected.

- Assess communications for verbal and nonverbal expressions of anxiety and fear about tests and/or potential or actual health problem.
- Be supportive of client and family.

Client Teaching
- Explain the procedure to the client (see Procedure). Explain that the radioactive gas is minimal.

VIDEO CAPSULE ENDOSCOPY (VCE)*

Normal Finding.   Normal mucosa of the small bowel

Description.   Video capsule endoscopy (VCE) is a noninvasive diagnostic procedure allowing visualization of the small bowel. A metal pill is swallowed. This pill contains a camera and a transmitter. Images are transferred to a receiver and hard drive. The client wears the hard drive within a beltpack during the study. The pill-isomer is powered for approximately 8 h by a battery contained within the pill.

The VCE is primarily used to evaluate gastrointestinal bleeding following a nondiagnostic upper and lower endoscopy and to diagnose Crohn's disease of the small bowel.

Purposes
- To determine origin of gastrointestinal bleeding when prior studies do not evidence upper GI tract or colon bleeding
- To determine whether chronic abdominal pain is due to small bowel disease
- To detect Crohn's disease

Clinical Problems
Positive findings: Crohn's disease, origin of GI bleeding, small bowel disease

---

*Written by Dr. Warren G. Butt, Gastroenterology-Stomach-Colon-Liver, Newark, Delaware.

Procedure

- Obtain a signed consent form.
- Withhold medications (e.g., antiinflammatory drugs) that cause small bowel ulceration. Ideally, these medications should be stopped 90 days prior to the test.
- Electrical leads are attached to the client's chest similar to ECG (EKG) leads.
- Pill is activated, then swallowed by the client.
- Client returns 8 h later to return the beltpack containing the receiver and hard drive.
- Pill passes uneventfully into the stool. The pill is not reused.

Factors Affecting Diagnostic Results

- Delayed or slowed GI motility may limit passage of the pill camera.
- Retained food content and bile may interfere with viewing.

Complications

- Small bowel strictures may prevent the pill passage. This may cause a bowel obstruction. To prevent this, a small bowel follow is sometimes used prior to VCE.

Nursing Implications

- Obtain a history of client's health problems.
- Record the medications that the client is taking. Note if a drug is an anti inflammatory agent.
- Record baseline vital signs. Maintain a chart for vital signs.

Client Teaching

- Explain the procedure to the client. Stress that he/she will be awake throughout the test.
- Instruct the client not to eat for 2 h after the pill camera is ingested.
- Explain to the client that normal activities of daily living may be performed during the test.
- Inform the client to return the beltpack after the test at a specified time.

X-RAY (CHEST, HEART, FLAT PLATE OF THE ABDOMEN, KIDNEY, URETER, BLADDER, SKULL, SKELETAL)

ROENTGENOGRAPHY, RADIOGRAPHY

Normal Findings.
Chest: Normal bony structure and normal lung tissue
Heart: Normal size and shape of the heart and vessel
Flat plate of abdomen: Normal abdominal structures
Kidney, ureter, bladder (KUB):   Normal kidney size and structure
Skull and skeletal: Normal structures

Description.   In the body there are four densities—air, water, fat, and bone—that will absorb varying degrees of radiation. Air has less density, causing dark images on the film, and bone has high density, causing light images. Bone contains a large amount of calcium and will absorb more radiation, allowing less radiation to strike the X-ray film; thus, a white structure is produced.

Today, X-ray studies cause only small amounts of radiation exposure because of the high quality of X-ray film and procedure. X-ray studies are requested primarily for screening purposes and are followed by other extensive diagnostic tests.

Purposes
- To identify bone structure and tissue in the body
- To detect abnormal size, structure, and shape of bone and body tissues

Clinical Problems

Test	Abnormal Findings
Chest	Atelectasis, pneumonias, tuberculosis, tumors, lung abscess, pneumothorax, sarcoma, sarcoidosis, scoliosis/kyphosis
Heart	Cardiomegaly, aneurysms, anomalies of the aorta
Abdominal (flat plate)	Abdominal masses, small bowel obstruction, abdominal tissue trauma, ascites

Test	Abnormal Findings
KUB	Abnormal size and structure of KUB, renal calculi, kidney and bladder masses
Skull	Head trauma (intracranial pressure, skull fractures), congenital anomalies, bone defects
Skeletal	Fractures, arthritic conditions, osteomyelitis

Procedure

Chest

- No food or fluid is restricted.
- A posteroanterior (PA) chest film is usually ordered with the client standing. An anteroposterior (AP) chest film could be ordered. A lateral chest film may also be ordered.
- Clothing and jewelry should be removed from the neck to the waist, and a paper or cloth gown should be worn.
- The client should take a deep breath and hold it as the X-ray is taken.

Heart

- No food or fluid is restricted.
- PA and left-lateral chest films are usually indicated for evaluating the size and shape of the heart.
- Clothing and jewelry should be removed from the neck to the waist, and a paper or cloth gown should be worn.
- Client instructions include body position and when to take a deep breath and hold it.

Abdomen and KUB

- No food or fluid is restricted.
- X-rays should be taken before an IVP or GI studies.
- Clothes are removed, and a paper or cloth gown is worn.
- Client lies in a supine position with arms away from the body on a tilted X-ray table.
- Testes should be shielded as an added precaution.

Skull

- No food or fluid is restricted.
- Remove hairpins, glasses, and dentures before the test.

- Various positions may be needed so that different areas of the skull can be X-rayed.

Skeletal

- Restrict food and fluids if fracture is suspected.
- Immobilize suspected fracture site.

Factors Affecting Diagnostic Results

- Radiopaque materials for IVP and GI studies administered within 3 days of routine X-rays (chest, flat plate of the abdomen, and KUB) could distort the pictures.

Nursing Implications
Client Teaching

- Inform the client that the X-ray test usually takes 10 to 15 min.
- Inform the client that there may be several X-rays taken, one or two chest films, or five skull films. The client may be asked to remain in the waiting room for 10 to 15 min after X-rays are taken to be sure the films are readable.
- Ask the female client if she is pregnant or if pregnancy is suspected. X-rays should be avoided during the first trimester of pregnancy. A lead apron covering the abdomen and pelvic area may be used.
- Explain that today's X-ray equipment and film are of good quality and decrease the exposure to radiation.

THREE

School Health Services: Education, Screening, and Testing*

Fundamental to the success of all children is good physical and mental health. The goal of school health services is to remove health barriers to learning. Health and learning go hand in hand: when one falters, so does the other. The school nurse holds a unique and important position to that end. He/she needs physical, mental, social, emotional, and ethical capabilities in addition to a professional and educational nursing background to ensure the health needs of all students.

The school nurse provides direct student health services; conducts health and wellness programs for school personnel; is involved in program planning, development, management, and evaluation; and provides health education and counseling for students and their families. This requires a community-wide approach to planning and implementation of services. The following must be considered in the approach:

- *Mortality* Trauma and violent causes, MVA, homicide, suicide, malignancy, infections—meningitis, pneumonia, and drug related
- *Morbidity* Data-reportable infections—Sexually Transmitted Diseases (STD), Human Immunodeficiency Virus (HIV), Attention Deficit Hyperactivity Disorder (ADHD), drug and alcohol abuse, teen pregnancy
- *Chronic disorders* Asthma, seizure disorders, diabetes, cystic fibrosis, cerebral palsy (CP), vision, hearing handicaps, mental disorders
- *Other* Pediculosis, scabies, ringworm, conjunctivitis, dental problems, nutritional, local conditions, managing environmental problems

---

*Written by Anne M. Biddle, RN, BSN, NCSN, School Nurse at Newark Charter School, Delaware

SCHOOL NURSE FUNCTIONS

A child-oriented focus with services based on identified student needs is key to a good health education program. Start by collecting data on local health problems see Figure 3–1. Once listed, prioritize and set goals and objectives and include parents and students at all levels. Networking with other community health workers enables sharing of successes and challenges with others' efforts. Good communication skills, legal and ethical knowledge, and familiarity with the budget process behoove the school nurse. As in business, the key is "knowing the student" so as to tailor a plan specific to the school and community.

Typically, the school health services offer a wide array of services in the course of the typical day, including the following:

- Health assessment
  - Staff education, that is, CPR/AED training
  - Employee health, including workman's compensation assessment
  - Work with community agencies to benefit children and parents, for example, Basket Brigade, Soap for Hope, CHADD
- Medical referral and follow up
- Vision screening/referral
- Hearing screening/referral
- Scoliosis screening/referral and follow up
- First aid
- Immunization review and referral
- Height, weight, BMI

$$\left(\frac{(\text{Weight (lb)} \times 703)}{(\text{height (in)})^2} \right)^{**}$$

**BMI for age

Overweight	Greater than 95th percentile
At risk for overweight	85–94th percentile
Normal	5–84th percentile
Underweight	Less than 5th percentile

Last Name	First and Middle Name	M	F	Date of Birth	*

SCHOOL HEALTH RECORD - STATE OF DELAWARE

Parent or Guardian	Address		Home Phone
Family Physician	Phone	Family Dentist	Phone
School Pupil is Attending 1	2	3	

ILLNESS AND HEALTH PROBLEMS

Chicken Pox	❏	Frequent Colds	❏	Diabetes	❏
Measles	❏	Frequent Tonsillitis	❏	Convulsive Disorders	❏
Mumps	❏	Hearing Difficulty	❏	Heart Trouble	❏
Rubella	❏	Speech Difficulty	❏	Nephritis	❏
Whooping Cough	❏	Vision Difficulty	❏	Orthopedic Difficulty	❏
Rheumatic Fever	❏	Allergies	❏	Menstrual Difficulty	❏
Tuberculosis	❏	Asthma	❏	Other	❏

INJURIES-SURGERY	**IMMUNIZATION RECORD (Dates)**		
		PRIMARY SERIES	BOOSTERS
	D.P.T.		
	D.T.		
	M.M.R.		x x x x x x x x x x
	Hep B		x x x x x x x x x x
	Polio (Oral)		
	Other		

VISION TESTING				W/O - Without Glasses W - With Glasses	**TUBERCULIN TEST**			**OTHER TESTS**		
Grade	Date	R	L	Comments	Date	Type	Result	Date	Type	Result
						HEARING TESTING		V - Normal Range X - Unsatisfactory		
					Grade	Date	R	L	Comments	

REFERRAL AND TESTS (Psychological, Mental, Hygiene, Speech, Social Service, Etc., Give Dates)	**DENTAL REFERRALS AND CARE**
	ORTHOPEDIC SCREENING AND FOLLOW UP

*Color Code
BLACK - Convulsive Disorder   YELLOW - Vision   ORANGE - Allergies, Other
RED - Cardiac   GREEN - Orthopedic   PINK - Kidney

FIGURE 3–1.   School Health Record.

- Administration of medication
- Special procedures (catheterization, blood glucose monitoring, peak flow meter, etc.)
- Teacher/nurse conferences
- Health and puberty education
- Individual health counseling
- Mental health and well-being
- Resource person to school/community, for example, dental care and public health clinics
- Evaluate nursing aspects of the school health program

HEARING SCREENING

Among the diagnostic testing that the school nurse performs is hearing screening. A pure tone audiometer that is calibrated annually is used in a quiet room—it is important to eliminate ambient noises in a room using heavy drapes, carpeting, and solid core doors. It is wise to test the audiometer preferably on oneself prior to testing others and to arrange the chairs such that the student cannot view the equipment. Screening should be performed at 1,000, 2,000, and 4,000 Hz with an intensity level of 20 dB (amplitude or loudness) at each frequency (sound cycles per second). This level can be increased to 25 dB if there appears to be a fair amount of extraneous noise. When the student fails to respond at any frequency in either ear, failure is noted and the student should be rescreened immediately and in 2 weeks if necessary. If both attempts result in failure, the student should be referred for appropriate follow-up and rescreened the following year. Excessive wax buildup is often a contributory cause of poor hearing. This is easily remedied with over-the-counter preparations for this purpose. Special equipment is available for students with significant limitations who are unable to test using the conventional method. These results are recorded on the School Health Record and the parent should be notified and advised to seek an ENT referral. It is protocol to follow up with the family to ensure adequate care of a suspected hearing loss.

Normal hearing range is from 1–15 dB, while slight hearing loss (16–25 dB) can cause missed consonants, and moderate loss (41–65 dB) results in missing most speech sounds. No speech sounds or normal conversation is heard with severe loss (65–95 dB) and profound loss, where no sounds are heard, is considered for values greater than 95 dB.

VISION SCREENING

Another test done routinely in the school is vision screening for acuity. The equipment used for screening include lighted charts, graduated cards, occluder, and a quiet room with 20 ft available between the student and the chart. One eye is covered, with both eyes kept open. If corrective lenses are usually worn, all testing should be done with the child wearing them. Some children learn to memorize the chart so it is wise to test backward, every other letters, and so forth. A reading under 20/50 should be referred or under 20/40 if the student complains of trouble seeing the board or other visual concerns. Family history of visual impairment is often a significant factor to consider. School nurses are in an excellent position to assist families in financial need in obtaining corrective lenses.

SCOLIOSIS: POSTURAL SCREENING

School-age children grow rapidly, particularly in middle school, which puts them at increased risk for developing scoliosis. School nurses are often the ones to detect this curvature of the spine. The screening procedure includes assessment of symmetry, gait, movement, pain, and the like.

- The nurse can take this time to ask if s/he carries a backpack—how is it carried, what is its weight, and so on. Students should be informed that they must not carry more than 15% of their body weight; packs should be above the waist and with a belt if possible. Now many ergonomically designed models are available and rolling backpacks are a boon to backs. Although poor posture or disproportioned backpacks do not cause scoliosis, the condition of those predisposed may be aggravated by these factors.

Suspected deviations must be referred for Phase II rescreening, and all results must be recorded on the students' health record. This test is done yearly on all students. Again, prevention and early detection are the keys to "getting it straight."

VACCINE REVIEW

Prior to school entry all children must have five DTaP vaccines (diphtheria, tetanus, acellular pertussis), four OPV (polio), four HIB (influenza), two MMR, one varicella (or proof of the disease) and three HBV (hepatitis B). Currently, the HBV is required prior to entry into seventh grade but is being given at birth routinely. A lead screening is also done and a PPD test for TB. If a student is at low risk for TB, a "paper screen" can be done by the school nurse. If all four answers are "no" as stated by parent/guardian, the student is considered to be at no risk and a PPD test is not necessary. This has become a great time and hassle saver for student, family, and nurse.

In high-risk populations, the flu shot, pneumococcal, and hepatitis A vaccines may also be given. The bacterial meningitis vaccine is highly recommended for high school seniors as college freshmen rate high in the risk of contracting this deadly disease. Pertussis boosters are being given at 11–12 years of age as this disease has also made a return in many areas. Human papillomavirus (HPV) vaccine is being given at the same age as well.

OBESITY AND DIABETES ASSESSMENT

Obesity has recently become a true epidemic in the school-age child. Reasons include sedentary lifestyles; more use of "screens" (computer, television, etc.); fast-food eating; and high fat, "empty calorie" eating. Hence it is vital to know more about diabetes than ever. Type 2 diabetes has reached epidemic proportions in our youth, which is a very unsettling fact. The American Diabetes Association (ADA) has cited the following parameters for diagnosing diabetes:

- Two fasting plasma glucose levels greater than 126 mg/dl if asymptomatic.
- Two random levels greater than 200 mg/dl if symptomatic.
- One high glucose level any time in someone who has diabetic symptoms.
- An oral glucose tolerance test showing a 2-h postprandial result of greater than 200 mg/dl.

School nurses are in an opportune position to assist students and families in healthy food selections, increased physical activity, and education about the hazards of poor choices.

In summary, school nursing begins with prevention of disease and organization of a plan. It is vital to "know the customer" (the student) and to tailor the care to the needs of the population. The population is not only the students in the school but the parents and families as well; hence good communication skills are a must. Health education covers physical, chronic and acute, as well as mental health, which requires continual updating, based on the needs of the community. Every year new disorders and treatments are discovered—staying abreast is the school nurse's responsibility. From child abuse to asthma to suicide to legal and environmental issues to bandages and beyond, the school nurse holds an awesome responsibility and plays a pivotal role in health maintenance and prevention.

REFERENCES

Gregory, EK (1998). *The Ear and Hearing: A Guide for School Nurses*. National Association of School Nurses, Inc.

Selekman, Janice (2006). *School Nurse: A Comprehensive Text*. Philadelphia: F.A. Davis

FOUR

Therapeutic Drug Monitoring (TDM)*

Selective drugs are monitored by serum and urine for the purposes of achieving and maintaining therapeutic drug effects and for preventing drug toxicity. In drugs with a wide therapeutic range (window), the difference between effective dose and toxic dose, are not usually monitored. Drug monitoring is important in maintaining a drug concentration–response relationship, especially when the serum drug range (window) is narrow, such as with digoxin and lithium. Therapeutic drug monitoring (TDM) is the process of following drug levels and adjusting them to maintain a therapeutic level. Not all drugs can be dosed and/or monitored by their blood levels alone.

Drug levels are obtained at peak time and trough time after a steady state of the drug has occurred in the client. Steady state is reached after four to five half-lives of a drug and can be reached sooner if the drug has a short half-life. Once steady state is achieved, the serum drug level is checked at the peak level (maximum drug concentration) and/or at trough/residual level (minimum drug concentration). If the trough or residual level is at the high therapeutic point, toxicity might occur. Careful assessment is needed by both physical and laboratory means.

TDM is required for drugs with a narrow therapeutic index or range (window); when other methods for monitoring drugs are noneffective, such as blood pressure (BP) monitoring; for determining when adequate blood concentrations are reached; for evaluating client's compliance to drug therapy; for determining whether other drugs have altered serum

---

*Revised and updated by Ronald J. Lefever, RPh., Pharmacy Services, Medical College of Virginia, Richmond, Virginia.

drug levels (increased or decreased) that could result in drug toxicity or lack of therapeutic effect; and for establishing a new serum-drug level when dosage is changed.

Drug groups for TDM include analgesics, antibiotics, anticonvulsants, antineoplastics, bronchodilators, cardiac drugs, hypoglycemics, sedatives, and tranquilizers. To effectively conduct TDM, the laboratory must be provided with the following information: the drug name and daily dosage, time and amount of last dose, time blood was drawn, route of administration, and client's age. Without complete information, serum drug reporting might be incorrect.

Drug	Therapeutic Range	Peak Time	Toxic Level
Acetaminophen (Tylenol)	10–20 mcg/ml	1–2.5 h	Greater than 50 mcg/ml Heptotoxicity: Greater than 200 mcg/ml
Acetohexamide (Dymelor)	20–70 mcg/ml (should be dosed according to blood glucose levels)	2–4 h	Greater than 75 mcg/ml
Alcohol	Negative		Mild toxic: 150 mg/dl Marked toxic: Greater than 250 mg/l
Alprazolam (Xanax)	10–50 ng/ml	1–2 h	Greater than 75 ng/ml
Amikacin (Amikin)	Peak: 20–30 mcg/ml	Intravenously: 0.5 h	Peak: Greater than 35 mcg/ml
	Trough: Equal or Less than 10 mcg/ml	0.5–1.5 h	Greater than 10 mcg/ml
Aminocaproic acid (Amicar)	100–400 mcg/ml	1 h	Greater than 400 mcg/ml
Aminophylline (see Theophylline)			
Amiodarone (Cordarone)	0.5–2.5 mcg/ml	2–10 h	Greater than 2.5 mcg/ml
Amitriptyline (Elavil) + nortriptyline (parent and active metabolite)	110–225 ng/ml	2–4 h (and up to 12 h)	Greater than 500 ng/ml

Drug	Therapeutic Range	Peak Time	Toxic Level
Amobarbital (Amytal)	1–5 mcg/ml	2 h	Greater than 15 mcg/ml Severe toxicity: Greater than 30 mcg/ml
Amoxapine (Asendin)	200–400 ng/ml	15 h	Greater than 500 ng/ml
Amphetamine:			
Serum	20–30 ng/ml		0.2 mcg/ml
Urine		Detectable in urine after 3 h; positive for 24–48 h	Greater than 30 mcg/ml urine
Aspirin (see Salicylates)			
Atenolol (Tenormin)	200–500 ng/ml	2–4 h	Greater than 500 ng/ml
Beta carotene	48–200 mcg/ml	Several weeks	Greater than 300 mcg/ml
Bromide	20–80 mg/dl		Greater than 100 mg/dl
Butabarbital (Butisol)	1–2 mcg/ml	3–4 h	Greater than 10 mcg/ml
Butalbital	10–20 mcg/ml		Greater than 40 mcg/ml
Caffeine	Adult: 3–15 mcg/ml Infant: 8–20 mcg/ml	0.5–1 h	Greater than 50 mcg/ml
Carbamazepine (Tegretol)	4–12 mcg/ml	6 h (range 2–24 h)	Greater than 9–15 mcg/ml
Chloral hydrate (Noctec)	2–12 mcg/ml	1–2 h	Greater than 20 mcg/ml
Chloramphenicol (Chloromycetin)	10–20 mg/l		Greater than 25 mg/l
Chlordiazepoxide (Librium)	1–5 mcg/ml	2–3 h	Greater than 5 mcg/ml
Chlorpromazine (Thorazine)	50–300 ng/ml	2–4 h	Greater than 750 ng/ml
Chlorpropamide (Diabinese)	75–250 mcg/ml	3–6 h	Greater than 250–750 mcg/ml

(continued)

Drug	Therapeutic Range	Peak Time	Toxic Level
Cimetidine (Tagamet)	Trough: 0.5–1.2 mcg/ml	1–1.5 h	Trough: Greater than 1.5 mcg/ml
Clonazepam (Klonopin)	10–60 ng/ml	2 h	Greater than 80 ng/ml
Clonidine (Catapres)	0.2–2.0 ng/ml (Hypotensive effect)	2–5 h	Greater than 2.0 ng/ml
Clorazepate (Tranxene)	0.12–1.0 mcg/ml	1–2 h	Greater than 1.0 mcg/ml
Codeine	10–100 ng/ml	1–2 h	Greater than 200 ng/ml
Cyclosporine	100–300 ng/ml	3–4 h	Greater than 400 ng/ml
Dantrolene (Dantrium)	1–3 mcg/ml	5 h	Greater than 5 mcg/ml
Desipramine (Norpramin)	125–300 ng/ml	4–6 h	Greater than 500 ng/ml
Diazepam (Valium)	0.5–2 mg/l 400–600 ng/ml Therapeutic	1–2 h	Greater than 3 mg/l Greater than 3000 ng/ml
Digitoxin (rarely administered)	10–25 ng/ml	Noticeable: 2–4 h Peak: 12–24 h	Greater than 30 ng/ml
Digoxin	0.5–2 ng/ml	PO: 6–8 h IV: 1.5–2 h	2–3 ng/ml
Dilantin (see Phenytoin)			
Diltiazem (Cardizem)	50–200 ng/ml	2–3 h	Greater than 200 ng/ml
Disopyramide (Norpace)	2–4 mcg/ml	2 h	Greater than 4 mcg/ml
Doxepin (Sinequan)	150–300 ng/ml	2–4 h	Greater than 500 ng/ml
Ethchlorvynol (Placidyl)	2–8 mcg/ml	1–2 h	Greater than 20 µg/ml
Ethosuximide (Zarontin)	40–100 mcg/ml	2–4 h	Greater than 150 mcg/ml
Flecainide (Tambocor)	0.2–1.0 mcg/ml	3 h	Greater than 1.0 mcg/ml
5-Flucytosine	Peak: 100 mcg/ml Trough: 50 mcg/ml		125 mcg/ml 125 mcg/ml
Fluoride			Greater than 15 µmol/l
Fluoxetine	90–300 ng/ml	2–4 h	Greater than 500 ng/ml

Drug	Therapeutic Range	Peak Time	Toxic Level
Flurazepam (Dalmane)	20–110 ng/ml	0.5–1 h	Greater than 1500 ng/ml
Folate	Greater than 3.5 mcg/ml	1 h	
Gentamicin (Garamycin)	Peak: 6–12 mcg/ml	IV: 15–30 min	Peak: Greater than 12 mcg/ml
	Trough: Less than 2 mcg/ml		Greater than 2 mcg/ml
Glutethimide (Doriden)	2–6 mcg/ml	1–2 h	Greater than 20 mcg/ml
Gold	1.0–2.0 mcg/ml	2–6 h	Greater than 5.0 mcg/ml
Haloperidol (Haldol)	5–15 ng/ml	2–6 h	Greater than 50 ng/ml
Hydromorphone (Dilaudid)	1–30 ng/ml	0.5–1.5 h	Greater than 100 ng/ml
Ibuprofen (Motrin, etc.)	10–50 mcg/ml	1–2 h	Greater than 100 mcg/ml
Imipramine (Tofranil) + desipramine (parent and active metabolite)	200–350 ng/ml	PO: 1–2 h IM: 30 min	Greater than 500 ng/ml
Isoniazid (INH, Nydrazid)	1–7 mg/ml (dose usually adjusted based on liver function tests)	1–2 h	Greater than 20 mg/ml
Kanamycin (Kantrex)	Peak: 15–30 mcg/ml	PO: 1–2 h	Peak: Greater than 35 mcg/ml
		IM: 30 min–1 h	Trough: Greater than 10 mcg/ml
Lead	Less than 20 mcg/ml		Greater than 80 mcg/ml
	Urine: Less than 80 mcg/24 h		Urine: Greater than 125 mcg/24 h
Lidocaine (Xylocaine)	1.5–5 mcg/ml	IV: 10 min	Greater than 6 mcg/ml
Lithium	0.8–1.2 mEq/l	0.5–4 h	Greater than 1.5 mEq/l
Lorazepam (Ativan)	50–240 ng/ml	1–3 h	Greater than 300 ng/ml

(continued)

Drug	Therapeutic Range	Peak Time	Toxic Level
Maprotiline (Ludiomil)	200–300 ng/ml	12 h	Greater than 500 ng/ml
Meperidine (Demerol)	0.4–0.7 mcg/ml	2–4 h	Greater than 1.0 mcg/ml
Mephenytoin (Mesantoin)	15–40 mcg/ml	2–4 h	Greater than 50 mcg/ml
Meprobamate (Equanil, Miltown)	15–25 mcg/ml	2 h	Greater than 50 mcg/ml
Methadone (Dolophine)	100–400 ng/ml	0.5–1 h	Greater than 2000 ng/ml or Greater than 0.2 mcg/ml
Methaqualone	1–5 mcg/ml		Greater than 10 mcg/ml
Methotrexate	Less than 0.1 µmol/l after 48 h	1–2 h	1.0×10^6 at 48 h
Methsuximide	Less than 1.0 mcg/ml	1–4 h	Greater than 40 mcg/ml
Methyldopa (Aldomet)	1–5 mcg/ml	3–6 h	Greater than 7 mcg/ml
Methyprylon (Noludar)	8–10 mcg/ml	1–2 h	Greater than 50 mcg/ml
Metoprolol (Lopressor)	75–200 ng/ml	2–4 h	Greater than 225 ng/ml
Mexiletine (Mexitil)	0.5–2 mcg/ml	2–3 h	Greater than 2 mcg/ml
Morphine	10–80 ng/ml	IV: immediately IM: 0.5–1 h SC: 1–1.5 h	Greater than 200 ng/ml
Netilmicin (Netromycin)	Peak: 0.5–10 mcg/ml Trough: Less than 4 mcg/ml	IV: 30 min	Peak: Greater than 16 mcg/ml Greater than 4 mcg/ml
Nifedipine (Procardia)	50–100 ng/ml	0.5–2 h	Greater than 100 ng/ml
Nortriptyline (Aventyl)	50–150 ng/ml	8 h	Greater than 200 ng/ml
Oxazepam (Serax)	0.2–1.4 mcg/ml	1–2 h	

Drug	Therapeutic Range	Peak Time	Toxic Level
Oxycodone (Percodan)	10–100 ng/ml	0.5–1 h	Greater than 200 ng/ml
Pentazocine (Talwin)	0.05–0.2 mcg/ml	1–2 h	Greater than 1.0 mcg/ml Urine: Greater than 3.0 mcg/ml
Pentobarbital (Nembutal)	1–5 mcg/ml	0.5–1 h	Greater than 10 mcg/ml Severe toxicity: Greater than 30 mcg/ml
Phenmetrazine (Preludin)	5–30 mcg/ml (urine)	2 h	Greater than 50 mcg/ml (urine)
Phenobarbital (Luminal)	15–40 mcg/ml	6–18 h	Greater than 40 mcg/ml Severe toxicity: Greater than 80 mcg/ml
Phenytoin (Dilantin)	10–20 mcg/ml	4–8 h	Greater than 20–30 mcg/ml Severe toxicity: Greater than 40 mcg/ml
Pindolol (Visken)	0.5–6.0 ng/ml	2–4 h	Greater than 10 ng/ml
Primidone (Mysoline)	5–12 mcg/ml	2–4 h	Greater than 12–15 mcg/ml
Procainamide (Pronestyl)	4–10 mcg/ml	1 h	Greater than 10 mcg/ml
Procaine (Novocain)	Less than 11 mcg/ml	10–30 min	Greater than 20 mcg/ml
Prochlorperazine (Compazine)	50–300 ng/ml	2–4 h	Greater than 1000 ng/ml
Propoxyphene (Darvon)	0.1–0.4 mcg/ml	2–3 h	Greater than 0.5 mcg/ml
Propranolol (Inderal)	Greater than 100 ng/ml	1–2 h	Greater than 150 ng/ml
Protriptyline (Vivactil)	50–150 ng/ml	8–12 h	Greater than 200 ng/ml
Quinidine	2–5 mcg/ml	1–3 h	Greater than 6 mcg/ml

(continued)

Drug	Therapeutic Range	Peak Time	Toxic Level
Ranitidine (Zantac)	100 ng/ml	2–3 h	Greater than 100 ng/ml
Reserpine (Serpasil)	20 ng/ml	2–4 h	Greater than 20 ng/ml
Salicylates (Aspirin)	10–30 mg/dl	1–2 h	Tinnitus: 20–40 mg/ml Hyperventilation: Greater than 35 mg/dl Severe toxicity: Greater than 50 mg/dl
Secobarbital (Seconal)	2–5 mcg/ml	1 h	Greater than 15 mcg/ml Severe toxicity: Greater than 30 µg/ml
Streptomycin	Peak: 5–20 mcg/ml		Greater than 40 mcg/ml
	Trough: Less than 5 mcg/ml		Greater than 40 mcg/ml
Sulfadiazine	100–120 mcg/ml		Greater than 300 mcg/ml
Sulfamethoxazole	90–100 mcg/ml		Greater than 300 mcg/ml
Sulfapyridine	75–90 mcg/ml		Greater than 300 mcg/ml
Sulfisoxazole	90–100 mcg/ml		Greater than 300 mcg/ml
Theophylline (Theodur, Aminodur)	10–20 mcg/ml	PO: 2–3 h IV: 15 min (depends on smoking or nonsmoking)	Greater than 20 mcg/ml
Thiocyanate	4–20 mcg/ml		Greater than 60 mcg/ml
Thioridazine (Mellaril)	100–600 ng/ml		Greater than 2000 ng/ml
	1.0–1.5 mcg/ml	2–4 h	Greater than 10 mcg/ml

Drug	Therapeutic Range	Peak Time	Toxic Level
Timolol (Blocadren)	3–55 ng/ml	1–2 h	Greater than 60 ng/ml
Tobramycin (Nebcin)	Peak: 5–10 mcg/ml	IV: 15–30 min	Peak: Greater than 12 mcg/ml
	Trough: 1–1.5 mcg/ml	IM: 0.5–1.5 h	Trough: Greater than 2 mcg/ml
Tocainide (Tonocard)	4–10 mcg/ml	0.5–3 h	Greater than 12 mcg/ml
Tolbutamide (Orinase)	80–240 mcg/ml	3–5 h	Greater than 640 mcg/ml
Trazodone (Desyrel)	500–2500 ng/ml	1–2 weeks	Greater than 4000 ng/ml
Trifluoperazine (Stelazine)	50–300 ng/ml	2–4 h	Greater than 1000 ng/ml
Trimethoprim/ Sulfame- thoxazole (TMP/SMX)	Peak: trimethoprim: Greater than 5 mcg/ml Peak: sulfamethoxazole Greater than 100 mcg/ml		
Valproic Acid (Depakene)	50–100 mcg/ml	0.5–1.5 h	Greater than 100 mcg/ml Severe toxicity: Greater than 150 mcg/ml
Vancomycin (Vanocin)	Peak: 20–40 mcg/ml	IV: Peak: 5 min	Peak: Greater than 80 mcg/ml
	Trough: 5–10 mcg/ml	IV: Trough: 12 h	
Verapamil (Calan)	100–300 ng/ml	PO: 1–2 h IV: 5 min	Greater than 500 ng/ml
Warfarin (Coumadin)	1–10 mcg/ml (dose usually adjusted by 1 to 2.5 × control)	1.5–3 days	Greater than 10 mcg/ml

HIV drugs are primarily dosed on the basis of the clients' viral load or CD4 counts. Many of these drugs have dosage adjustments for renal and/or hepatic impairment.

	Peak Time	Half-life
Combination HIV Drugs for Monitoring Antiretroviral		
Protease Inhibitors		
Lopinavir/ritonavir (Kaletra)	4 h	5–6 h
Nucleoside Analog Reverse Transcriptase Inhibitors (NRTIs)		
Abacavir/lamivudine/zidovudine (Trizivir)		
Lamivudine/zidovudine (Combivir)		
Single HIV Drugs for Monitoring		
Protease Inhibitors		
Amprenavir (Agenerase)	1–2 h	7–9.5 h
Indinavir (Crixivan)	0.8 h	2 h (hepatic impairment, 3 h)
Antiretroviral		
Stavudine (Zerit)	1–1.5 h	1.5 h (8 h in renal impairment)
Antiretroviral Protease Inhibitors		
Ritonavir (Norvir)	2–4 h	3–5 h
Guanosine Nucleoside Reverse Transcriptase Inhibitor		
Abacavir (Ziagen)		1.5 h
Nucleoside Reverse Transcriptase Inhibitors (NRTI)		
Didanosine (Videx)	0.25–1.5 h	1.5 h
Lamivudine (Epivir)		5–7 h (dose adjustment in renal impairment)
Zidovudine (Retrovir)	0.5–1.5 h	1 h (1.4–2.9 h in renal impairment)
Non-Nucleoside Reverse Transcriptase Inhibitor (NNRTI)		
Efavirenz (Sustiva)	3–5 h	40–55 h
Nevirapine (Viramune)	4 h	25–30 h

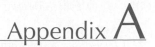

Health Problems with Laboratory and Diagnostic Tests

Various laboratory and diagnostic tests are ordered for diagnosing common clinical health problems. Forty common health problems with frequently ordered laboratory and diagnostic tests are listed.

1. **Alzheimer's disease**
   Laboratory tests: Amyloid beta protein, apolipoprotein, cerebrospinal fluid, ceruloplasmin, protein electrophoresis
   Diagnostic tests: CT of brain, MRI (brain), EEG, PET

2. **Anemia**
   Laboratory tests: Complete blood count (CBC), RBC indices, reticulocyte, iron, total iron-binding capacity (TIBC), ferritin, folic acid, vitamin B_{12}, haptoglobin (HP), erythrocyte sedimentation rate (ESR)
   Diagnostic tests: Bone marrow biopsy, Schilling test

3. **Angina pectoris**
   Laboratory tests: Troponins, creatine phosphokinase (CPK), anticardiolipin antibody antimyocardial antibody, homocysteine, lactate dehydrogenase isoenzymes, aspartate aminotransferase (AST), lipoproteins
   Diagnostic tests: Echocardiography, cardiac catheterization, stress exercise test, Holter monitor, ECG (EKG), ultrasonography (heart), PET, nuclear scan of the heart

4. **Anorexia nervosa**
   Laboratory tests: Electrolytes (especially potassium, sodium, chloride), transthyretin (prealbumin), thyroxine (T_4), triiodothyronine (T_3), estradiol, luteinizing hormone, lipoprotein

5. **Arthritis**

Laboratory tests: Antinuclear antibody (ANA), C-reactive protein (CRP), culture (synovial fluid), antistreptolysin O, complement (total), lupus test, rheumatoid factor (RF), ESR, uric acid

Diagnostic tests: X-ray of the bone

6. **Asthma**

Laboratory tests: Arterial blood gases (ABGs), culture (sputum), CBC

Diagnostic tests: Pulmonary function tests, pulse oximetry, chest X-ray

7. **Breast cancer**

Laboratory tests: Breast cancer tumor tests (BRCA 1 and BRCA 2), cancer tumor markers (CA 15-3 and CA 27.29 most common; also CA 50, CA 125), carcinoembryonic antigen (CEA), Her-2/neu oncogene, estrogen, estradiol, prolactin, progesterone, follicle-stimulating hormone (FSH)

Diagnostic tests: Mammography, biopsy (stereotactic–breast), ultrasonography, MRI

8. **Cerebrovascular accident (CVA)**

Laboratory tests: CBC, serum cholesterol, cerebrospinal fluid (CSF)

Diagnostic tests: CT brain scan, nuclear brain scan, MRI, cerebral angiography, PET, oculoplethysmography

9. **Cholecystitis (acute)**

Laboratory tests: CBC, direct bilirubin, serum alkaline phosphatase

Diagnostic tests: Gallbladder and biliary ultrasound, CT of the gallbladder, cholangiogram, nuclear gallbladder scan

10. **Cirrhosis of the liver**

Laboratory tests: Liver enzyme tests: alkaline phosphatase (ALP), gamma-glutamyl transferase (GGT), alanine aminotransferase (ALT/SGPT), 5'nucleotidase (5'N); total and direct bilirubin; serum protein; serum albumin; prealbumin assay; CBC; platelet aggregation; prothrombin time (PT); serum electrolytes; plasma ammonia; antimitochondrial antibody; zinc; zinc protoporphyrin; antismooth muscle antibody (ASTHMA)

Diagnostic tests: Nuclear liver scan, CT of the liver, liver biopsy, hepatic angiography, biopsy

11. **Colorectal cancer**
    Laboratory tests: CEA, serum electrolytes, fecal analysis for occult blood
    Diagnostic tests: Barium enema, sigmoidoscopy, colonoscopy, biopsy
12. **Congestive heart failure (CHF)**
    Laboratory tests: CBC, serum electrolytes, serum and urine osmolality
    Diagnostic tests: X-ray of heart and chest, ECG/EKG, Cerebral vascular pressure (CVP), pulmonary artery catheter (monitoring PCWP), echocardiography
13. **Cystic fibrosis**
    Laboratory tests: Chloride (sweat), sputum culture, electrolytes, D-xylose absorption test, trypsin
    Diagnostic tests: Chest X-rays, pulmonary function tests
14. **Cystitis**
    Laboratory tests: Urinalysis, culture (urine), BUN, serum creatinine, CBC
    Diagnostic tests: Cystoscopy, cystometry, ultrasound (kidney), CT (kidney), nuclear scan (kidney)
15. **Deep-vein thrombophlebitis (DVT)**
    Laboratory tests: CBC, PT, PTT/APTT
    Diagnostic tests: Doppler ultrasonography, venography
16. **Diabetes mellitus (DM)**
    Laboratory tests: CBC, serum/blood FBS (fasting blood sugar or blood glucose) and postprandial blood sugar (PPBS or feasting blood sugar), glucose self-monitoring, hemoglobin A_1c, insulin and insulin antibody, glucagon serum electrolytes, serum acetone, ABGs, oral glucose tolerance test, serum BUN
17. **Eclampsia (toxemia) of pregnancy**
    Laboratory tests: CBC, electrolytes, glucose, creatinine, BUN, uric acid, albumin (urine), protein (quantitative), PTT international ratio (INR), lipoproteins
    Diagnostic tests: Blood pressure monitoring
18. **Emphysema**
    Laboratory tests: ABGs, serum alpha-1-antitrypsin
    Diagnostic tests: Chest X-ray, pulmonary function tests, nuclear lung scan, thoracoscopy

19. **Endocarditis**
    Laboratory tests: Blood cultures, WBC count, RBC indices, ESR, ANA, C_3 and C_4 complements, CRP, RF, creatinine
    Diagnostic tests: Echocardiography, ECG/EKG

20. **Gynecologic problems**
    Laboratory tests: Estrone (E_1), estrogen, estradiol (E_2), prolactin
    Diagnostic tests: Biopsy, cervicography, colposcopy, hysteroscopy

21. **Hepatitis**
    Laboratory tests: Hepatitis A (HAV) antibody, hepatitis profile, hepatitis B surface antigen (HbsAG), CBC, bilirubin (total, direct, indirect, urine), urobilinogen
    Diagnostic tests: CT (liver), ultrasound (liver)

22. **Hypertension**
    Laboratory tests: Electrolytes, BUN, creatinine, BUN/creatinine ratio, aldosterone, renin, catecholamines, thyroid tests, urinalysis
    Diagnostic tests: Blood pressure monitoring

23. **Lung cancer**
    Laboratory tests: ABGs, sputum cytology, serotonin
    Diagnostic tests: Chest X-ray, bronchoscopy, CT of lungs lung biopsy, MRI, mediastinoscopy

24. **Meningitis**
    Laboratory tests: Cultures: cerebrospinal fluid (CSF), sputum, and viral, WBC, electrolytes
    Diagnostic tests: CT scan, spinal puncture, X-ray of the skull

25. **Multiple sclerosis (MS)**
    Laboratory tests: CSF analysis
    Diagnostic tests: MRI, CT scan, EMG, EEG

26. **Myocardial infarction—acute (AMI)**
    Laboratory tests: Cardiac enzymes: CPK and CPK isoenzymes (CPK-MB), aspartate aminotransferase (AST/SGOT), lactic dehydrogenase (LDH) and LDH isoenzymes with LDH_1 greater than LDH_2; CBC; lipoproteins: cholesterol, triglycerides, LDL, HDL; serum electrolytes; PT, PTT/APTT; serum and urine myoglobin; serum/blood glucose; ESR; AGBs; AMA; homocysteine, troponins
    Diagnostic tests: ECG/EKG 12 leads, thallium myocardial imaging, ECG/EKG, cardiac angiography (cardiac catheterization), X-ray of heart and chest, exercise/stress testing, PET, pacemaker monitoring

27. **Osteoporosis**
    Laboratory tests: Serum calcium, serum phosphorus, serum ALP, protein electrophoresis
    Diagnostic tests: X-ray of bone, bone density scan
28. **Pancreatitis (acute)**
    Laboratory tests: Serum and urine amylase, serum lipase
    Diagnostic tests: CT and ultrasound of the pancreas
29. **Peptic ulcer**
    Laboratory tests: Serum electrolytes; *Helicobacter pylori;* pepsinogen
    Diagnostic tests: Upper GI series, gastric analysis studies, gastric acid stimulation test, esophagogastroduodenoscopy
30. **Pharyngitis/sinusitis**
    Laboratory tests: Culture of the pharynx, culture from nasal secretions, CBC
    Diagnostic tests: Sinus CT, X-ray (facial area), sinus endoscopy
31. **Pneumonia**
    Laboratory tests: CBC, sputum culture, blood culture, ABGs
    Diagnostic tests: Chest X-ray, pulmonary function tests, nuclear lung scan
32. **Pregnancy and fetal distress**
    Laboratory tests: Alpha fetoprotein, E_1, estriol (E_3), estetrol (E_4), fetal hemoglobin, ferritin, human chorionic gonadotropin, methemoglobin, pregnanediol, progesterone
    Diagnostic tests: Fetal nonstress test, contraction stress test, fetoscopy
33. **Prostatic disorders (cancer, Benign prostatic hypertrophy (BPH), prostatitis)**
    Laboratory tests: Prostate-specific antigen (PSA), total and free % PSA, acid phosphatase (ACP)/prostatic acid phosphatase (PAP), CBC, ALP, CA 15-3, urinalysis
    Diagnostic tests: Digital examination, ultrasonography, biopsy
34. **Pulmonary embolism (PE)**
    Laboratory tests: CBC, PT, PTT/APTT, ESR, plasminogen
    Diagnostic tests: Chest X-ray, nuclear lung (perfusion) scan, pulmonary angiography, CT, MRI, ECG, venography
35. **Renal failure (RF)**
    Laboratory tests: Serum BUN, serum creatinine, urinalysis, serum and urine osmolality, ABGs, anti-GBM, BUN/creatinine ratio

Diagnostic tests: Kidney, Ureter and bladder (KUB) X-ray, nuclear renal scan, renal angiography

36. **Rheumatoid arthritis (RA)**

    Laboratory tests: CBC, RF, ANA, antimitochondrial, CRP, complements 3 and 4, sed rate or ESR, protein electrophoresis

    Diagnostic tests: Synovial fluid analysis, X-ray of joints, nuclear bone scan

37. **Systemic lupus erythematosus (SLE or lupus)**

    Laboratory tests: Anticardiolipin antibodies (ACA), CBC, sed rate or ESR, ANA, anti-DNA, lupus erythematosus cell test (LE cell test), CRP, urinalysis, complements 3 and 4

    Diagnostic tests: Kidney biopsy

38. **Thyroid disorders**

    Laboratory tests: Thyroid antibodies (TA), thyroid-stimulating hormone (TSH), T_4, T_3

    Diagnostic tests: CT (neck), nuclear scan of the thyroid, ultrasound (thyroid), radioactive iodine (RAI) uptake

39. **Tuberculosis**

    Laboratory tests: Culture of sputum for acid-fast (AF) bacteria, tuberculin skin tests (Mantoux test), urinalysis

    Diagnostic tests: X-ray and CT of the chest

40. **Ulcerative colitis**

    Laboratory tests: CBC, serum electrolytes, sed rate (ESR)

    Diagnostic tests: Barium enema

Laboratory Test Values
for Adults and Children

Laboratory tests and their reference values for adults and children are listed alphabetically, including types of specimens and color-top tubes. Reference values differ from laboratory to laboratory, so nurses should refer to the published laboratory values used in each hospital or private laboratory for any differences. Note: mcg/ml is the same as mg/l; mcg is the same as mcg (microgram).

Test	Specimen (Color-top Tube)	Reference Values
Acetaminophen	Serum (Red)	*Adult and Child:* Therapeutic: 5–20 mcg/ml, 31–124 µmol/l (SI units); toxic: greater than 50 mcg/ml, greater than 305 µmol/l (SI units); greater than 200 mcg/ml—possible hepatotoxicity
Acetone	Serum (Red) or plasma (Green)	*Adult and Child:* 0.3–2.0 mg/dl, 51.6–344 µmol/l (SI units), ketones: 2–4 mg/dl; qualitative will show negative. *Newborn:* slightly higher than adult
Acid phosphatase	Serum (Red)	*Adult:* less than 2.6 ng/ml; 0–5 U/l range; varies according to the method used; 0.2–13 IU/l (SI units) *Child:* 6.4–15.2 U/l

(continued)

Test	Specimen (Color-top Tube)	Reference Values
Activated partial thromboplastin time (APTT)	Plasma (Blue)	*Adult:* 20–35 s or seconds
Adenovirus antibody	Serum (Red)	Negative
Adrenocortico-tropic hormone (ACTH)	Plasma (Green)	*Adult:* 7–10 AM: 8–80 pg/ml; 4 PM: 5–30 pg/ml; 10 PM–12 midnight: less than 10 pg/ml
Alanine amino-transferase (ALT or SGPT)	Serum (Red)	*Adult and Child:* 10–35 U/l; 4–36 U/l (SI units). *Infant:* could be twice as high *Elderly:* Slightly higher than adult
Albumin	Serum (Red)	*Adult:* 3.5–5.0 g/dl, 52%–68% of total protein *Child:* 4.0–5.8 g/dl *Newborn:* 2.9–5.4 g/dl *Infant:* 4.4–5.4 g/dl
Alcohol	Serum (Red) or plasma (Green)	*Adult or Child:* 0% alcohol influence: greater than 0.10%. Alcohol toxicity: greater than 0.25%
Aldolase (ALD)	Serum (Red)	*Adult:* less than 6 U/l; 22–59 mU/l at 37°C (SI units) *Child:* 6–16 U/dl *Infant:* 12–24 U/dl
Aldosterone	Serum (Red) or plasma (Green)	*Adult:* less than 16 ng/dl (fasting); 4–30 ng/dl (sitting position) *Child:* (3–11 years): 5–70 ng/dl *Pregnancy:* 2 to 3 times higher than adult
	Urine	*Adult:* 6–25 mcg/24 h
Alkaline phosphatase (ALP)	Serum (Red)	*Adult:* 42–136 U/l; ALP[1]: 20–130 U/l; ALP[2]: 20–120 U/l *Elderly:* slightly higher *Infant and Child (0–12 years):* 40–115 U/l *Older child:* (13–18 years): 50–230 U/l
Alpha₁ antitrypsin	Serum (Red)	*Adult and Child:* 78–200 mg/dl, 0.78–2.0 g/l *Newborn:* 145–270 mg/dl

Test	Specimen (Color-top Tube)	Reference Values	
Alpha fetoprotein (AFP)	Serum (Red)	*Nonpregnancy:* less than 15 ng/ml	
		Pregnancy:	
		Weeks of Gestation	*ng/ml*
		8–12	0–39
		13	6–31
		14	7–50
		15	7–60
		16	10–72
		17	11–90
		18	14–94
		19	24–112
		20	31–122
		21	19–124
(AFP)	Amniotic fluid	*Weeks of Gestation*	*mcg/ml*
		15	5.5–31
		16	5.7–31.5
		17	3.8–32.5
		18	3.6–28
		19	3.7–24.5
		20	2.2–15
		21	3.8–18
Amikacin	Serum (Red)	*Adult:* Therapeutic, peak: 15–30 mg/l; trough: less than 10 mg/l; toxic: greater than 35 mg/l	
Amino acid	Urine	200 mg/24 h	
Ammonia	Plasma (Green)	*Adult:* 15–45 mcg/dl, 11–35 µmol/l (SI units)	
		Child: 29–70 mcg/dl; 29–70 µmol/l (SI units)	
		Newborn: 64–107 mcg/dl	
Amylase	Serum (Red)	*Adult:* 60–160 Somogyi U/dl, 30–170 U/l (SI units)	
		Elderly: could be slightly high	
	Urine	*Adult:* 4–37 U/l/2 h	
Amyloid beta protein precursor (Alzheimer's marker)	CSF	450 units/l	

(continued)

Test	Specimen (Color-top Tube)	Reference Values
Angiotensin-converting enzyme (ACE)	Serum (Red) or plasma (Green)	*Adult* greater than 20 years 8–67 U/l *Child:* usually not performed
Anion gap	Serum (Red)	10–17 mEq/l
Antibiotic sensitivity test (C & S)	Culture	*Adult and Child:* sensitive or resistant to antibiotic
Anticardiolipin antibodies (ACA)	Serum (Red)	Negative
Antidiuretic hormone (ADH)	Plasma (Lavender)	Adult: 1–5 pg/ml; 1–5 ng/l
Anti-DNA	Serum (Red)	*Adult:* less than 1:85 *Child:* less than 1:60–1:70
Antiglomerular basement membrane (Anti-GBM)	Serum (Red)	Negative
Antimitochondrial antibody (AMA)	Serum (Red or Gray)	*Adult:* Negative: 1:5–1.10 dilution Intermediate level: 1:20–1:80 dilution Strongly suggestive of biliary cirrhosis: greater than 1:80 Positive for biliary cirrhosis: greater than 1:160
Antimyocardial antibody (AMA)	Serum (Red)	None detected
Antinuclear antibodies (ANA)	Serum (Red)	*Adult and Child:* negative
Antiparietal cell antibody (APCA)	Serum (Red)	Negative: 0–1:120 titer Positive: 1:180 titer
Antiscleroderma antibody (Scl-70)	Serum (Red)	Negative: less than 20 units Positive: greater than 25 units
Antismooth muscle antibody (ASTHMA)	Serum (Red)	Negative: less than 1:20 titer Positive: greater than 1:20 titer

Test	Specimen (Color-top Tube)	Reference Values
Antisperm antibody	Semen Blood	*Adult*: negative for agglutinating antibody.
	Serum (Red)	Moderately positive: 50%
		Strongly positive: 100%
Antistreptolysin O (ASO)	Serum (Red)	*Adult:* less than 100 IU/ml
		Newborn: same as mother
		2–5 years: less than 100 IU/ml
		12–19 years: less than 200 IU/ml
Apolipoproteins (Apo)	Plasma (Lavender)	Apo A-1: see test
		Apo B: see test
	Serum (Red)	Ratio Apo A-1/Apo B: see test
Arterial blood gases (ABGs)	Blood	*Adult:* pH: 7.35–7.45; $Paco_2$: 35–45 mm Hg; PaO_2: 75–100 mm Hg; HCO_3: 24–28 mEq/l; BE: –2 to +2
		Child: pH: 7.36–7.44; others are same as adult
Ascorbic acid	Plasma (Gray)	*Adult and Child:* 0.6–2.0 mg/dl, 34–114 μmol/dl (SI units)
	Serum (Red)	0.2–2.0 mg/dl
Aspartate aminotransferase (AST) (SGOT)	Serum (Red)	*Adult and Child: average range:* 8–38; *5*–40 U/l (Frankel), 4–36 IU/l, 16–60 U/ml 30°C (Karen), 8–33 U/l 37°C (SI units). Female lower than male. Exercise increases levels
		Elderly: slightly higher
		Newborn: four times the normal
Atrial natriuretic hormone (ANH)	Plasma (Lavender)	*Adult:* 20–77 pg/ml; 20–77 ng/l (SI units)
Barbiturate	Serum (Red)	*Phenobarbital*
		Adult and Child: therapeutic: 15–40 mg/l; toxic: greater than 40 mg/l
		Amobarbital
		Adult and Child: therapeutic: 3–12 mg/l; toxic: greater than 12 mg/l
Bence-Jones protein	Urine	*Adult and Child:* negative to trace

(continued)

Test	Specimen (Color-top Tube)	Reference Values
Beta₂ microglobulin	Blood (Lavender)	*Adult*: less than 2 mcg/dl; 1.0–2.4 mg/l (SI units)
	Serum (Red)	*Elderly:* 0.25 mg/dl
	Urine	*Adult*: less than 120 mcg/24 h
Bilirubin	Serum (Red)	Total: *Adult:* 0.1–1.2 mg/dl, 1.7–20.5 µmol/l (SI units)
		Child: 0.2–0.8 mg/dl
		Newborn: 1–12 mg/dl, 17.1–205 µmol/l (SI units)
		Direct: *Adult:* 0.0–0.3 mg/dl, 1.7–5.1 µmol/l (SI units)
		Indirect: *Adult:* 0.1–1.0 mg/dl, 1.7–17.1 µmol/l (SI units)
	Urine	*Adult and Child:* negative to 0.02 mg/dl
Bioterrorism infectious products (Anthrax, Botulism, Smallpox)	Culture: blood, sputum stool	*Adult and Children:* negative
Bleeding time	Blood	*Adult:* Ivy method: 3–7 min; Duke method: 1–3 min
Blood urea nitrogen (BUN)	Serum (Red)	*Adult:* 5–25 mg/dl
		Elderly: slightly higher
		Child: 5–20 mg/dl
		Newborn: 5–15 mg/dl
Blood urea nitrogen/ creatinine ratio	Serum (Red)	BUN: creatinine 10:1 to 20:1 Average: 15:1
Brain natriuretic peptide (BNP)	Plasma (Lavender)	*Adult:* Desired: less than 100 pg/ml; less than 100 ng/l (SI units)
		Positive: greater than 100 pg/ml; greater than 100 ng/l (SI units)
Breast cancer genetic (BRCA-1 and BRCA-2)	Blood (Lavender or Blue)	*Adult:* negative

Test	Specimen (Color-top Tube)	Reference Values
Breast cancer tumor prognostic markers	Breast tissue	*Adult*: 6 markers; see test
Bromide	Serum (Red)	*Adult and Child:* 0 Therapeutic: less than 80 mg/dl; toxic: greater than 100 mg/dl
Calcitonin (hCT)	Serum (Red)	*Adult:* Male: less than 40 pg/ml or ng/l; female: less than 25 pg/ml or ng/l *Child:* less than 70 pg/ml; less than 70 ng/l (SI units)
Calcium (Ca)	Serum (Red)	*Adult:* 4.5–5.5 mEq/l, 9–11 mg/dl, 2.3–2.8 mmol/l (SI units). *Ionized Ca:* 4.25–5.25 mg/dl; 2.2–2.5 mEq/l, 1.1–1.24 mmol/l *Child:* 4.5–5.8 mEq/l, 9–11.5 mg/dl *Newborn:* 3.7–7.0 mEq/l, 7.4–14.0 mg/dl *Infant:* 5.0–6.0 mEq/l, 10–12 mg/dl
	Urine	*Adult:* low calcium diet: less than 150 mg/24 h; average calcium diet: 100–250 mg/24 h; high calcium diet: 250–300 mg/24 Normal:
Cancer tumor markers (CA 15–3, CA 19–9, CA 27.29, CA 50, CA 125)	Serum (Red)	CA 15–3: less than 30 units/ml; less than 30 kU/l (SI units) CA 19–9: less than 37 units/ml; less than 37 kU/l (SI units) CA 27.29: less than 37 units/ml; less than 37 kU/l (SI units) CA 50: less than 17 units/ml; less than 17 kU/l (SI units) CA 125: less than 35 units/ml; less than 35 kU/l (SI units)
Candida antibody test	Serum (Red)	Negative Positive: greater than 1.8 titer
Cannabinoid (Marijuana)	Urine	Negative: less than 50 mg/ml

(continued)

Test	Specimen (Color-top Tube)	Reference Values
Carbamazepine	Serum (Red)	*Adult:* Therapeutic: 4–12 mg/ml; toxic: greater than 12–15 mg/ml
Carbon dioxide combining power (CO_2)	Serum (Red) or plasma (Green)	*Adult:* 22–30 mEq/l, 22–30 mmol/l (SI units) *Panic Range:* less than 15 mEq/l and greater than 45 mEq/l *Child:* 20–28 mEq/l
Carbon monoxide (CO) blood carboxy hemoglobin	Blood (Lavender)	*Adult and Child:* Nonsmoker: less than 2.5% saturation of Hb; smoker: average (1–2 pk): 4%–5% saturation of Hb; heavy: 5%–12% saturation of Hb; life threatening: greater than 15% saturation of Hb
Carcinoembryonic antigen (CEA)	Plasma (Lavender)	*Adult:* nonsmokers: less than 2.5 ng/ml; smokers: less than 5.0 ng/ml; neoplasm: greater than 12 ng/ml; inflammatory: greater than 10 ng/ml
Cardiovascular disease genetic test	Plasma (Lavender) Serum (Red)	Negative: no angiotensinogen gene
Carotene	Serum (Red)	*Adult:* 60–200 mcg/dl (varies with diet) *Child:* 40–130 mcg/dl
Catecholamines	Serum: see test Urine	*Adult:* total: less than 100 mcg/24 h, 0–14 mcg/dl (random) Epinephrine: less than 20 mcg/24 h Norepinephrine: less than 100 mcg/24 h *Child:* less than adult due to weight differences
Cerebrospinal	Spinal	*Adult:* pressure: 75–175 mm H_2O; WBC: 0–8 µl; protein: 15–45 mg/dl; glucose: 40–80 mg/dl *Child:* pressure: 50–100 mm H_2O; WBC: 0–8 µl; protein: 14–45 mg/dl; glucose: 35–75 mg/dl
Ceruloplasmin (Cp)	Serum (Red)	*Adult and Child:* 18–45 mg/dl, 180–450 mg/l (SI units) *Infant:* less than 23 mg/dl

Test	Specimen (Color-top Tube)	Reference Values
Chlamydia	Serum (Red)	*Adult: Normal titer:* less than 1:16 *Positive titer:* greater than 1:64
Chloride (Cl)	Serum (Red)	*Adult:* 95–105 mEq/l, 95–105 mmol/l (SI units) *Child:* 98–105 mEq/l *Newborn:* 94–112 mEq/l *Infant:* 95–110 mEq/l
Cholesterol	Serum (Red)	*Adult:* less than 200 mg/dl; moderate risk: 200–240 mg/dl; high risk: greater than 240 mg/dl *Child:* 2–19 years: 130–170 mg/dl; moderate risk: 171–184 mg/dl; high risk: greater than 185 mg/dl *Infant:* 90–130 mg/dl
Cholinesterase (pseudocho-linesterase)	Blood, plasma (Green)	*Adult and Child:* 0.5–1.0 mg/dl, 6–8 IU/l *Adult and Child:* 3–8 units, 8–18 IU/l 37°C
Clot retraction	Blood (Red)	*Adult and Child:* 1–24 h
Cold agglutinins (CA)	Serum (Red)	*Adult and Child:* 1–8 antibody titer; positive: greater than 1:16 titer
Complement: Total	Serum (Red)	*Adult:* 75–160 kU/l (SI units)
Complement C₃	Serum (Red)	*Adult:* *Male:* 80–180 mg/dl *Female:* 76–120 mg/dl *Elderly:* slightly higher
Complement C₄	Serum (Red)	*Adult:* 15–45 mg/dl
Coombs' direct	Blood (Lavender)	*Adult and Child:* negative
Coombs' indirect	Serum (Red)	*Adult and Child:* negative
Copper (Cu)	Serum (Red)	*Adult:* male: 70–140 mcg/dl; female: 80–155 mcg/dl; pregnancy: 140–300 mcg/dl *Child:* 30–190 mcg/dl *Adolescent:* 90–240 mcg/dl *Newborn:* 20–70 mcg/dl
	Urine	*Adult:* 0–60 mcg/24 h Wilson's disease: greater than 100 mcg/24 h
Corticotropin	Plasma (Green)	*Adult:* 8–10 AM: up to 80 pg/ml

(continued)

Test	Specimen (Color-top Tube)	Reference Values
Cortisol	Plasma (Green)	*Adult:* 8–10 AM: 5–23 mcg/dl; 4–6 PM: 3–13 mcg/dl *Child:* 8–10 AM: 15–25 mcg/dl; 4–6 PM: 5–10 mcg/dl
	Urine	*Adult:* 24–105 mcg/24 h
C-Peptide	Serum (Red)	*Adult:* Fasting: 0.8–1.8 ng/ml; 0.27–63 mmol/l (SI units)
C-Reactive Protein (CRP)	Serum (Red)	*Adult:* 0; positive: greater than 1:2 titer
Creatine phosphokinase (CPK)	Serum (Red)	*Adult:* male: 5–35 mcg/ml, 30–180 IU/l; female: 5–25 mcg/ml, 25–150 IU/l *Child:* male: 0–70 IU/l 30°C; female: 0–50 IU/l 30°C *Newborn:* 65–580 IU/l at 30°C
CPK isoenzymes	Serum (Red)	*Adult:* CPK-MM: 94%–100% (muscle); CPK-MB: 0%–6% (heart); CPK-BB: 0% (brain)
Creatinine (Cr)	Serum (Red)	*Adult:* 0.5–1.5 mg/dl, 45–132.5 umol/l (SI units) *Elderly:* slightly lower *Child:* 0.4–1.2 mg/dl *Newborn:* 0.8–1.4 mg/dl *Infant:* 0.7–1.7 mg/dl
	Urine	*Adult:* 0.9–1.9 g/24 h
Creatinine clearance	Urine	*Adult:* male: 85–135 mg/min; female: 85–120 ml/min *Elderly:* slightly lower *Child:* males slightly higher
Cross-match	Blood (Red)	*Adult and Child:* compatible
Cryoglobulins	Serum (Red)	*Adult:* negative *Child:* negative
Cultures	Various specimens	*Adult and Child:* negative or no pathogen
Cytomegalovirus (CMV) antibody	Serum (Red)	*Adult and Child:* negative to less than 0.30
D-Dimer test	Blood (Blue)	Negative for D-Dimer fragments Positive: greater than 250 ng/ml; greater than 250 mcg/l (SI units)

Test	Specimen (Color-top Tube)	Reference Values
Dexamethasone suppression test	Plasma Urine	*Adult:* Cortisol: less than 5 mcg/dl; 17-OHCS: less than 4 mg/5 h (greater than 50% reduction of plasma cortisol and urine 17-OHCS)
Diazepam (Valium)	Serum (Red)	*Adult:* therapeutic: 0.5–2.0 mg/l, 400–600 ng/ml; toxic: greater than 3 mg/l, greater than 3,000 ng/ml
Digoxin	Serum (Red)	*Adult and Child:* therapeutic: 0.5–2.0 ng/ml, 0.5–2 nmol/l (SI units); toxic: greater than 2 ng/ml *Infant:* therapeutic: 1–3 ng/ml; toxic: greater than 3.5 ng/ml
Dilantin (Phenytoin)	Serum (Red)	*Adult:* therapeutic: 10–20 mcg/ml; toxic: greater than 20 mcg/ml *Child:* toxic: greater than 15–20 mcg/ml
Diltiazem (Cardizem)	Serum (Red)	*Adult:* therapeutic: 50–200 ng/ml; toxic: greater than 200 ng/ml
Disseminated intravascular coagulation (DIC)	Plasma (Blue)	*Adult:* platelet, PT, APTT, fibrinogen, thrombin time, fibrin split products, and plasma paraprotamine
D-Xylose absorption test	Blood (Gray)	25 g: 25–75 mg/dl/2 h; 5 g: 8–28 mg/dl/2 h
	Urine	25 g: greater than 3.5 g/5 h; greater than 5 g/24 h; 5 g: 1.2–2.4 g/5 h
Encephalitis virus antibody	Serum (Red)	less than 1:10
Enterovirus group	Serum (Red)	Negative
Erythrocyte sedimentation rate (ESR, sed rate)	Blood (Lavender)	*Adult:* Westergren method: less than 50 years, male: 0–15 mm/h; female: 0–20 mm/h; greater than 50 years, male: 0–20 mm/h; female: 0–30 mm/h Wintrobe method: male: 0–9 mm/h; female: 0–15 mm/h *Child:* 0–20 mm/h *Newborn:* 0–2 mm/h

(continued)

Test	Specimen (Color-top Tube)	Reference Values	
Estetrol (E$_4$)	Plasma (Red)	*Pregnancy:*	
		Weeks of Gestation	*pg/ml*
		20–26	140–210
		30	350
		36	900
		40	Greater than 1,050
	Amniotic fluid	*Weeks of Gestation*	*ng/ml*
		32+	0.8
		40+	13.0
Estradiol (E$_2$)	Serum (Red)	*Female:* follicular phase: 20–150 pg/ml; midcycle phase: 100–500 pg/ml; luteal phase: 60–260 pg/ml; menopause: less than 30 pg/ml	
		Child: less than 30 pg/ml; 6 months to 10 years: 3–10 pg/ml	
		Male: 15–50 pg/ml	
Estriol (E$_3$)	Serum (Red)	*Pregnancy:*	
		Weeks of Gestation	*ng/dl*
		25–28	25–165
		29–32	30–230
		33–36	45–370
		37–38	75–420
		39–40	95–450
	Urine	*Weeks of Gestation*	*ng/dl*
		25–28	6–28
		29–32	6–32
		33–36	10–45
		37–40	15–60
Estrogen	Serum (Red)	*Adult:* early menstrual cycle: 60–200 pg/ml; midcycle: 120–440 pg/ml; late cycle: 150–350 pg/ml; postmenopause: less than 30 pg/ml; male: 12–34 pg/ml	
		Child: 1–6 years: 3–10 pg/ml; 8–12 years: less than 30 pg/ml	

Test	Specimen (Color-top Tube)	Reference Values
	Urine	*Adult:* preovulation: 5–25 mcg/24 h; follicular phase: 24–100 mcg/24 h; luteal phase: 22–80 mcg/24 h; postmenopause: 0–10 mcg/24 h; male: 4–25 mcg/24 h
		Child: less than 12 years: 1 mcg/24 h; greater than 12 years: same as adult
Estrone (E$_1$)	Serum (Red)	*Adult: Female:* follicular phase: 30–100 pg/ml; ovulatory phase: greater than 150 pg/ml; luteal phase: 90–160 pg/ml; postmenopausal: 20–40 pg/ml
		Male: 10–50 pg/ml
		Child (1–10 years old): less than 10 pg/ml
	Urine	*Female:* follicular phase: 4–7 mcg/24 h; ovulatory phase: 11–30 mcg/24 h; luteal phase: 10–22 mcg/24 h; postmenopausal: 1–7 mcg/24 h
Ethosuximide	Serum (Red)	*Adult:* therapeutic: 40–100 mcg/ml; toxic: greater than 100 mcg/ml
		Child: therapeutic: 2–4 mg/kg day toxic: same as adult or higher
Factor assay	Plasma (Blue)	See Factor Assay in text
Febrile agglutinins	Serum (Red)	*Adult and Child:*
		Brucella: less than 1:20
		Tularemia: less than 1:40
		Salmonella: less than 1:40
		Proteus: less than 1:40
Fecal fat	Stool	Quantitative: *Adult:* 2–7 g/24 h 7–25 mmol/day (SI units)
		Child (less than 1 year old): 1.0 g/24 h
Ferritin	Serum (Red)	See Ferritin in text
Fetal hemoglobin (HbF)	Blood (Lavender, Green)	*Adult:* 0%–2%
		Child: Newborn: 60%–90% 1–5 months: less than 70%; 6–9 months: less than 5% 1 year: less than 2%

(continued)

Test	Specimen (Color-top Tube)	Reference Values
Fibrin degradation products (FD)	Blood (Blue)	*Adult:* 2–10 mcg/ml
Fibrinogen	Plasma (Blue)	*Adult and Child:* 200–400 mg/dl *Newborn:* 150–300 mg/dl
Folic acid (Folate)	Serum (Red)	*Adult and Child:* 3–16 ng/ml, greater than 2.5 ng/ml (RIA)
	Blood (Lavender)	*Adult:* 200–700 ng/ml
Follicle-stimulating hormone (FSH)	Serum (Red)	*Adult:* follicular phase: 4–30 mU/ml; midcycle: 10–90 mU/ml; luteal phase: 4–30 mU/ml; postmenopause: 40–170 mU/ml; male: 4–25 mU/ml *Child:* prepubertal: 5–12 mU/ml
FTA-ABS	Serum (Red)	*Adult and Child:* negative
Fungal organisms	Various specimens	*Adult and Child:* negative
Gamma-glutamyl transferase (GGT)	Serum (Red)	*Adult and Child:* average: 0–45 IU/l; male: 4–23 IU/l, 9–69 U/l at 37°C (SI units); female: 3–13 IU/l, 4–33 U/l at 37°C (SI units) *Elderly:* slightly higher *Newborn:* 5× higher *Premature:* 10× higher
Gastrin	Serum (Red) or plasma (Lavender)	*Adult:* fasting: less than 100 pg/ml; nonfasting: 50–200 pg/ml
Gentamicin	Serum (Red)	*Adult:* therapeutic, peak: 6–12 mcg/ml; trough: less than 2 mcg/ml; toxic: greater than 12 mcg/ml
Glucose fasting (FBS)	Serum (Red)	*Adult:* 70–110 mg/dl; 3.9–6.1 mmol/l (SI units) *Elderly:* 70–120 mg/dl; 3.9–6.7 mmol/l (SI units) *Panic value:* less than 40 mg/dl, greater than 700 mg/dl *Child:* 60–100 mg/dl; 3.3–5.5 mmol/l (SI units) *Newborn:* 30–80 mg/dl; 1.7–4.4 mmol/l (SI units)

Test	Specimen (Color-top Tube)	Reference Values
Glucose (PPBS)	Blood/plasma (Gray)	*Adult*: Serum and Plasma: less than 140 mg/dl/2 h, less than 7.8 mmol/l (SI units)
	Serum (Red)	Whole blood: less than 120 mg/dl/2 h; less than 6.7 mmol/l (SI units)
		Elderly: Serum: less than 160 mg/dl; less than 8.9 mmol/l (SI units)
		Whole blood: less than 140 mg/dl; less than 7.8 mmol/l (SI units)
		Child: Serum: less than 140 mg/dl; less than 6.7 mmol/l (SI units)
Glucagon	Plasma (Lavender)	*Adult:* 50–200 pg/ml, 50–200 ng/l (SI units)
		Newborn: 0–1750 pg/ml
Glucose-6-phosphate dehydrogenase (G6PD)	Blood (Green or Lavender)	*Adult and Child:* quantitative test: 8–18 IU/g Hb, 125–281 U/dl packed RBC, 251–511 U/dl (cells)
Glucose tolerance test (OGTT)	Serum (Red) Blood (Gray)	see test; Reference Values
Growth hormone (GH or hGH)	Serum (Red)	*Adult:* male: less than 5 ng/ml; female: less than 10 ng/ml
		Child: less than 10 ng/ml
Haptoglobin (Hp)	Serum (Red)	*Adult and Child:* 60–270 mg/dl, 0.6–2.7 g/l (SI units)
		Newborn: 0–10 mg/dl
		Infant: 1–6 months: 0–30 mg/dl
Helicobacter pylori	Serum (Red)	Negative
Hematocrit (Hct)	Blood (Lavender)	*Adult:* male: 40%–54%; female: 36%–46%
		Child: 1–3 years: 29%–40%; 4–10 years: 31%–43%
		Newborn: 44%–65%
Hemoglobin (Hb or Hgb)	Blood (Lavender)	*Adult:* male: 13.5–18 g/dl; female: 12–15 g/dl
		Child: 6 months–1 year: 10–17 g/dl; 5–14 years: 11–16 g/dl
		Newborn: 14–24 g/dl

(continued)

Test	Specimen (Color-top Tube)	Reference Values
Hemoglobin A₁c	Plasma (Lavender, Green)	*Adult: Nondiabetic:* 2%–5%; *diabetic control:* 2.5%–6%; *diabetic uncontrolled:* greater than 8.0%; *Child: Nondiabetic:* 1.5%–4%
Hemoglobin electrophoresis	Blood (Lavender)	*Adult:* Hb A₁: 95%–98% total Hb; A₂: 1.5%–4%; F: less than 2%; C: 0%; D: 0%; S: 0% *Child:* Hb F: 1%–2% after 6 months *Newborn:* Hb F: 50%–80% total Hb *Infant:* Hb F: 8%
Hepatitis A virus	Serum (Red)	Negative
Hepatitis B surface antigen (HB$_s$Ag)	Serum (Red)	*Adult and Child:* negative
Herpes simplex virus antibody	Serum (Red)	Negative: less than 1:10 Positive: greater than 1:10 Positive greater than 1:10 to 1:500
Heterophile antibody	Serum (Red)	*Adult and Child:* normal: less than 1:28 titer; abnormal: 1:56
Hexosaminidase (A and B)	Serum (Red) Amniotic fluid	Total: 5–20 U/l 55%–80% *Elderly:* slightly higher
Homocysteine	Blood (Lavender or Green)	*Adult:* 4–17 µmol/l (fasting)
Human chorionic gonadotropin (hCG)	Serum (Red)	*Adult:* nonpregnant: less than 0.01 IU/ml Pregnant:

Weeks of Gestation	Values (IU/ml)
1	0.01–0.04
2	0.03–0.10
4	0.10–1.0
5–12	10–100
13–25	10–30
26–40	5–15

| | Urine | *Adult:* Nonpregnant: negative; pregnant: 1–12 weeks: 6,000–500,000 IU/24 h |

Test	Specimen (Color-top Tube)	Reference Values	
Human immuno-deficiency virus (HIV), AIDS virus	Serum (Red)	*Adult and Child:* seronegative	
Human leukocyte antigen (HLA)	Serum (Green)	Histocompatibility match or non-match	
Human placental lactogen (HPL)	Serum (Red)	*Nonpregnant female:* less than 0.5 mcg/ml	
		Pregnant female	
		Weeks of Gestation	*Reference Values*
		5–7	1.0 mcg/ml
		8–27	less than 4.6 mcg/ml
		28–31	2.4–6.0 mcg/ml
		32–35	3.6–7.7 mcg/ml
		36–term	5.0–10.0 mcg/ml
		Male: less than 0.5 mcg/ml	
17-OHCS	Urine	*Adult:* average: 2–12 mg/24 h; male: 3–12 mg/24 h; female: 2–10 mg/24 h	
		Elderly: lower than adult	
		Child: 2–4 years: 1–2 mg/24 h; 5–12 years: 6–8 mg/24 h	
		Infant: less than 1 mg/24 h	
5-HIAA	Urine	*Adult:* random sample: negative; quantitative: 2–10 mg/24 h	
Immunoglobulins (Ig)	Serum (Red)	*Adult:* total Ig: 900–2,200 mg/dl; IgG: 650–1,700 mg/dl; IgA: 70–400 mg/dl; IgM: 40–350 mg/dl; IgD: 0–8 mg/dl; IgE: 0–120 mg/dl	
		Child: 6–16 years: total Ig: 800–1,700; IgG: 700–1,650 mg/dl; IgA: 80–230 mg/dl; IgM: 45–260 mg/dl; IgE: less than 62 U/ml	

(continued)

Test	Specimen (Color-top Tube)	Reference Values
Insulin	Serum (Red)	*Adult:* 5–25 µU/ml, 10–250 µIU/ml *Panic Value:* less than 5 µU/ml
Insulin antibody test	Serum (Red)	less than 4% serum binding of beef or pork
International normalized ratio (INR)	Plasma (Blue)	For anticoagulant therapy: 2.0–3.0 INR
Iron	Serum (Red)	*Adult:* 50–150 mcg/dl, 10–27 µmol/l (SI units) *Child:* 6 months–2 years: 40–100 mcg/dl *Newborn:* 100–250 mcg/dl *Elderly:* 60–80 mcg/dl
Iron-binding capacity (IBC; TIBC)	Serum (Red)	*Adult and Child:* 250–450 mcg/dl *Newborn:* 60–175 mcg/dl *Infant:* 100–135 mcg/dl
Ketone bodies	Urine	*Adult and Child:* negative
17-Ketosteroids (17-KS)	Urine	*Adult:* male: 5–25 mg/24 h; female: 5–15 mg/24 h *Elderly:* 4–8 mg/24 h *Child:* 1–3 years: less than 2 mg/24 h; 3–6 years: less than 3 mg/24 h; 7–10 years: less than 4 mg/24 h; 10–12 years: less than 5–6 mg/24 h *Adolescent:* male: 3–15 mg/24 h; female: 3–12 mg/24 h
Lactic acid	Blood (Green)	*Adult: arterial* blood: 0.5–2.0 mEq/l, 11.3 mg/dl, 0.5–2.0 mmol/l (SI units); *venous* blood: 0.5–1.5 mEq/l, 8.1–15.3 mg/dl, 0.5–1.5 mmol/l (SI units); *panic:* greater than 5 mEq/l, greater than 45 mg/dl, greater than 5 mmol/l (SI units)
Lactic dehydrogenase (LD or LDH)	Serum (Red)	*Adult:* 100–190 IU/l, 70–250 U/l *Child:* 50–150 IU/l *Newborn:* 300–1,500 IU/l

Test	Specimen (Color-top Tube)	Reference Values
LDH isoenzymes	Serum (Red)	*Adult:* LDH$_1$: 14%–26%; LDH$_2$: 27%–37%; LDH$_3$: 13%–26%; LDH$_4$: 8%–16%; LDH$_5$: 6%–16%
Lactose	Serum/plasma (Gray)	less than 0.5 mg/dl
	Urine	12–40 mg/dl
Lactose	Serum/plasma (Gray)	*Adult and Child:* less than 0.5 mg/dl, less than 14.5 μmol/l (SI units)
	Urine	12–40 mg/dl
Lactose test tolerance	Serum/plasma (Gray)	Tolerance: FBS + 20–50 mg/dl; intolerance: less than 20 mg/dl
Latex allergy test	Serum (Red)	Negative: less than 0.35 international units/ml Positive: 0.35+ international units/ml
Lead	Blood (Brown)	*Adult:* 10–20 mcg/dl; acceptable: 20–40 mcg/dl, toxic: greater than 80 mcg/dl *Child:* less than 20 mcg/dl, toxic: greater than 50 mcg/dl
Lecithin/sphin-gomyelin ratio (L/S)	Amniotic fluid	*Adult:* 1:1 before 35 weeks' gestation; L: 6–9 mg/dl; S: 4–6 mg/dl 4:1 after 35 weeks' gestation L: 15–21 mg/dl; S: 4–6 mg/dl
Legionnaire's antibody	Serum (Red)	Negative
Leucine amino-peptidase (LAP)	Serum (Red)	*Adult:* 8–22 μU/ml, 12–33 IU/l, 20–50 U/l at 37°C (SI units)
Leukoagglutinin test	Blood (Lavender) Serum (Red)	Negative: No dye uptake
Lidocaine	Serum (Red)	*Adult:* therapeutic: 1.5–5.0 mcg/ml; toxic: greater than 6 mcg/ml
Lipase	Serum (Red)	*Adult:* 20–180 IU/l, 14–280 mU/ml, 14–280 U/l (SI units) *Child:* 20–136 IU/l *Infant:* 9–105 IU/l
Lipoproteins	Serum (Red)	*Adult:* total lipids: 400–800 mg/dl, 4–8 g/l (SI units) Cholesterol: 150–240 mg/dl

(continued)

Test	Specimen (Color-top Tube)	Reference Values
		Triglycerides: 10–190 mg/dl
		Phospholipids: 150–325 mg/dl
		LDL: 60–130 mg/dl; HDL: 29–77 mg/dl; low-risk HDL: greater than 46 mg/dl
Lithium	Serum (Red)	*Adult:* therapeutic: 0.5–1.5 mEq/l; toxic: greater than 1.5 mEq/l; lethal: greater than 4.0 mEq/l
Lupus erythe-matosus (LE) cell test	Blood (Green or Red)	*Adult and Child:* No LE cells
Luteinizing hormone (LH)	Serum (Red)	*Serum:* Adult: female: follicular phase: 5–30 mIU/ml; midcycle: 50–150 mIU/ml; luteal phase: 2–25 mIU/ml. Postmenopausal: 40–100 mIU/ml. Male: 5–25 mIU/ml. Child: 6–12 years: less than 10 mIU/ml; 13–18 years: less than 20 mIU/ml
		Urine: Adult: female: follicular phase: 5–25 IU/24 h; midcycle: 30–90 IU/24 h; luteal phase: 2–24 IU/24 h; postmenopausal: greater than 40 IU/24 h. Male: 7–25 IU/ml
Lyme disease test	Serum (Red)	less than 1:256
Lymphocytes (T and B) assay	Blood (Lavender)	T cells: 60%–80%; 600–2,400 cells/μl
		B cells: 4%–16%; 50–250 cells/μl
Magnesium (Mg)	Serum (Red)	*Adult:* 1.5–2.5 mEq/l, 1.8–3.0 mg/dl
		Child: 1.6–2.6 mEq/l
		Newborn: 1.4–2.9 mEq/l
Malarial smear	Blood (Lavender)	*Adult and Child:* negative
Methemoglobin (hemoglobin M, HbM)	Blood (Lavender or Green)	Normal: less than 1.5% of total Hgb; 0.06–0.24 g/dl; 9.2–37.0 μmol/l (SI units)
		Positive: greater than 20%–70%
		Lethal: greater than 70%
Mumps antibody	Serum (Red)	*Adult and Child:* Negative: less than 1:8 titer; Positive: greater than 1:8

Test	Specimen (Color-top Tube)	Reference Values
Myoglobin	Serum (Red)	Serum: *Adult:* 12–90 ng/ml; Urine: Negative: less than 20 ng/ml
Nifedipine (Procardia)	Serum (Red)	*Adult:* therapeutic: 50–100 ng/ml; toxic: greater than 100 ng/ml
N-Telopeptide cross-links (Ntx)	Serum (Red)	*Female:* 6.2–19 mM BCE/l *Male:* 5.4–24.2 mM BCE/l
	Urine	*Female:* 5.0–65 mM BCE/l creatinine *Male:* 3.0–51 mM BCE/l creatinine
5-Nucleotidase	Serum (Red)	*Adult:* less than 17 U/l
Occult blood	Feces	*Adult and Child:* negative
Opiates	Serum and Urine	Negative (see text)
Osmolality	Serum (Red)	*Adult:* 280–300 mOsm/kg H_2O *Child:* 270–290 mOsm/kg H_2O *Panic value:* less than 240 mOsm/kg and greater than 320 mOsm/kg
	Urine	*Adult and Child:* 50–1,200 mOsm/kg H_2O *Newborn:* 100–600 mOsm/kg H_2O
Osteocalcin	Serum (Red)	*Female:* Premenopausal: 0.5–7.8 ng/ml; 0.5–7.8 mcg/l (SI units)
	Check with the institution	Postmenopausal: 1.2–11 ng/ml; 1.2–11 mcg/l (SI units) Male: 1.5–11.5 ng/ml: 1.5–11.5 mcg/l (SI units)
Ova and parasites	Feces	*Adult and Child:* negative
Parathyroid hormone (PTH)	Serum (Red)	*Adult:* C-terminal/midregion: 50–330 pg/ml; intact/midregion: 11–54 pg/ml; N-terminal: 8–24 pg/ml
Partial thrombo-plastin time (PTT)	Plasma (Blue)	*Adult:* 60–70; APTT: 20–35
Parvovirus B 19 antibody	Serum (Red)	Negative to IgG and IgM antibodies to parvovirus B 19
Pepsinogen 1	Serum (Red)	*Adult:* 124–142 ng/ml; 124–142 ug/l (SI units) *Child:* See test in book; Reference Values

(continued)

Test	Specimen (Color-top Tube)	Reference Values
Phenylalanine	Serum (Red)	*Child:* 0.5–2.0 mg/dl
Phenylketonuria	Urine	*Child:* negative
Phospholipids	Serum (Red)	*Adult:* 150–325 mg/dl
Phosphorus (P)	Serum (Red)	*Adult:* 1.7–2.6 mEq/l, 2.5–4.5 mg/dl, 0.78–1.52 mmol/l (SI units)
		Child: 4.5–5.5 mg/dl
		Infant: 4.5–6.7 mg/dl
		Elderly: slightly lower than adult
Platelet aggregation and adhesions	Blood (Blue)	*Adult:* aggregation in 3–5 min
Platelet antibody test	Blood (Blue)	*Adult:* negative
Platelet count	Blood (Lavender)	*Adult and Child:* 150,000–400,000 µl, 0.15–0.4 × 10^{12}/l (SI units)
		Premature: 100,000–300,000 µl
		Newborn: 150,000–300,000 µl
		Infant: 200,000–475,000 µl
Porphobilinogen	Urine	*Adult and Child:* random, negative quantitative: 0–2 mg/24 h
Porphyrins:		
Coproporphyrins	Urine	*Adult:* random: negative or 3–20 mcg/dl; quantitative: 15–160 mcg/24 h
		Child: 0–80 mcg/24 h
Uroporphyrins	Urine	*Adult:* random: negative; quant: less than 30 mcg/24 h
		Child: 10–30 mcg/24 h
Potassium (K)	Serum (Red)	*Adult:* 3.5–5.3 mEq/l, 3.5–5.0 mmol/l (SI units)
		Child: 3.5–5.5 mEq/l
		Infant: 3.6–5.8 mEq/l
	Urine	*Adult:* 25–120 mEq/24 h
Prealbumin assay	Serum (Red)	*Adult:* 17–40 mg/dl; *Female:* 18 mg/dl; *Male:* 21.6 mg/dl
		Child: 2–3 years: 16–28 mg/dl
		Newborn: 10–11.5 mg/dl

Test	Specimen (Color-top Tube)	Reference Values
Pregnanediol	Urine	*Adult:* female: proliferative phase: 0.5–1.5 mg/24 h; luteal phase: 2–7 mg/24 h; postmenopause: 0.1–1.0 mg/24 h; male: 0.1–1.5 mg/24 h

Pregnancy:

Weeks of Gestation	mg/24 h
10–19	5–25
20–28	15–42
28–32	25–49

Child: 0.4–1.0 mg/24 h

Test	Specimen (Color-top Tube)	Reference Values
Pregnanetriol	Urine	*Adult:* male: 0.4–2.4 mg/24 h; female: 0.5–2.0 mg/24 h *Child:* 0–1.0 mg/24 h *Infant:* 0–0.2 mg/24 h
Primidone	Serum (Red)	*Adult:* therapeutic: 5–12 mcg/ml; toxic: greater than 12–15 mcg/ml *Child:* less than 5 years: therapeutic: 7–10 mcg/ml; toxic: greater than 12 mcg/ml
Procainamide	Serum (Red)	*Adult:* therapeutic: 4–10 mcg/ml; toxic: greater than 10 mcg/ml
Progesterone	Serum (Red) or plasma (Lavender)	*Adult:* Female: follicular phase: 0.1–1.5 ng/ml; 20–150 ng/dl; luteal phase: 2–28 ng/ml; 250–2,800 ng/dl; postmenopausal: less than 1.0 ng/ml; less than 100 ng/dl. Pregnancy: first trimester: 9–50 ng/ml; second trimester: 18–150 ng/ml; third trimester: 60–260 ng/ml. Male: less than 1.0 ng/ml; less than 100 ng/dl
Prolactin	Serum (Red) or plasma (Lavender)	*Adult:* follicular phase: 0–23 ng/ml; luteal phase 0–40 ng/ml; male: 0.1–20 ng/ml. Pituitary tumor: greater than 100–300 ng/ml; pregnancy: trimester: 1st: less than 80 ng/ml; 2nd: less than 160 ng/ml; 3rd: less than 400 ng/ml

(continued)

Test	Specimen (Color-top Tube)	Reference Values
Propranolol (Inderal)	Serum (Red)	*Adult:* therapeutic: 50–100 ng/ml; toxic: greater than 500 ng/ml
Prostate-specific antigen (PSA)	Serum (Red)	Male: normal: 0–4 ng/ml BPH: 4–19 ng/ml; prostate CA: 10–120 ng/ml
Prostate specific antigen Total PSA Free PSA % Free PSA		Normal: 2.5–4.0 ng/ml Normal: greater than 1.0 ng/ml Normal: greater than 26%
Protein (total)	Serum (Red)	*Adult:* 6.0–8.0 g/dl *Child:* 6.2–8.0 g/dl *Premature:* 4.2–7.6 g/dl *Newborn:* 4.6–7.4 g/dl *Infant:* 6.0–6.7 g/dl
Protein electrophoresis Albumin Globulin	Serum (Red)	*Adult:* 3.5–5.0 g/dl *Child:* 4.0–5.8 g/dl *Adult:* 1.5–3.5 g/dl
Protein	Urine	*Adult:* random: 0–5 mg/dl; 25–150 mg/24 h
Prothrombin time	Plasma (Blue)	*Adult:* 11–13 s PT: 1.5–2.0 times the control in seconds
Quinidine	Serum (Red)	*Adult:* therapeutic: 2–5 mcg/ml; toxic: greater than 5 mcg/ml
Rabies antibody test	Serum (Red)	*Adult:* negative, IFA less than 1:16
Rapid plasma reagin (RPR)	Serum (Red)	*Adult and Child:* nonreactive
Red blood cell (RBC) indices	Blood (Lavender)	*Adult:* RBC count: $4.6–6.0 \times 10^{12}$ (million/µl) MCV: 80–98 cubic microns (cuu) or fl (SI units) MCH: 27–31 pg MCHC: 32%–36% or 0.32–0.36 g/dl

Test	Specimen (Color-top Tube)	Reference Values
		Child: RBC: $3.8–5.5 \times 10^{12}$
		MCV: 82–92 cuμ or fl
		MCH: 27–31 pg
		MCHC: 32%–36% or 0.32–0.36 g/dl
		Newborn: RBC: $4.8–7.2 \times 10^{12}$
		MCV: 96–108 cuμ or fl
		MCH: 32–34 pg
		MCHC: 32%–33% or
		0.32–0.33 g/dl
		RDW (coulter S): 11.5–14.5
Renin	Plasma (Lavender)	*Adult:* 30 min supine:
		0.2–2.3 ng/ml; upright:
		1.6–4.3 ng/ml; restricted salt diet:
		4.1–10.8 ng/ml
Reticulocyte count	Blood (Lavender)	*Adult:* 0.5%–1.5% of all RBCs, 25,000–75,000 μl
		Child: 0.5%–2.0% of all RBCs
		Newborn: 2.5%–6.5% of all RBCs
		Infant: 0.5%–3.5% of all RBCs
Rheumatoid factor (RF)	Serum (Red)	*Adult:* less than 1:20 titer, 1:20–1:80 positive for rheumatoid conditions; greater than 1:80 for rheumatoid arthritis
		Elderly: slightly increased
Rh typing	Blood (Lavender or Red)	*Adult and Child:* Rh+ and Rh–
Rotavirus antigen	Blood and Feces	Negative
Rubella antibody detection	Serum (Red)	*Adult:* less than 1:8. Rubella exposure and immunity: 1:32–1:64 titer; definite immunity: Greater than 1:64
Rubeola antibodies	Serum (Red)	Negative: less than four fold titer
		Positive: greater than four fold titer
Salicylate aspirin	Serum (Red or Green)	*Adult:* therapeutic: 5 mg/dl (headache), 10–30 mg/dl rheumatoid arthritis; mild toxic: greater than 30 mg/dl; severe toxic: greater than 50 mg/dl; lethal: greater than 60 mg/dl

(continued)

Test	Specimen (Color-top Tube)	Reference Values
		Child: mild toxic: greater than 25 mg/dl
		Elderly: mild toxic: greater than 25 mg/dl
Semen analysis	Semen	*Adult:* 50–150 million/ml
Serotonin	Plasma (Lavender)	*Adult:* 50–175 ng/ml; 10–30 mcg/dl; 0.29–1.15 μmol/l (SI units)
Sickle cell test	Blood (Lavender)	*Adult and Child:* 0 sickle cells
Sodium (Na)	Serum (Red)	*Adult and Child:* 135–145 mEq/l, 135–145 mmol/l (SI units)
		Infant: 134–150 mEq/l
	Urine	*Adult and Child:* 40–220 mEq/l/24 h
T$_3$ (Triiodothyronine)	Serum (Red)	*Adult:* 80–200 ng/dl
		Child: 5–10 years 95–240 ng/dl; 10–15 years 80–210 ng/dl
		Newborn: 40–215 ng/dl
T$_4$ (Thyroxine)	Serum (Red)	*Adult:* 4.5–11.5 mcg/dl. T$_4$ RIA: 5–12 mcg/dl; free T$_4$: 1.0–2.3 ng/dl
		Child: 1–6 years: 5.5–13.5 mcg/dl; 6–10 years 5–12.5 mcg/dl
		Newborn: 11–23 mcg/dl
		Infant: 1–4 months: 7.5–16.5 mcg/dl; 4–12 months: 5.5–14.5 mcg/dl
Testosterone	Serum or plasma (Red or Green)	*Adult:* male: 0.3–1.0 mcg/dl, 300–1,000 ng/dl; female: 0.03–0.1 mcg/dl, 30–100 ng/dl
		Child: male: 12–14 years: greater than 0.1 mcg/dl, greater than 100 ng/dl
Theophylline	Serum (Red)	*Adult and Child:* therapeutic: 5–20 mcg/ml, 28–112 μmol/l (SI units); toxic: greater than 20 mcg/ml
		Elderly: 5–18 mcg/ml; toxic: greater than 20 mcg/ml
		Newborn: 3–12 mcg/ml; toxic: greater than 13 mcg/ml
Thyroid antibodies	Serum (Red)	*Adult:* negative or less than 1:20

Test	Specimen (Color-top Tube)	Reference Values
Thyroid-binding globulin (TBG)	Serum (Red)	*Adult:* 10–36 mcg/dl
Thyroid-stimulating hormone (TSH)	Serum (Red)	*Adult:* 0.35–5.5 µIU/ml, less than 10 µU/ml, less than 10^3 IU/l (SI units), less than 3 ng/ml *Newborn:* less than 25 µIU/ml (third day)
Tobramycin	Serum (Red)	*Adult:* therapeutic: peak: 5–10 mcg/ml; trough: less than 2 mcg/ml; toxic: greater than 12 mcg/ml
Torch test	Serum (Red)	*Child:* negative
Toxoplasmosis antibody test	Serum (Red)	*Adult and Child:* negative or less than 1:4, past exposure: 1:4–1:64; acute infection: greater than 1:424
T_3 resin-uptake	Serum (Red)	*Adult:* 25%–35% uptake
Transferrin	Serum (Red)	*Adult:* 200–430 mg/dl; 2–4.3 g/l (SIunits) *Pregnancy (full term):* 300 mg/dl; 3.0 g/l (SI units) *Newborn:* 125–275 mg/dl; Transferrin saturation: 20%–50%
Triglycerides	Serum (Red)	*Adult:* 12–29 years 10–140 mg/dl; 30–39 years 20–150 mg/dl; 40–49 years 30–160 mg/dl; greater than 50 years 40–190 mg/dl *Child:* 5–11 years 10–135 mg/dl *Infant:* 5–40 mg/dl
Troponins Cardiac troponin 1	Blood (Green) Serum (Red)	Cardiac troponin 1: Normal: 0.1–0.5 ng/ml; 0.1 mcg/l (SI units) Positive myocardial injury: greater than 2.0 ng/ml; 2.0 mcg/l (SI units)
Cardiac troponin T		Cardiac troponin T: Normal: less than 0.2 ng/ml; less than 0.2 mcg/l (SI units)

(continued)

Test	Specimen (Color-top Tube)	Reference Values
Uric acid	Serum (Red)	*Adult:* male: 3.5–8.0 mg/dl; female; 2.8–6.8 mg/dl *Panic Value:* greater than 12 mg/dl *Elderly:* 3.5–8.5 mg/dl *Child:* 2.5–5.5 mg/dl
	Urine	*Adult:* 250–750 mg/24 h (normal diet)
Urinalysis	Urine	*Adult, Child, and Newborn:* See urinalysis in text
Urobilinogen	Urine	*Adult and Child:* Random: negative or less than 1.0 Ehrlich units, 2 h: 0.3–1.0 Ehrlich units, 24 h: 0.5–4.0 mg/24 h, 0.09–4.23 µmol/24 h (SI units)
Valproic acid	Serum (Red)	*Adult and Child:* Therapeutic: 50–100 mcg/ml; toxic: greater than 100 mcg/ml
Vanillylmandelic acid (VMA)	Urine	*Adult and Child:* 1.5–7.5 mg/24 h *Adolescent:* 1–5 mg/24 h
VDRL	Serum (Red)	*Adult and Child:* negative
Verapamil (Calan)	Serum (Red)	*Adult:* therapeutic: 100–600 mcg/l; toxic: greater than 600 mcg/l
Viral culture		Negative
Vitamin A	Serum (Red)	See text
Vitamin B$_{12}$	Serum (Red)	*Adult:* 200–900 pg/ml
West Nile virus antibodies	Serum (Red) CSF	Negative
White blood cells (WBCs)	Blood (Lavender)	*Adult:* Total: 4,500–10,000 µl *Child:* 2 years 6,000–17,000 µl *Newborn:* 9,000–30,000 µl
WBC differential: neutrophils (total) Segments Bands	Blood (Lavender)	*Adult:* 50%–70%, 2,500–7,000 µl *Child:* 1 year 32% *Newborn:* 61% *Adult:* 50%–65%, 2,500–6,500 µl *Adult:* 0%–5%, 0–500 µl
Eosinophils		*Adult:* 1%–3%, 100–300 µl
Basophils		*Adult:* 0.4%–1%, 40–100 µl
Monocytes		*Adult:* 4%–6%, 200–600 µl *Child:* 1–12 years 4%–9%

Test	Specimen (Color-top Tube)	Reference Values
Lymphocytes		*Adult:* 25%–35%, 1,700–3,500 µl *Child:* 6 years: 42%, 12 years: 38% *Infant:* 60% *Newborn:* 61%
Zinc	Plasma (Navy blue) Urine	*Adult:* 60–150 mcg/dl, 11–23 µmol/l (SI units) 150–1250 mcg/24 h
Zinc Protoporphyrin	Plasma (Lavender, Green)	*Adult and Child:* 15–77 mcg/dl, 0.24–1.23 µmol/l (SI units); Average: less than 35 µg/dl

CT and MRI Contrast

The most common diagnostic tests performed are the CT and MRI scans. Computed tomography (CT) uses an X-ray beam (ionized radiation) that gives a cross-sectional and two-dimensional images of the shape and structure of organs. The CT test is frequently prescribed in emergency situations, such as to determine the presence of hemorrhagic stroke or a clinical problem such as an acute appendicitis. CT can differentiate between blood from air and soft tissue from tumors. CT scan can be performed with or without iodinated contrast media (dye).

Magnetic resonance imaging (MRI) produces a cross-sectional images similar to CT, but does not use ionizing radiation and is free to the exposure of X-rays. MRI uses magnetic properties of hydrogen atoms short-radiowave pulses to create image from multiple angles. It can differentiate between edema and tumor. MRI excels in diagnosing pathologic problems associated with Central nervous system (CNS) disorders, e.g., hemorrhage, edema, cerebral infarction, subdural hematoma, multiple sclerosis, and tumors. If an emergency situation occurs during imaging, the client must be moved from the MRI room so that resuscitation equipment can be used. Metal objects cannot be present within the body or within the vicinity when using MRI. MRI testing is more expensive than CT testing.

	CT	*MRI*
Purposes	• To screen for coronary disease; head, liver, and renal lesions; tumors; edema; abscesses; infection; metastatic diseases; vascular diseases; stroke; bone destruction • To locate foreign objects in soft tissues, e.g., eye • To detect hemorrhagic stroke • To direct placement of drainage tubes	• To detect central nervous system lesions, vascular problems (blood flow, hemorrhage), cardiac perfusion problems; tumor; or edema • To diagnose demyelinating diseases, e.g., MS • To distinguish tumors or other lesions from normal tissues
General procedure	• CT may or may not use IV iodinated contrast media (dye) • NPO for 4 h if IV contrast media is given • Client should remain still or motionless during the procedure • The CT scanner produces a narrow X-ray beam, which gives a two-dimensional view • Increase water intake following CT with contrast media to eliminate dye from the kidneys	• Remove metal objects before the MRI scan • There should be *no* metal in body, e.g., wire, shrapnel or metal replacement (knee) • With closed MRI, client lies on a narrow table with a cylinder-type scanner that can rotate around the body • An open MRI may be available if the client is claustrophic • A noniodinated contrast media, gadolinium, IV, may be ordered
Caution	• Allergic reaction to IV iodinated contrast media (dye). Cortisone or antihistamine drug may be given prior to administering contrast media • CT is *not* advised if the woman is pregnant • Oral hypoglycemic agents (antidiabetic drug), such as glycophage, are contraindicated if iodinated contrast media is used	• Injury due to a metal object • Potential thermal burns (some transdermal drug patches, e.g., nicotine scopolamine if worn during the MRI might cause thermal burns) • Use of noniodinated contras: media (gadolinium) may be contraindicated if kidney dysfunction is present

BIBLIOGRAPHY

Adams RM (1995). *School Nurse's Survival Guide*. Paramus, NJ: Prentice Hall.

AIDS in humans dates to 1930, researcher finds (2000, February 2). *The News Journal,* A4.

Angelidis PA (1994). MR image compression using a wavelet transform coding algorithm. *Magnetic Resonance Imaging,* 12(7): 1111–1112.

Availability of rapid HIV test extended (2003, March 10). *Nursing Spectrum,* 12(5): 32.

Barrick B, Vogel S (1996). Application of laboratory diagnostics in HIV testing. *Nursing Clinics of North America,* 31(1): 41–45.

Bartholet J (2000, January 17). The years. *Newsweek,* 32–37.

Barzoloski-O'Connor B (2003, June 16). SARS—The latest menacing microbe. *Nursing Spectrum,* 12(12PA): 16–18.

Bernstein AD, et al. (2000). The revised naspe/BPEG generic code for antibradycardia, adaptive-rate and multisite pacing. *PACE,* 25: 260–264.

Black JM, Matassarin-Jacobs E (1997). *Luckmann and Sorensen's Medical–Surgical Nursing.* 5th ed. Philadelphia: WB Saunders.

Blood health by the numbers (2002). *The Cleveland Clinics,* 4(12): 4.

Brown, R (2006, July 13). 1-Pill HIV cocktail approved by FDA. *The News Journal.*

Bynum R (1999, August 31). Drop in deaths from AIDS slows. *The New Journal,* A5.

Carter T (2003, March 4). Studies say sex not main cause in Africa. *The Washington Times,* A-1, A-11.

Cassetta RA (1993). AIDS: Patient care challenges nursing. *The American Nurse,* 25: 1, 24.

Cassetta RA (1993). The new faces of the epidemic. *The American Nurse,* 25: 16.

CDC revises AIDS definition (1993). *The American Nurse,* 25: 20.

CDC. HIV/AIDS Surveillance Report (2001). 13(2).

CDC. Surveillance of health care personnel with HIV/AIDS, as of December, 2001 (Updated 2003, January 27). Division of Health Care Quality Promotion National Center for Infectious Diseases, pp 1, 2. www.cdc.gov/ncidod/hip/BLOOD/hivpersonnel.htm

CDC. Need for sustained HIV prevention among men who have sex with men (2002, March 11). National Center for HIV, STD and TB Prevention Division of HIV/AIDS Prevention, pp 1–3. www.cdc.gov/hiv/pubs/facts/msm.htm

CDC. FAQ'S: Frequently asked questions about HIV and HIV testing (2003, June 16). National HIV Testing Resources, CDC National Prevention Information Network (NPIN), pp 1–4. www.hivtest.org/subindex.cfm?FuseAction=FAQ

CDC. National Prevention in Formation Network (NPIN) (2003, June 16). National HIV Testing Resources. www.hivtest.org/subindex.cfm?FuseAction=Spotlight

CDC. Rapid HIV testing of women in labor and delivery (2003, April 25). CDC for HIV, STD, and TB Prevention. Divisions of HIV/AIDS Prevention, pp 1–3. www.cdc.gov/hiv/pubs/rt-women.htm

Chernecky CC, Krech RL, Berger BJ (1993). *Cholesterol Uptake in Laboratory Tests and Diagnostic Procedures*. Philadelphia: Saunders. 1: 7, 8.

Chernecky CC, Berger BJ, eds. (2004). *Laboratory Tests and Diagnostic Procedures*. 4th ed. Philadelphia: WB Saunders.

Cholesterol Uptake (1988). 1(6): 7, 8.

Cose E (2000, January 17). A cause that crosses the color line. *Newsweek,* 49.

Cowley G (2000, January 17). Fighting the disease: What can be done. *Newsweek,* 38.

Crandall BF, Kulch P, Tabsh K (1994). Risk assessment of amniocentesis between 11 and 15 weeks: Comparison to later amniocentesis controls. *Prenatal Diagnosis,* 14: 913–939.

C-Sections recommended for HIV positive pregnant women (1999, October/November). *AWHONN Lifelines,* 3(5): 17.

Curry JC (1994). Interpreting laboratory data. In: Muma RD, Lyons BA, Borucki MJ, Pollard RB, eds. *HIV Manual for Health Care Professionals*. Norwalk, CT: Appleton & Lange, pp 111–122.

Delbeke D, Martin WH (2001). Positron emission tomography imaging in oncology. *The Radiologic Clinics of North America,* 39(5): 883–918.

DeLorenzo L (1993). The changing face of AIDS. *The Nursing Spectrum,* 2: 19.

Dershem B, Agruss J, Schwelnus E (2006, October 9). Tips to avoid blood redraws. *Nursing Spectrum,* 15(21).

DeVita VT Jr, Hellman S, Rosenberg SA (1992). *AIDS: Etiology, Diagnosis, Treatment and Prevention*. 3rd ed. Philadelphia: Lippincott.

Ellenbogen KA, Thames MD (1997). New insights into pacemaker syndrome gained from hemodynamic, humoral and vascular responses during ventriculo-atrial pacing. *American Journal of Cardiology,* 79: 1226–1229.

Enfuvirtide (Fuzeon) for HIV infection (2003, June 23). *The Medical Letter,* 45(1159): 49, 50.

Epstein JD (1998, September 19). Dupont AIDS drug gets FDA approval. *The News Journal,* A1, A8.

Esch JF, Frank SV (2001, June). Drug resistance and nursing practice. *AJN,* 101(6): 30–36.

Fahey FH (2001). Positron emission tomography instrumentation. *Radiologic Clinics of North America,* 39(5): 919–930.

Fahey JL, Nishanian P (1997). Laboratory diagnosis and evaluation of HIV infection. In: Fahey JL, Flemmig DS, eds. *AIDS/HIV Reference Guide for Medical Professionals*. 4th ed. Baltimore: Wilkins and Wilkins, pp 232–242.

Fischbach FT (2004). *A Manual of Laboratory Diagnostic Tests*. 7th ed. Philadelphia: Lippincott.

Fisher M, Prichard JW, Warach S (1995). New magnetic resonance techniques for acute ischemic stroke. *Journal of the American Medical Association,* 274(11): 908–911.

Flake KJ (2000). HIV testing during pregnancy: Building the case for voluntary testing. *AWHONN Lifelines,* 4C: 13–16.

Flemmig DS, Johiro AK (1997). HIV counseling and testing. In: Fahey JL, Flemmig DS, eds. *AIDS/HIV Reference Guide for Medical Professionals*. 4th ed. Baltimore: Wilkins and Wilkins, pp 57–74.

Food and Drug Administration (1995). Mammography quality deadline. *FDA Medical Bulletin,* 25(1): 3.

Francois Xavier Bagnoud Center. National Pediatric and Family Resource Center and AETC National Resource Center (2003, May 15). HIV and pregnancy: Managing mother and baby, train the trainer slide set. University of Medicine and Dentistry of NJ. www.aidsetc.org/

Froelicher ES (1994). Usefulness of exercise testing shortly after acute myocardial infarction for predicting 10 year mortality. *American Journal of Cardiology,* 74: 318–323.

Fulcher AS, Turner MA (2002). MR cholangiopancreatography. *Radiologic Clinics of North America,* 40(6): 1363–1376.

Garg K (2002). CT of pulmonary thromboembolic disease. *The Radiologic Clinics of North America,* 40(1): 111–122.

Gebbie KM (2001, June). Privacy: The patient's right. *AJN,* 101(6): 69, 71, 72.

Gerberding JL (1992). HIV transmission to providers and their patients. In: Sande MA, Volberding PA, eds. *The Medical Management of AIDS*. 3rd ed. Philadelphia: Saunders, pp 54–64.

Gorman C (1997, January 6; 1996, December 30). The disease detective. *Time,* 148(29): 56–62, 63.

Grady C (1992). HIV disease: Pathogens and treatment. In: Flaskerud JH, Unguarski PJ, eds. *HIV/AIDS: A Guide to Nursing Care*. 2nd ed. Philadelphia: Saunders, pp 30–53.

Guzman ER, Rosenberg JC, Houlihan C (1994). A new method using vaginal ultrasound and transfundal pressure to evaluate the asymptomatic incompetent cervix. *Obstetrics and Gynecology,* 83(2): 248–252.

Handbook of Diagnostic Tests. 3rd ed. (2003). Philadelphia: Lippincott Williams, and Wilkins.

Haney DQ (2000, January 31). Virus levels linked to AIDS transmission. *The News Journal,* A3.

Hardy CE, Helton GJ, Kondo C, et al. (1994). Usefulness of magnetic resonance imaging for evaluating great-vessel anatomy after arterial switch operation for D-transposition of the great arteries. *American Heart Journal,* 128: 326–332.

Henry JB (2001). *Clinical Diagnosis and Management by Laboratory Methods.* 12th ed. Philadelphia: WB Saunders.

Henry J Kaiser Family Foundation (2002, July). The HIV/AIDS epidemic in the United States. HIV/AIDS Policy Fact Sheet (developed as part of AIDS at 20: A National HIV/AIDS Policy Initiative: Joint initiative of the Henry J. Kaiser Family Foundation and the Ford Foundation. www.kff.org/AIDSat20

High triglyceride (2002). *Mayo Clinic Health Letter,* 20(9): 7.

HIV/AIDS Surveillance Reports (June, 1999). Atlanta: Centers for Disease Control and Prevention. 11(1).

Hoefner BM (2005, December). Serum tumor markers, pp 20, 22–24. www.mlo-online.com.

Homocysteine (2002). *Mayo Clinic Health Letter,* 20(9): 6.

Improving bone density (2003). *Mayo Clinic Health Letter,* 21(2): 7.

Is it the "new cholesterol"? About homocysteine (2000). *The Cleveland Clinics,* 2(6): 4, 5.

Iskandrian AE, Chaudhry FA (2000). Stress echocardiography and stress nuclear testing, Part I. *A Journal of Cardiovascular Ultrasound and Allied Technology,* 17(5): 463–469.

Itchhaporia D, Cerqueira MD (1995). New agents and new techniques and nuclear cardiology. *Current Opinion in Cardiology,* 10(6): 650–655.

Jaffe MS (1996). *Medical–Surgical Nursing Care Plans: Nursing Diagnoses & Interventions.* 3rd ed. Stamford, CT: Appleton & Lange.

Johnsen C (1999, June 1). Hepatitis C: The shadow epidemic. *Nursing Spectrum,* 8(11): 14–16.

Johnson D, Silverstein-Currier J, Sanchez-Keeland L (1999). Building barriers to HIV: Protecting women through contraception and infection prevention. *Advance for Nurse Practitioners,* 7(5): 40–44.

Johnson LL, Lawson MA (1996). New imaging techniques for assessing cardiac function. *Critical Care Clinics,* 12(4): 919–937.

Kalichman SC (2003). *The Inside Story on AIDS: Experts Answer Your Questions.* American Psychological Association: Washington, DC.

Kanal E, Shaibani A (1994). Firearm safety in the MR imaging environment. *Radiology,* 193: 875–876.

Kaplan A, Jack R, Opheim KE, et al. (1995). *Clinical Chemistry. Interpretation and Techniques.* 4th ed. Baltimore: Williams & Wilkins.

Kee JL, Paulanka B, Purnell, L (2004). *Fluids and Electrolytes with Clinical Applications.* 7th ed. New York: Delmar Publishers.

Kee JL (2005). *Laboratory and Diagnostic Tests with Nursing Implications.* 7th ed. NJ: Prentice-Hall Health.

Kee JL, Hayes ER (2006). *Pharmacology: A Nursing Process Approach.* 5th ed. Philadelphia: Saunders.

Keeys, MU (1994). Nuclear cardiology stress testing. *Nursing 94,* 24(1): 63, 64.

Kirton CA, Talotta D, Zwolski V, eds. (2001). *Handbook of HIV/AIDS Nursing.* St. Louis: Mosby.

Knoben JE, Anderson PO (1993). *Clinical Drug Data.* 7th ed. Hamilton, IL: Drug Intelligence Publications.

Kurytka D (1996). Advances in HIV/AIDS care. *The Nursing Spectrum,* 5(26): 6.

LeBlond RF, DeGowin RL, Brown DD (2004). *DeGowin's Diagnostic Examination.* 8th ed. New York: McGraw-Hill.

Leonard T (2006, June 4). Misery likely to continue for many more decades. *Sunday News Journal.*

Locher AW (1996, July/August). Ethics, women with HIV, and procreation: Implications for nursing practice. *Journal of Obstetric, Gynecologic and Neonatal Nursing,* 25(6): 465–469.

Mallery S, VanDam J (2000). Advances in diagnostic and therapeutic endoscopy. *Medical Clinics of North America,* 84(5): 1059–1079.

Masland T, Norland R (2000, January 17). 10 Orphans. *Newsweek,* 42–45.

Maule WF (1994). Screening for colorectal cancer by nurse endoscopists. *New England Journal of Medicine,* 330(3): 183–184.

McClatchey KD, ed. (1994). *Clinical Laboratory Medicine.* Baltimore: Williams & Wilkins.

McClatchey KD, ed. (2002). *Clinical Laboratory Medicine.* 2nd ed. Philadelphia: Lippincott, Williams, and Wilkins.

McGhic AI (2001). *Handbook of Non-invasive Cardiac Testing.* New York: Oxford University Press.

McGuinness G, Naidich DP (2002). CT of airways disease and bronchiectasis. *The Radiologic Clinics of North America,* 40(1): 3–19.

Mellico KD (1993). Interpretation of abnormal laboratory values in older adults. Part I. *Journal of Gerontological Nursing,* 19(1): 39–45.

Mennemeyer ST, Winkelman JW (1993). Searching for inaccuracy in clinical laboratory testing using Medicare data: Evidence for prothrombin time. *Journal of the American Medical Association,* 269: 1030–1033.

Mettler FA (1996). *Essentials of Radiology.* Philadelphia: WB Saunders.

Moran BA (2000). Maternal infections. In: Mattson S, Smith JE, eds. *Core Curriculum for Maternal-Newborn Nursing.* 2nd ed. Philadelphia: WB Saunders, 419–448.

Moulton-Barrett R, Triadafilopoulos G, Michener R, et al. (1993). Serum C-bicarbonate in the assessment of gastric *Helicobacter pylori* urease activity. *American Journal of Gastroenterology,* 88(3): 369–373.

Myers MC, Page MD (1996). Caring for the laboring woman with HIV infection on AIDS. In: Martin EJ, ed. *Intrapartum Management Modules.* 2nd ed. Baltimore: Wilkins and Wilkins, pp 451–486.

Nanda NC, Miller A, Puri VK, et al. (2000). Assessment of myocardial perfusion by power contrast agent. *A Journal of Cardiovascular Ultrasound and Allied Technology,* 17(5): 457–460.

National Center for HIV, STD, and TB Prevention. Divisions of HIV/AIDS Prevention (2003, April 13). HIV and AIDS: are you at risk? pp 1–5. www.cdc.gov/hiv/pubs/brochure/astrisk.htm

National Committee for Clinical Laboratory Standards (1995). *How to define, determine, and utilize reference intervals in the clinical laboratory, approved guidelines.* NCCLS Document C-28-A. 25(4).

N-High Sensitivity C-Reactive Protein Announcement (2000). DE: *Dade-Behring.*

Noble D (1993). Controversies in the clinical chemistry laboratory. *Analytical Chemistry,* 84(6): 797–800.

Norris MKG (1993). Evaluating serum triglyceride levels. *Nursing 93,* 23(5): 31.

Nuzhat AA, Shah JN, Kochman ML (2002). Endoscopic ultrasonography and endoscopic retrograde cholangiopancreatography imaging for pancreaticobiliary pathology: The gastroenterologist's perspective. *Radiologic Clinics,* 40(6): 1377–1396.

Nyamath A, Flemmig DS (1997). Prevention consideration for women. In: Fahey JL, Flemmig, DS, eds. *AIDS/HIV Reference Guide for Medical Professionals.* 4th ed. Baltimore: Wilkins and Wilkins, pp 232–242.

Office of Communications and Public Liaison Treatment of HIV Infection (2002, January). *Fact Sheet* from National Institute of Allergy and Infectious Diseases. National Institutes of Health, U.S. Department of Health and Human Services, p 11. (Updated June 6, 2003.) www.niaid.nih. gov/factsheets/treat-hiv.htm

Overmoyer B (1999). Breast cancer screening. *The Medical Clinics of North America,* 83(6): 1443–1466.

Pagana KD, Pagana TJ (2005). *Mosby's Diagnostic and Laboratory Test Reference.* 7th ed. St. Louis: CV Mosby.

Pavlovich-Davis SJ (2003, February 10). Human growth hormone—Pharmaceutical fountain of youth? *Nursing Spectrum,* 12(3PA): 16–18.

Peterson KJ, Solie CJ (1994). Interpreting laboratory values in chronic renal insufficiency. *American Journal of Nursing,* 94(5): 56B, 56E, 56H.

Peterson KL, Nicod P (1997). *Cardiac Catheterization Methods, Diagnosis, and Therapy.* Philadelphia: WB Saunders.

Porembka, DT (1996). Transesophageal echocardiography. *Critical Care Clinics,* 12(4): 875–903.

Preston DC, Shapiro BE (2002, May). Needle electromyography: Fundamentals, normal and abnormal patterns. *The Neurologic Clinics of North America,* 20(2): 361–396.

Purvis A (1997, January 6; 1996, December 30). The global epidemic. *Time,* 148(29): 76–78.

Rakel RE (1996). *Saunders' Manual of Medical Practice*. Philadelphia: WB Saunders.

Ravel R (1995). *Clinical Laboratory Medicine*. 6th ed. Chicago: Year Book.

Remer EM, Baker ME (2002). Imaging of chronic pancreatitis. *The Radiologic Clinics of North America*, 40(6): 1229–1242.

Romancyzuk AN, Brown JP (1994). Folic acid will reduce risk of neural tube defects. *American Journal of Maternal Child Nursing*, 19(6): 331–334.

Ross, E (2002, July 9). New medicine effective against drug-resistant HIV: T-20 studies show treatment could save lives. Conference: Barcelona, Spain. News Journal, Wilmington, DE.

Rotello LS, Radin EJ, Jastremski MS, et al. (1994). MRI protocol for critically ill patients. *American Journal of Critical Care*, 3(3): 187–190.

Sayad DE, Clarke GD, Peshock RM (1995). Magnetic resonance imaging of the heart and its role in current cardiology. *Current Opinion in Cardiology*, 10(6): 640–649.

Schnell ZB, Leeuwen AM, Kranpitz TR (2003). *Davis's Comprehensive Handbook of Laboratory and Diagnostic Tests with Nursing Implications*. Philadelphia: FA Davis.

Selekman J (2006). *School Nurse: A Comprehensive Test*. Philadelphia: FA Davis.

Selig PM (1996). Pearls for practice: Management of anticoagulation therapy with the international normalized ratio. *Journal of the American Academy of Nursing Practitioners*, 8(2): 77–80.

Sipes C (1995, January/February). Guidelines for assessing HIV in women. *MCN: The American Journal of Maternal Child Nursing*, 20(1): 29–33.

Smart SC, Sagar KB (2000). Diagnostic and prognostic use of stress echocardiography in stable patients. *A Journal of Cardiovascular Ultrasound and Allied Technology*, 17(5): 465–473.

Smith S, Forman D (1994). Laboratory analysis of cerebrospinal fluid. *Clinical Laboratory Science*, 7(4): 32–38.

Spinner A (2006, September 25). Less stress, more nursing care for infants. *Nursing Spectrum*, 15(21).

Strimike C (1996). Understanding intravascular ultrasound. *American Journal of Nursing*, 96(6): 40–43.

Stringer M, Librizzi R (1994). Complications following prenatal genetic procedures. *Nursing Research*, 43(2): 184–186.

Sutton D (1995). Angiography. In: Sutton D, Young JWR. *A Concise Textbook of Clinical Imaging*. 2nd ed. St. Louis: CV Mosby.

TB Facts for Health Care Workers (1993). Atlanta, GA: Department of Health and Human Services, Public Health Service, Centers for Disease Control and Prevention, National Center for Prevention Services, Division of Tuberculosis Elimination.

Thacker SB (2003, May 2). HIPPA privacy rule and public health: Guidance from CDC and Human Services. *MMWR*, 52(1): 1–12.

The Ear and Hearing: A Guide for School Nurses (1998). NY: National Association of School Nurses, Inc.

The Ear and Hearing, A Guide for School Nurses (1998). *National Association of School Nurses, Inc.*

Thompson E, Detwiler DS, Nelson CM (1996). Dobutamine stress echocardiography: A new, noninvasive method for detecting ischemic heart disease. *Heart & Lung,* 25(2): 87–97.

Thompson L (1995). Percutaneous endoscopic gastrostomy. *Nursing 95,* 25(4): 62–63.

Tietz NW ed. (1997). *Clinical Guide to Laboratory Tests.* 3rd ed. Philadelphia: Saunders.

Topol EJ, Holmes DR, Rogers WJ (1991). Coronary angiography after thrombolytic therapy for acute myocardial infarction. *Annual of Internal Medicine,* 114(10): 877–885.

Trzcianowska H, Martensen E (2001, June). HIV and AIDS: Separating fact from fiction. *AJN,* 101(6): 53–59.

Ungvarski PJ (2001, June). The past 20 years of AIDS. *AJN,* 101(6): 26–29.

U.S. Food and Drug Administration (2002, Nov 7). FDA approves new rapid HIV test kit. *FDA News (PO2-49),* pp 1, 2. www.fda.gov/bbs/topics/NEWS/2002/NEW00852.html

Vannier MW, Marsh JL (1996). Three-dimensional imaging surgical planning, and image-guided therapy. *Radiologic Clinics of North America,* 34(3): 545–561.

Virtual colonoscopy: Not quite as good as the "real" thing (2002). *The Cleveland Clinics,* 4(12): 1, 6.

Vitamin C (2000). *The Cleveland Clinics,* 2(6): 7.

Wallach J (1998). *Handbook of Interpretation of Diagnostic Tests.* Philadelphia: Lippincott-Raven.

Ward DE (1999). *The AmFAR AIDS Handbook: The Complete Guide to Understanding HIV and AIDS.* New York: W W Norton.

Washington JA (1993). Laboratory diagnosis of infectious diseases. *Infectious Disease Clinics of North America,* 7(2): 13.

Weiner S (2003, June 2). School nurse—Never a dull moment. *Nursing Spectrum,* 12(11PA): 10.

Whole-body CT: Looking for trouble (2003). *The Cleveland Clinics,* 5(7): 1, 7.

Wilbourn AJ (2002). Nerve conduction studies: Types, components, abnormalities, and value in localization. *The Neurologic Clinics of North America,* 20(2): 305–338.

Wilde P, Hartnell GC (1995). Cardiac imaging. In: Sutton D, Young JWR. *A Concise Textbook of Clinical Imaging.* 2nd ed. St. Louis: CV Mosby.

Willard S (2000, December 18). AIDS in the older adult: Aging raises unique treatment concerns. *Advance for Nurses (Greater Philadelphia edition),* 2(25): 11–13.

Williams AB (2001, June). Adherence to HIV regimens: 10 vital lessons. *AJN,* 101(6): 37–44.

Williamson MR (1996). *Essentials of Ultrasound*. Philadelphia: WB Saunders.

Woeste S (2005, July). Diagnosing prostate cancer. *LabMedicine*, 36(7): 399, 400.

Wofson AB, Paris PM (1996). *Diagnostic Testing in Emergency Medicine*. Philadelphia: WB Saunders.

Womack C, Thomas JD (1996). Easing the way through an MRI. *RN*, 59(10): 34–37.

Wong ND, Vo W, Abrahamson D, et al. (1994). Detection of coronary artery calcium by ultrafast computed tomography and its relation to clinical evidence of coronary artery disease. *American Journal of Cardiology*, 73: 223–227.

Zanotti KM, Kennedy AW (1999). Screening for gynecologic cancer. *The Medical Clinics of North America*, 83(6): 1467–1476.

Zaret BL, Wackers FJ (1993). Nuclear cardiology. *New England Journal of Medicine*, 329(12): 855–863.

Zubal IG (1996). The evolution of imaging devices: A constant challenge with combining progress. In: *Yearbook of Nuclear Medicine*. St. Louis: CV Mosby.

Zurlinden J (2002, April 8). HIV update. *Nursing Spectrum*, 11(7PA).

INDEX